SELF AND NOT-SELF

SELF AND NOT-SELF

CELLULAR IMMUNOLOGY BOOK ONE

SIR MACFARLANE BURNET
O.M., F.R.S., Nobel Laureate

MELBOURNE UNIVERSITY PRESS
CAMBRIDGE UNIVERSITY PRESS
1969

PUBLISHED BY

MELBOURNE UNIVERSITY PRESS
Carlton 3053, Victoria, Australia

AND

THE SYNDICS OF THE CAMBRIDGE UNIVERSITY PRESS
Bentley House, 200 Euston Road, London N.W.1
American Branch: 32 East 57th Street, New York, N.Y.10022

© SIR F. MACFARLANE BURNET 1969

Library of Congress Catalogue Card Number: 69-12162

Dewey Decimal Classification Number: 576.23

Standard Book Numbers:

MUP $\begin{cases} 522\ 83928\ 2 \text{ clothbound} \\ 522\ 83926\ 6 \text{ paperback} \end{cases}$

CUP $\begin{cases} 521\ 07521\ 1 \text{ clothbound} \\ 521\ 09558\ 1 \text{ paperback} \end{cases}$

Printed in Great Britain
at the University Printing House, Cambridge
(Brooke Crutchley, University Printer)

CONTENTS

Preface		*page* vii
1	The history of immunological ideas	3
2	The general character of immune phenomena	21
3	The thymus in relation to the origin and differentiation of lymphoid cells	57
4	The immunocyte: its definition, recognition and distribution	74
5	The nature of antibody	98
6	The origin of immune pattern	125
7	The role of macrophages, eosinophils and other auxiliary agents in relation to adaptive immunity	147
8	The immunocyte and its response to specific stimulation	163
9	Antibody production	189
10	Immunological unresponsiveness	213
11	The integration and deployment of immune responses	232
12	Autoimmune disease as a breakdown in immunological homeostasis	255
13	Immunological surveillance and the evolution of adaptive immunity	286
Epilogue		309
Bibliography		311
Index		313

PLATES *between pages* 80–1

PREFACE

When I wrote *Cellular Immunology*, I had two objectives. The first was simply to provide a readable and accurate account of the clonal selection theory of immunity. I feel rightly or wrongly that this brought immunology for the first time into full relationship with the general development of biology and that many people interested in one or other aspect of biology might appreciate an account of modern immunology in terms of these ideas. The second was to provide for my fellow immunologists a technical justification for the interpretations I have put on the phenomena we study. By dividing the work into two parts the second requirement could be covered by adding a technical restatement with documentation in the form of Book II without necessarily providing it for readers primarily interested in the general approach.

Self and Not-Self is identical with Book I of the complete *Cellular Immunology*. It is written as an essay for readers interested, as biologists of one sort or another, in immunology but not necessarily concerned directly with immunological research. Only occasional references are made to the workers on whose findings the discussion is based and little or no mention is made of work in fields which seem to have no special relevance to the central theme. The primary object is to present a current version of clonal selection theory which could form a satisfactory background for reading or investigation in immunology.

Experience in lecturing and discussion over the past few years has made me very much aware of the difficulty many students and even some investigators find in grasping the nature of the selective approach. I have therefore deliberately presented the general concept from different points of view and at different levels of elaboration. I hope that the central theme that gives the title *Self and Not-Self* to the book is everywhere well to the fore. The need and the capacity to distinguish between what is acceptable as self and what must be rejected as alien is the evolutionary basis of immunology.

Preface

No book can ever be completely up to date, and here and there I find attitudes that I should like to modify. In particular my ideas about the evolution of immunity have developed in somewhat different fashion since the manuscript was completed.

The work was commenced some years ago, but the book has been written essentially as a post-retirement activity since I left the Hall Institute in 1965. I am indebted to the University of Melbourne for a Rowden White Fellowship over the period, to Professor Rubbo for providing office space in the School of Microbiology, to the Wellcome Trustees who have made it possible for me to employ a secretary, and to a grant from Merck Sharp and Dohme Research Laboratories, New Jersey, to cover stationery and other office expenses. I owe a special debt of gratitude to Mrs L. Nillson who has carried out many retypings and assisted in all other aspects of its production with intelligence, accuracy and cheerfulness.

F. M. BURNET

September 1968

SELF AND NOT-SELF

1 The history of immunological ideas

The history of immunological ideas must have begun when people began to realize that a man or a child with a pock-marked face did not take smallpox again. No doubt it was also old wives' knowledge that other recognizable childhood infections struck once only, but the virulence of smallpox in the eighteenth century in Europe, when it was one of the main causes of death in childhood, gave it pre-eminence. The history of variolization as a deliberate attempt to provoke immunity and of its replacement at the end of the century by Jenner's 'vaccination' with cowpox is known to all. For all its practical importance there was no possible basis at that time for any significant theoretical ideas about the way in which protection was achieved.

The first approach to a general method of immunization against an infectious disease came with Pasteur's work (1880) on the protection of fowls against chicken cholera by inoculation with 'attenuated virus'; in this case, old cultures of the micro-organism called *Pasteurella aviseptica*. To explain his results, Pasteur suggested that the immunizing infection 'exhausted' something necessary for the proliferation *in vivo* of the virulent culture.

With the recognition around this time of the universality of bacteria and the existence of specifically pathogenic types, a new problem began to be recognized—the normal resistance of animals against most bacteria. Apparently related to this was the capacity of blood held outside the body to resist putrefaction much longer than most organic materials. Freshly drawn blood was able to kill at least some types of bacteria and gradually the idea of special agents in the blood adapted to defend the body against bacterial invasion gave birth to the concept of specific antibodies. Concurrently, however, there developed an alternative way of looking at the defence against bacteria as a function of the white cells of the blood. The classical controversy between cellular and humoral theories of natural immunity flourished from about 1884, when Metchnikoff described his researches on phagocytic cells in the crustacean *Daphnia*, until 1903, when Almroth Wright's ideas on opsonins began gradually to lead to a recognition of the complexity of the processes concerned and the importance of more than one type of cell and many humoral factors.

The future course of immunological theory, as something concerned with a much wider field than immunity against infection, was laid down in 1898 by Bordet's recognition of immune lysis of foreign red cells followed in 1904 by Landsteiner's discovery of the ABO blood groups. From this time onward there was a steady increase in interest in the immunological behaviour of cells and body fluids and soon a realization of the fact that only *foreign* material was antigenic added an important new problem for understanding.

With von Behring's discovery of potential therapeutic agents against diphtheria and tetanus in 1895 and Ehrlich's subsequent studies on the nature of antitoxin, it was inevitable that the main stream of immunological thought for the first forty years of this century should be concerned with the problem of antibody. How was it possible for the body to produce something which would neutralize specifically any one of a large group of poisonous substances against which it had been immunized? Ehrlich's side-chain theory was the first serious attempt to explain the origin of antibody. It was based on a primitive picture of a living protoplasmic molecule which carried a variety of side-chains by which food molecules could be taken in and which could equally serve as receptors for the attack of damaging substances like bacterial toxins. If the molecule was not 'lethally' damaged it responded by an overproduction of the receptors involved with their liberation into the blood as antitoxin. The theory was obviously designed to deal with toxins and antitoxins and depended, of course, on there being available in the body pre-formed molecular groupings which could unite specifically with what we should now call antigenic determinants.

When Landsteiner developed methods of studying artificial antigens made by the chemical union of small molecules—haptens— to carrier proteins, it soon became evident that there were far too many possible types of antibody to allow each to be accepted as representing a pre-formed receptor on molecules or cells liable

The history of immunological ideas

to attack by the antigen. By 1930 it was clear that antibodies were associated with serum globulins and, independently, Breinl and Haurowitz, Alexander and Mudd all suggested that antibody might represent globulin which had been synthesized in contact with antigen and, in so doing, had taken on a complementary steric configuration which would ensure that, on renewed contact with the antigen, a firm union could occur. This was the first form of what Lederberg subsequently called the 'instructive' theory of antibody formation.

The whole initial concept of immunity was in relation to infectious disease in man or his domestic animals. Pasteur was trained as a chemist, but once he had shown the potentiality of immunization with attenuated pathogens the central objectives of immunological research were defined for the next sixty or seventy years. Immunology was one of the practically important aspects of medical bacteriology and almost all those concerned in its advance were medically trained. There were, of course, other interests in immune processes that went much wider than their applicability to the cure or prevention of disease. The specificity of immunity called for laboratory study of its basis and led to serological methods both for the classification of pathogenic micro-organisms and for retrospective diagnosis of the infecting organism. The triumphs of immunology were practical ones: the production of antitoxins against tetanus and diphtheria and, later, toxoids for active immunization; a variety of bacterial vaccines, most of which have suffered a progressive diminution in reputation with the years, and eventually immunization against poliomyelitis and other virus diseases.

THE BIOCHEMICAL APPROACH

The theoretical approach over most of the period was at a rather superficial level and it is probably correct to say that not until Pauling became interested in immunology around 1940 was there any effective association of immunology with the developing principles of biochemistry. The concepts of Ehrlich, for instance, were *ad hoc* constructions with only a minimal relevance to the chemical form in which they were cast. Landsteiner's work in the 1930s was of immense importance in establishing a chemical basis for the specificity of immune pattern and almost automatically suggested that antibodies were produced in the body by some impression of complementary pattern on normal serum globulin during the process of its synthesis.

The development of quantitative methods by Heidelberger about this time largely substituted the techniques of the biochemist for the medical immunologists' methods of titration to a limit dilution. When mixtures of a soluble purified antigen with a corresponding antiserum reacted to produce a precipitate, Heidelberger was concerned to know the amounts of the two reagents in the precipitate in terms of milligrams or micrograms. This provided immunological information in what a chemist could regard as a meaningful fashion. Antibodies were clearly proteins and with the rapid development of an understanding of the polypeptide structure of proteins and, in particular, of the potential ways in which the basic polypeptide chain could be folded to give secondary and tertiary structure, Pauling was able to give a relatively precise formulation to what has since become known as the classical instructive theory of antibody formation. All theories must be produced within the limitations of contemporary knowledge. In 1940 there was hardly a hint of the part played by nucleic acid in coding the amino acid sequence of polypeptide chains and very little conception of the complexity of γ-globulin and other proteins. The essence of Pauling's concept was that, as synthesized, a polypeptide chain had no inbuilt compulsion to adopt any specific type of folding and intramolecular bonding. A vast variety of arrangements were thermodynamically all equally admissible, normal γ-globulin representing a random mixture of the various possible three-dimensional configurations. When, however, the newly synthesized polypeptide chain was brought into contact with the steric patterns of parts of the antigenic molecule or particle, it would develop a stable configuration in a pattern complementary to that of the antigen. Secondary hydrogen bonding between the coils in their new position then stabilized the structure. When the antigen was in one way or another separated and made available to mould another polypeptide chain, a cavity appropriate to fit firmly with the antigenic determinant on a subsequent occasion was left imprinted on the antibody molecule.

The biochemical approach

Much of this picture of the nature of antibody has been retained. Most writers conceive the two combining sites of a single antibody molecule to be cavities formed by amino acid residues so distributed as to provide a complementary steric pattern to the corresponding antibody. It is more than possible that this is too naïve a concept but from the point of view of providing an acceptable picture of how antigen and antibody react it has been valuable. Where the instructive approach has proved insufficient is its failure (*a*) to conform to the new understanding of the nature of protein synthesis, (*b*) to provide an interpretation of immune tolerance and (*c*) to account for the changing character of a given antibody during the course of immunization. Another aspect of antibody which has become very prominent recently is its heterogeneity. With every refinement for the physical separation of related protein molecules, it has become more and more evident that each antiserum is made up of a heterogeneous population of molecules with the one common feature of a recognizably specific capacity for union with the antigen in question.

THE APPEARANCE OF SELECTION THEORIES

In the period between 1940 and 1955 there was rapid technical advance in immunology as in other biological sciences. The Second World War had a major influence in two directions, due to the immense practical importance of blood transfusion and plastic surgery in dealing with war casualties. The ABO blood groups had been discovered many years before but now there was a much greater volume of laboratory work going on in this field. As a result, the Rh groups and their clinical significance were discovered in 1940. The various immunological disorders associated with pregnancy and transfusion now became matters of major interest and, in particular, underlined what Medawar called the 'uniqueness of the individual'. In the field of transplantation it was discovered and rediscovered that while plastic surgery could deal almost without limitation with the patient's own tissues, most attempts to use any other person's skin or other tissue to replace deficiencies were wholly unsuccessful. The time was ripe to emphasize the importance of 'self' and 'not-self' for immunology and to look for the ways in which recognition of the difference could be mediated. In due course, the concept of tolerance and the experimental demonstration of acquired immunological tolerance became known to all immunologists and immediately raised grave difficulties for 'instructive' theories.

New experimental work on antibodies themselves greatly complicated the picture. In human beings it became clear that there were three main types of antibody-carrying immunoglobulins (Ig G, Ig M, Ig A), each with their own physical characteristics and with at least one distinguishing antigenic quality. In all mammals examined there are at least three such types and wherever intensive search has been made, as in mice or human beings, a complex of antigenic groups and subgroups has been found. The elaboration of this field has depended first on the application of simple electrophoresis (Tiselius), then on the refinement of antigen-antibody precipitin reactions that becomes possible when the reactions take place in agar (Ouchterlony, 1948) and finally on the combination of both techniques in immunoelectrophoresis (Williams and Grabar, 1955).

This work has no direct bearing on the nature of the combining site—which in fact has only been directly studied in Ig G antibodies—but there is a good deal to suggest that the combining site may be the same for any type of immunoglobulin. Clearly the situation was far more complex than Pauling had envisaged in 1940, and over the last decade the main theoretical discussion on immunity has been concerned with the possibility of replacing instructive theories of the Pauling type by selective theories of antibody formation. The two types of approach are similar in principle to what has occurred in another contemporary field, the acquisition by a bacterial culture of 'adaptive' capacity to resist an antibiotic or to ferment a sugar against which it is normally inactive. In the one field we ask whether the antibiotic impresses some change on a small proportion of bacteria so that they produce descendants genetically resistant (instructive approach) or whether in any large population there will be so many mutants of all sorts that some will be resistant to the antibiotic and in its presence will be able to proliferate selectively. In the field of antibody production, selective theories endow a unique quality on the genetic mechanism of antibody-producing cells and the forms ancestral to them. Within that population by some process, which may be accelerated somatic mutation or some operationally similar random re-assortment of pre-existent patterns, cells develop each of which can produce one of a vast number of different patterns of antibody. It is a further necessary postulate of selective (or genetic) theories that each cell, each *immunocyte*, must also possess receptors (or 'fixed antibody') which on contact with antigen of one particular type will cause the cell to proliferate selectively.

The first suggestion that a selective theory of antibody production was possible came from Jerne in 1955. In the course of studies of the production of antibody against bacteriophage, he found an unusual type of antibody present in small amounts in normal serum. It is well known to all serologists that for almost any sort of antigen very refined tests will show 'traces' of antibody in most normal sera and sometimes surprisingly large amounts. Jerne felt that these traces were real pre-existent antibody and speculated that the first step in the production of antibody was the union of antigen with appropriate molecules of natural antibody. The complex was then taken up by macrophages of the reticulo-endothelial system and stimulated them to produce more antibody of the same pattern as had been drawn into them by union with the antigen. It was left uncertain how the original normal antibodies had arisen and no reasonable analogy was available to indicate how or why an accidentally chosen cell should produce replicas of a protein taken into its cytoplasm. There are still supporters of a modified version of Jerne's theory but most of them would now assume that the uptake of the antigen–antibody complex was merely the first step in processing the *antigen* into a suitable form for its basic function of stimulating lymphoid cells of the same clone that had produced the natural antibody.

One of the principal virtues of Jerne's natural selection theory was that it offered an interpretation of the failure of the body to make antibody against its own constituents—its natural tolerance. It was regarded as self-evident that any natural globulins capable of reacting with cell components accessible to the circulation would be eliminated from the plasma. This did not, however, deal particularly adequately with the phenomenon of neonatal tolerance

The history of immunological ideas

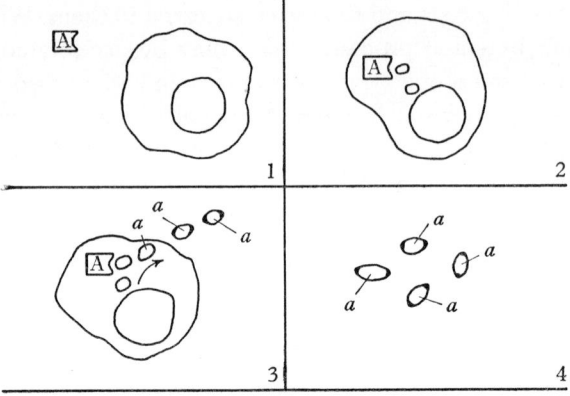

Fig. 1. The instructive theory of Pauling (1940) and his predecessors. Non-specific polypeptide chains are moulded after synthesis to take on specific immune pattern by physical contact with antigen.

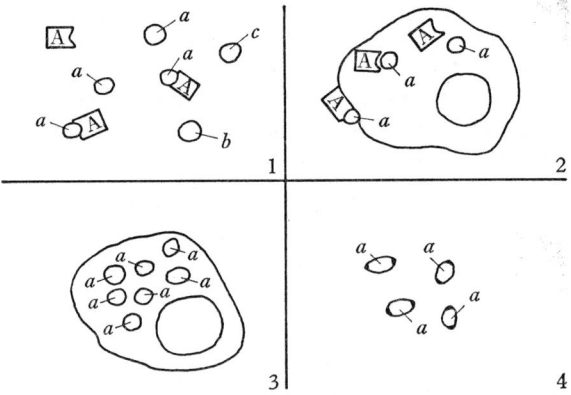

Fig. 2. The natural selection theory (Jerne, 1955). 'Natural antibody' unites with antigen; the complex is ingested by a phagocytic cell and more antibody is produced to the pattern of that ingested.

Figs 1–4. A series of diagrams to show in oversimplified form the essential features of four concepts of the process of antibody formation.

which had recently been demonstrated by Billingham, Brent and Medawar (1953) and had provoked widespread interest. It seemed that if a foreign antigen were implanted early enough, an animal would fail to become immunized and would subsequently be incapable of producing antibody or its equivalent against the antigen.

The appearance of selection theories

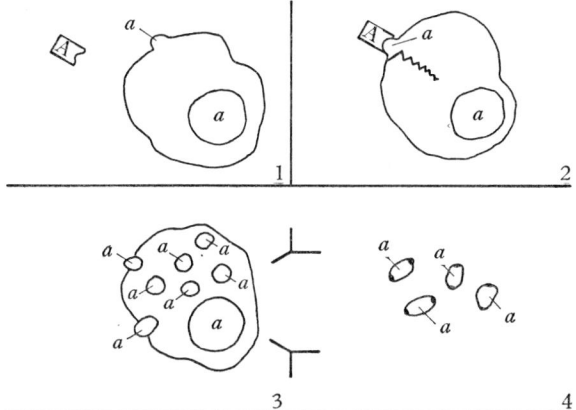

Fig. 3. The clonal selection theory (Burnet, 1957). Stem cells by a process of randomized somatic genetic change develop different immune patterns, one only being expressed for each cell and clone. Contact with the corresponding antigen provokes antibody formation or other specific response.

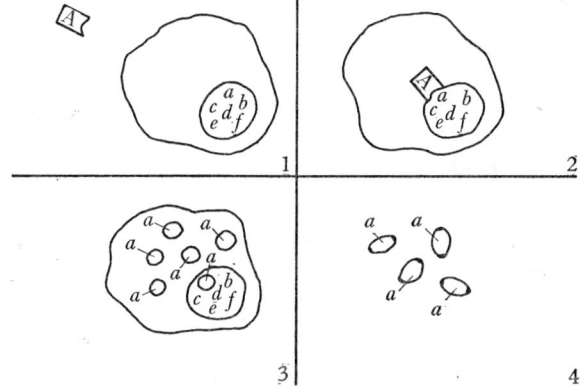

Fig. 4. Subcellular selection theory (Lederberg, 1959). Each cell has preexistent capacity to produce large numbers of antibody patterns. Entry of antigen selects the appropriate pattern for expression.

The situation subsequently became more complex, but it was very largely from consideration of the implications of immune tolerance that concepts of cellular (or clonal) selection approaches began to develop. In 1957 Talmage and Burnet suggested independently that it was more satisfactory to consider the process primarily in terms of clones of lymphoid cells. The implications of this view were stated *in extenso* by Burnet in 1959 and since then the approach has been widened and modified with increasing knowledge until it has reached the form with which this book is concerned.

THE CLONAL SELECTION THEORY OF IMMUNITY

In its original form this clonal selection theory of immunity postulated a randomization of pattern amongst differentiating lymphoid cells in embryonic life, so that each lymphoid cell in the body carried one immunological pattern expressed either as a 'receptor' or as the specificity of the antibody produced by the cell or its descendants. Subject to the possibility of mutation, the pattern was transmitted by somatic inheritance to all descendants giving rise to large numbers of clones of cells, each with a distinct immunological specificity.

The novel features of the approach were all related to a concentration of attention on the behaviour of cells as units rather than on the process of antibody synthesis. The basic concept was of the immunologically competent cell—a term now replaced by 'immunocyte'—that is, a cell which is susceptible to specific stimulation by contact with the appropriate antigenic determinant. On this hypothesis the result of such contact will depend on two major factors, the effective concentration of antigen in the cell's environment and the avidity of union between antigenic determinant and the combining site on the cell receptors. Factors dependent on the local environment of the immunocyte and its physiological state will presumably also play a part. The main possibilities of reaction are (*a*) destruction, especially if physiologically immature, (*b*) proliferation without essential change of character—to what we would now call memory cells and (*c*) proliferation and antibody production as a clone of plasma cells.

It was immediately evident that such an approach provided an alternative mechanism by which the amount and type of antibody and immunocytes could be adjusted to the current needs of the body. It also provided the simplest possible interpretation of how the body's own constituents are shielded from immunological attack.

At the time of writing it is probably correct to say that most experimental immunologists are averse from supporting any comprehensive statement of immunological theory. There is a general feeling that current activity in the elucidation of the molecular structure of the immunoglobulins will within a few years provide a solid background not now in existence against which theoretical concepts with some hope of being definitive may be developed.

This must be accepted but it seems that already the major decision between instructive and selective theories has been made. It is now mainly a matter of working out what mechanism is concerned in generating the diverse genetic patterns which govern the production of the vast repertoire of specific antibodies which can be produced more or less on demand.

My own preference has been to look to somatic mutation for the origin of this diversity, but there can be no doubt that genetic influences of the normal sort are important. With the development of ways by which the individualities of immunoglobulin molecules could be recognized irrespective of their specificity as antibodies, it became clear that complex inheritable genetic information from more than one source in the genome was converging to determine the structure of antibody. When the first complete sequences of amino acids in one set of the polypeptide chains that make up Ig G were established in 1965–6, a much more direct approach to the problem of genetic origins lay open. Already it seems virtually certain that the evolution of the immunoglobulin molecule has involved several successive duplications of a primitive cistron coding for 100–110 amino acids. Many immunochemists have been impressed with the probable resemblance between the processes which have produced the haemoglobins and the emerging evolutionary history of the immunoglobulins.

There can be no doubt that in part any antibody, any immunoglobulin, is produced by the interaction of a number of genetic units. There is wide sympathy for the view not yet elaborated in detail that there is a store, as it were, of genetic information which can be drawn on to provide a very large number of combinations each of which can code for a functioning antibody molecule. Somatic mutation is still a curiously unpopular concept amongst biologists and many would look to genetic processes (in the normal sense) to provide all the necessary variety of antibody pattern.

There is no sort of unanimity on the matter. None can be possible till much more structural information is accumulated. It is, however, not quite pure guesswork to suggest that both (germinal) genetic and somatic genetic processes play an important role and that in broad terms the former can be compared to the coarse adjustment and the latter to the fine adjustment of a microscope. Again relying on an intuitive sense of what is biologically likely in the absence of relevant data, one would expect genetic effects to be more important in small short-lived animals like mice, and somatic mutation to play a much greater part in large long-lived animals like men.

Whatever the eventual assignment of responsibility for antibody diversity, there is a quality about immunological phenomena which calls for a random process by which antibody patterns are distributed, as it were, to immunocytes and established for the descendant clone by strict phenotypic restriction.

The other important feature that has been revealed by the structural studies of immunoglobulin light chains is the much greater diversity of the N terminal 107 residues than of the other half of the chain. Circumstantial evidence points strongly toward 'labile' sectors of this type in both chains being concerned with the formation of the combining sites and therefore with the specificity of the antibody. For the present it is probably true to say that technical achievement is not yet adequate to support the speculations on the nature of specificity.

There have also been a number of attempts to devise a quasi-instructive theory in which the choice amongst some tens of thousands of potentialities in each cell is actually made by the antigenic determinant. Theories of this general character are easy to endow with *ad hoc* qualifications which make them almost impossible to disprove. The main virtue of the clonal selection theory is that it can be disproved immediately it can be shown that from a single cell (or its operational equivalent) three or more unrelated primary antibodies can be produced to nominated antigens.

In parallel with the ideas on the nature of the relationship between antigen and antibody and the gradual elaboration of the complexity and heterogeneity of the immunoglobulins, the cells responsible for antibody production have also been the subject of much discussion. One of the most fruitful lines of experimental advance since 1957 has been the development of technical methods by which single cells or pure clones derived from a single cell can be studied immunologically, and these techniques have now brought a much clearer understanding of the interrelationships of the cells concerned. In parallel with these single-cell studies there has been a steady growth in the understanding of the cytological character of the various cell populations available for experimental transfer and manipulation.

Any attempt to disprove or modify a clonal selection theory would necessarily have to make much use of these new techniques, and it is in fact the ability of the theory to absorb in natural fashion the various concepts as they arose from the new experimental approaches that has been its main claim to validity. It is worth while therefore in this historical introduction to devote a few pages to the significance of the new techniques that have been developed in recent years for handling immunologically significant cells.

THE CELLULAR ASPECTS OF IMMUNITY

The first set of cells to be considered as producers of antibody were the macrophages of Metchnikoff or the reticulo-endothelial system of Aschoff, both defined by their capacity to take in foreign particulate matter or macromolecular dyes. With the prevalent instructive view of antibody formation it seemed reasonable that the cells taking up the antigen should be those making the corresponding antibody. It was evident that two important sites for antibody production were spleen and lymph nodes, in both of which cells of the reticulo-endothelial system were numerous; so also were lymphocytes and plasma cells, while there were also smaller numbers of mast cells and a variety of supporting cells. In each site, activity associated with artificial immunization was evidenced by the appearance of germinal centres (reaction centres, secondary follicles) in the primary lymph follicles of lymph nodes and spleen, and of plasma cells at the periphery of the lymph follicles and in the red pulp of the spleen and the medullary cords of lymph nodes. On the necessary but unprovable and improbable assumption that the three cell types were completely distinct it was felt that either the macrophage, the lymphocyte or the plasma cell must be the producer of antibody.

In 1948 Fagraeus showed conclusively that antibody production was correlated with the presence of plasma cells, and since then there has been no serious alternative to the view that antibodies and immunoglobulins are predominantly secreted by plasma cells and the intermediate cells of the lymphoblast to plasma cell series. The application of all the modern methods of cytological study leads to the same conclusion. Electron micrographs show abundant rough endoplasmic reticulum in plasma cells and special methods have identified globulin and antibody between the lamellae. The numerous polyribosomes and the active nucleolus also indicate a rapid synthesis of protein and are responsible for the characteristic staining of the plasma cell by the Unna–Pappenheim method.

The first of the direct histochemical methods to be adapted to immunological experimentation was Coons's 'fluorescent antibody' approach (Coons et al. 1942). There are relatively simple ways of attaching fluorescent dyes to soluble proteins using the same principles that Landsteiner applied in binding antigenic determinants of known character to carrier proteins. If a semi-purified antibody is labelled in this fashion with fluorescein and used to stain a thin section of fresh tissue, there will be a precipitation of antibody at any site where the corresponding antigen is present in adequate concentration. The most important antigen for such experiments is paradoxically enough antibody itself or, more correctly, immunoglobulin. If human tissues are to be studied, purified antibodies are prepared from rabbits immunized each with a pure solution of one of the antigenically distinguishable human immunoglobulins and linked to a suitable fluorescent dye. Any cell in a tissue section which is secreting significant amounts of the appropriate immunoglobulin will be 'stained' and the fluorescent areas can be recognized microscopically with appropriate illumination. All studies are in agreement that plasma cells are the predominant producers of each of the defined immunoglobulins. By suitable refinement using treatment first with antigen then with specific fluorescent antiserum (the sandwich technique) it can also be shown that in an immunized animal many plasma cells are producing antibody of corresponding specificity.

A few years later, autoradiographic techniques were introduced and soon concentrated on the use of tritiated thymidine as a marker by which the lineage of a given cell could be traced. If a cell in the process of duplicating its DNA before mitosis is exposed to labelled thymidine, this is rapidly taken up and incorporated into the DNA of the chromosomes. Owing to the conservative quality of DNA replication, the thymidine taken up is retained by the nucleus and distributed approximately equally to any descendant nuclei. The location and amount of label is determined by overlaying thin sections or smears with photographic film. After processing and staining, the number of silver grains associated with a cell nucleus is a measure of the amount of label present. Subject to a variety of technical safeguards, cells showing nuclear label are lineal descendants of cells which at the time the tritiated thymidine was administered were actively synthesizing DNA. The application of this technique to immunological problems is only limited by the ingenuity and dexterity of the experimenter, and many results will be discussed in later chapters.

Other radioisotopic techniques have also been applied, one of the most important being to provide labelled amino acids to a cell population in order to show by subsequent measurement of activity in specific antibody that antibody was being actually synthesized by the cells during the time the labelled amino acids were present in the system.

From these and other types of experiment it became clear that Fagraeus was correct in ascribing antibody production predominantly to immature and mature plasma cells.

It is still uncertain to what extent other morphological cell types are associated with antibody. When appropriate antisera against the different immunoglobulins are used to detect cells carrying or producing the antigens in question, the strongest reactions to each type are given by plasma cells, but there is frequently a general glow over germinal centres and on scattered reticular cells. There are some small cells, not morphologically different from small lymphocytes, which may be present in thoracic duct fluid, that show strong staining for γ-globulin in their thin rim of cytoplasm;

the significance of these lymphokinocytes is unknown. Quite recently it has been found that many lymphocytes can produce at least small amounts of immunoglobulins and, in suitable material, actual production of antibody can be demonstrated.

Perhaps the most important available generalization on which all interpretations must be based is that antigen is taken up by cells that do not produce antibody—macrophages of various types—and that antibody is produced by plasma cells that contain no detectable antigen. There are two tenable interpretations that will have to be discussed. The first is that within some of the macrophages the antigen is broken down to give rise to a certain number of antigenic determinant–RNA complexes which have a special capacity to stimulate competent lymphoid cells to which they are transferred. The second (which does not necessarily exclude the first) is that the main immunological function of the reticulo-endothelial system is to reduce the concentration of circulating antigen to a level low enough for an effective response by the antibody-producing mechanism.

With the statement of the clonal selection theory it seemed immediately evident that the theory would be disproved if it were shown that a single cell could regularly produce more than two antibodies. With the increasing information about immunoglobulin types and the as yet unexcluded possibilities of interchange of immunological information between cells, we should nowadays be sceptical about so simple an approach. Nevertheless, for one reason or another, the last decade has seen great activity in devising ways of demonstrating and measuring antibody production from single cells and in seeking to demonstrate cells producing more than one type of antibody after immunization with multiple antigens.

For obvious reasons, very sensitive assay methods must be available if the antibody produced by a single cell isolated in a droplet of fluid is to be measured. Neutralization of bacterial viruses and immobilization of bacterial flagella have both been successfully used. As is usually the case with biological experiments the results are not in themselves decisive but they have contributed valuable new information.

A less direct but more fruitful approach was devised by Jerne and Nordin, who showed that single cells could produce sufficient haemolytic antibody against foreign red cells to allow the development of a plaque-counting technique. If a mouse is making antibody after an injection of sheep red cells four days previously, most of the antibody-producing cells are in the spleen. Their number can be obtained by emulsifying known numbers of spleen cells with a suspension of sheep red cells in melted agar. The agar is poured and, after setting, incubated for 30 minutes during which any antibody diffuses from the cell and attaches to adjacent red cells. By flooding the plate with guinea-pig serum (complement) the areas where antibody is attached to red cells become visible as clear areas (plaques) of haemolysis. By appropriate artifices, similar plaques can be used to measure the number of cells producing other antibodies and from 1964 onwards the technique became standard in most immunological laboratories.

Two other methods of handling single cells for quite different purposes have also been significant for immunological theory. The first was developed in my laboratory by Boyer (1960), who found that when adult fowl leucocytes were placed on the chorioallantois of chick embryos, rather large opaque foci developed whose number was proportional to the numbers of leucocytes added. The evidence subsequently obtained is interpreted as showing that an adult immunocyte reactive against an antigenic determinant of the recipient membrane will initiate a focal lesion in which both host and donor cells are involved. It is in fact a typical graft-versus-host reaction.

The second is a by-product of studies on the recovery of mice lethally irradiated and subsequently given bone-marrow cells from normal animals. Such mice take up to thirty days to die in the absence of treatment. Till and McCulloch found that if such mice were given a small dose of bone-marrow cells intravenously and killed five to ten days later, their spleens showed discrete white masses of cells a millimetre or two in diameter. Irradiated mice receiving no further treatment showed only shrunken spleens without nodules. Again, the number of these foci was proportional to the number of bone-marrow cells administered and each was predominantly a clone derived from a single initiating cell. Just as in the foci of the chorioallantoic membrane, these nodules are open to the entry of circulating cells and the idea that they are 'clones' must be used very circumspectly.

THE CONTRIBUTION OF IMMUNOPATHOLOGY

Running in parallel with experimental immunology has been a growing interest in immunopathology and, as has been the case in many fields of medicine, pathological findings have thrown much light on the normal functioning of the immune mechanism.

For fairly obvious reasons, acquired haemolytic anaemia was the first autoimmune disease to be clearly recognized. Many other human diseases in which there is at least a major autoimmune component are now known and similar conditions have been recognized in mice and dogs. One's first reaction to autoimmune disease is that it must represent a disturbance in the development of natural tolerance and almost all who have written on the nature of immune tolerance have been influenced by ideas drawn from pathology.

Of even greater influence on the development of immunology has been the progressive understanding of the nature of the myeloma proteins, Bence Jones protein and of the conditions with which they are associated. As soon as electrophoretic methods were applied to these pathological sera it became clear that there was a great excess of a homogeneous population of immunoglobulin molecules. In Waldenström's words these were 'monoclonal gammopathies' in which the myeloma protein is operationally and perhaps absolutely equivalent to antibody produced by a single clone of immunocytes. As will be shown in later pages, this realization not only gave a great impetus to chemical studies on immunoglobulins but was also probably the most potent factor in bringing about a more tolerant attitude to the clonal selection theory.

We can omit in this outline other interesting leads from pathology, particularly in relation to the thymus, but mention must be made of congenital agammaglobulinaemia. This was a by-product of the antibiotic treatment of ailing infants. It was of special importance in showing that a normal complement of lymphocytes could be present without plasma cells and that while antibody production failed to occur, a variety of skin hypersensitivities could develop, measles ran a normal course with subsequent immunity and skin homografts could be rejected. No theoretical approach to immunology could subsequently be complete unless this dissociation of immune functions could be covered.

2 The general character of immune phenomena

THE FUNCTIONS OF THE IMMUNE RESPONSE IN VERTEBRATES

Evolutionary considerations

Until the early 1950s it was implicit in medical and microbiological thought that immunity was concerned wholly with defence against micro-organismal infection. Various clinical and laboratory phenomena such as anaphylaxis which, though obviously immunological in character had no bearing on protection against infection, were well known but could be interpreted as artefacts arising from unbiological contrivance or circumstance. In recent years this attitude has changed, perhaps mainly because of the upsurge of interest in tissue transplantation in surgery. Tissue grafting is something unknown in nature, so at first sight it is hard to understand how an impressively large and self-consistent body of scientific knowledge could have been accumulated around something that from the evolutionary standpoint was meaningless. There are, however, two very important natural mammalian situations which in significant ways are analogous to an experimental graft of foreign tissue, pregnancy and cancer. A pregnancy represents the implantation of foreign tissue in the uterus—it is in most respects formally equivalent to grafting skin from an F_1 mouse (AB) on to an individual of one or other of the pure line parent strains AA and BB from which it was derived. The AB skin graft on an AA recipient is foreign in respect of its B component and will be rejected. The AB foetus in an AA mother thrives. Clearly, some special mechanism must have been evolved to allow placental reproduction.

A cancer results from the multiplication of cells within the body which are alien in the sense that they are not adequately subject to the controls that ensure the morphological integrity of the body. It is now realized that most malignant cells are antigenically distinguishable from related normal cells of the animal in which the tumour has arisen, but the difference in histocompatibility antigens is always slight. There is a steadily increasing opinion that the immunological difference between normal and malignant cells is biologically and even clinically very important. In addition there is a still more important point which depends on the fact that a spontaneous tumour initially at least retains the essential antigenic character of the host. If it arises in a mouse of pure line strain A, it will behave on transplantation very like a piece of A's normal tissue. It will 'take' in almost 100 per cent of mice of strain A or in F_1 hybrids obtained by mating A mice with any other pure line strain. It will be rejected like a foreign skin graft in any other type of host.

There are no populations of genetically uniform mammals in nature. Given the general properties of the evolutionary population, every naturally occurring individual will differ in its inheritance from every other individual. There is, however, no *a priori* reason why two animals of the same species should not accept transplants from one another. This can, in fact, be done in insects and in many types of embryonic or immature vertebrates. The characteristic incompatibility of mammalian skin grafts is of relatively late evolutionary origin. One of the possible reasons for the existence of this immunological individuality within a vertebrate species can be put succinctly by saying that, in its absence, cancer could be a contagious disease.

Evolution, therefore, may have moulded immune mechanisms for other reasons than defence against micro-organisms. Invertebrates require just as effective means of countering infections as vertebrates but they produce no antibodies. Amongst the lower vertebrates, the hagfish shows no evidence of an immune response to any of the standard tests but a more advanced cyclostome, the lamprey, shows for the first time the attributes of the immune mechanism which is present in all higher forms. It appears, therefore, that at an early stage in vertebrate evolution a need arose for some mechanism beyond what had been developed against bacterial infection in the invertebrates. Discussion of the vertebrate, and specifically the mammalian, immune mechanism leads almost inevitably to the conclusion that it is more basically concerned with the control of tissue integrity and reaction against recognized anomaly in tissues than in defence against micro-organisms and the production of antibody. One can imagine that with the emergence of the new tissue-controlling mechanism new possibilities of effective defence arose and thereafter the two interrelated functions evolved together.

A third type of immunological phenomenon distinct from either of these categories, though in curious ways related to both, is currently described as 'delayed hypersensitivity'. The tuberculin reaction is the classical example but there are, in addition, various types of skin hypersensitivity to natural or synthetic chemicals and clear indications that many of the manifestations of chronic infectious or autoimmune disease are based on the same type of reaction.

There are, then, three main biological functions of the immune system to be considered: tissue control as exemplified by the rejection of foreign skin grafts, tissue reactions that are not mediated by antibody such as the tuberculin reaction, and antimicrobial functions such as protection by antiviral antibody or the production of antitoxin in diphtheria and similar bacterial infections.

Transplantation immunity

Transplantation immunity is usually demonstrated by skin grafting. It is well known that a plastic surgeon can graft a piece of skin from any part of his patient's body to any other part. If, however, he attempts to borrow skin from a donor—for example, to make good skin lost in very extensive burns—the best he can hope for is that the borrowed skin will be retained for a little over a week. By fourteen to twenty days it will have been completely rejected. There are three exceptions to this rule which, in themselves, almost define the processes involved:

(*a*) When two people are identical twins they will accept and retain skin grafts from each other. Identical twins arise by the splitting of the fertilized ovum after the first division, with the two cells both going on to normal development. The twins have exactly the same genetic endowment.

(*b*) Very rarely twins are found who are clearly not identical but differ from ordinary two-egg twins by sharing *in utero* a blood supply from fused placentas. Despite the fact that the twins are genetically distinct, arising from two separately fertilized ova, blood cells of all types move freely between the two embryos and they are born with this mixed blood condition. If one is genetically blood group O and the other group A, each will have the same mixture of O and A cells and retain the mixture for life. Such twins will also accept and retain reciprocal skin grafts.

(c) There is an extremely rare condition in which a baby is born with a thymus which fails to develop. Such infants have virtually no lymphocytes in their blood, are extremely prone to infection and, even with the best of medical care, usually die within two years. If a child with this condition is grafted with a piece of unrelated skin the graft heals satisfactorily and is retained as long as the child survives.

Clinical observations of this sort would never have been made without the background of years of work on experimental skin grafting with pure line strains of mice, rats and hamsters. For the present, however, we can use the clinical findings to introduce the essential features of tissue immunity.

In the first place we have the demonstration that for a tissue to be rejected it must be recognizably *different* and that the differences involved are genetic in origin. By rigid and prolonged inbreeding, pure lines of mice can be obtained, each member of which is genetically equivalent to any other. The standard test for such genetic purity is to interchange skin grafts. All should be retained.

Genetic identity is not, however, a *necessary* condition for skin graft acceptance. The intermingling of placental blood of two dissimilar twins is a natural experiment which shows that tolerance of another individual's tissues is possible if the body has experienced the presence of the foreign cells from a period early in embryonic life. From this deduction the whole topic of *immunological tolerance* has developed and in a sense the present hope that organ transplantation will one day be regularly possible.

When the thymus fails to develop, lymphocytes are few or absent and standard antigens fail to provoke antibody formation. If one removes the thymus from baby mice on the first day of life, broadly similar changes result. In particular, such mice will accept skin from foreign strains of mice and even from rats. The implication is clear that an immunological process is concerned in skin graft rejection and that the presence of lymphocytes is essential.

In summary, studies of transplantation of skin and other tissues in experimental animals supported by such findings in man as have been mentioned have provided the following conclusions:

(*a*) Skin rejection requires the recognition by the recipient that the graft contains antigenic determinants not present in the recipient's cells. All antigenic determinants are genetically controlled. They may change by mutation in the germ cells or by somatic mutation.

(*b*) Recognition that an antigenic determinant is foreign requires that it shall not have been present in the body during embryonic life. Conversely, any foreign cells introduced early enough in life will be accepted as if they were the body's own cells for as long as they persist. There is more than one explanation of tolerance but the existence of the phenomenon was the stimulus that led to the conception of the clonal selection approach to immunity.

(*c*) Skin rejection requires the action of lymphoid cells. It can be accelerated by the presence of specific antibodies but these are probably not necessary for the reaction.

(*d*) If a mouse of strain A is grafted with skin B and rejects it in 10 days, a second graft of B on the same animal will be rejected more rapidly. The effect is specific, not being shown against skin from unrelated strains, and represents a typical secondary immune response.

(*e*) The reverse of skin rejection is the so-called graft-versus-host reaction which occurs when mature lymphoid cells are introduced into a recipient of another strain which, for one or other reason, is unable to destroy the cells. They can react in various ways against the host, particularly when introduced into very young recipients. These are liable to die with the expressively named 'runt disease'.

(*f*) There are several phenomena which seem to establish that there are in normal lymphocyte populations a proportion of cells which are immediately capable of recognizing and reacting against foreign tissue antigens.

Delayed hypersensitivity reactions

In 1891 Koch described the tuberculin reaction by which a guinea-pig actively infected with tuberculosis responded to a subcutaneous injection of a sterile filtrate from a tubercle bacillus culture. There was a sharp rise of temperature and the development of severe inflammation and necrosis at the site of the injection. In normal guinea-pigs there was virtually no reaction of any sort. With purified reagents and small intradermal injections the same reaction in the form of the Mantoux test is widely used in human medicine. In experimental animals it has become the prototype of *delayed hypersensitivity* reactions.

Such reactions, which in various more or less similar forms may be given by a wide variety of antigens, reach their peak around 24 hours after injection in most of the commonly studied examples. There are, however, some much slower reactions of otherwise similar quality which are seen in the lepromin and Kveim tests for leprosy and sarcoidosis respectively. All such delayed reactions are clearly differentiated both from the acute Arthus reactions seen in experimental animals immunized with standard soluble antigens and with acute allergic responses such as are seen when hay fever patients are tested with the incriminated pollen extract. The latter may for the present be dismissed as resulting from the fixation of a special type of antibody in the tissues of the skin and its reaction with the antigen. Delayed hypersensitivity has proved more difficult to interpret, and since the rejection of foreign tissues is basically due to very similar processes, there has been a big surge of new interest in the phenomenon.

It has not been possible to show that circulating antibody is in any way involved in delayed hypersensitivity though the possible activity of antibody adsorbed to the surface of leucocytes or macrophages has not been finally excluded. Most immunologists regard as the main key to the nature of delayed hypersensitivity the fact that if a very large mass of lymphoid cells is transferred from a sensitized guinea-pig to a normal one, the recipient also becomes reactive within a few hours. When an injection of antigen is made into the skin the response is essentially the same in the passively sensitized recipient as in the actively sensitized animal. What is observed is redness and swelling of the reaction site represented histologically by dilatation and stasis in small blood vessels and a vigorous migration of mononuclear cells which, as they pass through the walls of small venules and capillaries, appear to be mainly small lymphocytes. As they pass away from the capillary into the tissues they become larger and most would be called histiocytes.

There are many unsolved aspects of this reaction. What stimulates the movement of cells through the vessel wall? What proportion of the migrating cells have a specific immune relationship to the antigen deposited in the tissues? How does contact of antigen with cell give rise to the vascular responses we observe? In addition, delayed hypersensitivity has served as a central point from which many related experimental phenomena have been developed, only one or two of which need be mentioned in this orienting approach.

Transplantation immunity as demonstrated in experiments with skin grafts may well be a slightly modified delayed hypersensitivity response. Histologically the early stage of rejection is shown by a local accumulation of mononuclear cells including lymphocytes and plasma cells. Homograft immunity can be transferred to another animal by lymphoid tissue cells but not by serum. Finally, if we have an animal A which has developed homograft immunity against B, an intradermal inoculation of A's lymphocytes into B's skin will give a reaction of the same quality as a delayed hypersensitivity reaction.

In the field of clinical immunology there has been much recent interest in the reactions of human blood lymphocytes in the presence of kidney bean phytohaemagglutinin and certain antigens. It has been known for many years that a variety of plant extracts, particularly from leguminous seeds, could agglutinate red cells, and sometimes showed useful specificity for one or other of the ABO human blood groups. As a logical development from this work, such phytohaemagglutinins were used to separate leucocytes from red cells in blood. The addition of the extract to citrated or heparinized blood caused rapid clumping and sedimentation of red cells, leaving leucocytes in suspension in the supernatant fluid.

It had been well known that blood leucocytes held under ordinary tissue culture conditions did not proliferate. Cultures made from leucocytes obtained by the use of phytohaemagglutinin, however, rather surprisingly showed large numbers of mitoses that resulted from the enlargement and then division of small lymphocytes. The next step was the observation of Pearmain and his colleagues in New Zealand that tuberculin or PPD added to blood lymphocytes from tuberculin-positive individuals produced enlargement and mitoses but not cells from non-reactors. The present position which could readily be changed by a few intelligently planned experiments suggests that the phenomenon may be a measure of the range of delayed hypersensitivity reactions shown by the donor of cells.

Immunity against micro-organismal infection

The third broad area of immune function is in many ways the most obvious and, by far, of the greatest practical importance. We can prevent diphtheria, tetanus, poliomyelitis and whooping cough, smallpox and yellow fever with almost complete certainty by a simple application of immunological principles. Yet, looked at from the evolutionary angle, there are puzzling features. In underdeveloped regions, which included Europe until a little over a hundred years ago, by far the greatest concentration of mortality was in infants around the time that their maternally transmitted immunity had disappeared. Once the period from 6 months to 5 years had been survived, children had usually sufficient immunity to the common pathogens to be immune to them for life. It appears that the best evolutionary solution to the problem of survival in a heavily contaminated environment is to accept the unprotected state for the first impact of any particular infection and provide the survivors with a solid immunity that will render an otherwise dangerous pathogen harmless. The classical example is yellow fever. European children brought up in a country where the disease was prevalent might suffer from other diseases but never, as adolescents or adults, from yellow fever. Unprotected adults such as the European soldiers brought to the West Indies during the Napoleonic wars had an appalling death rate from yellow fever.

The mechanism of protection against second or subsequent attacks of infectious disease is not quite as clear now as it seemed twenty years ago. In virus diseases it was regarded as self-evident that antibody persisting in circulation plus the capacity to produce further antibody at short notice were the protective agents. The fact that children with congenital agammaglobulinaemia who can produce no detectable antibody show a normal course during an attack of measles and have a solid subsequent immunity was disconcerting. There are indications that other virus diseases do not behave so normally as measles in these children but the nature of measles immunity remains unexplained. The main disability in agammaglobulinaemic children is the occurrence of repeated bacterial infection of the respiratory tract, which suggests that long-held ideas about pneumococcal infections and the part played by antibody in their control are probably correct. Nothing discovered since the great days of research on pneumonia in the 1930s has diminished the importance of the opsonizing function of antibody in allowing control of bacterial infections.

THE THEORETICAL APPROACH

In the immediately preceding sections, I have outlined the range of phenomena with which this book is concerned and in the rest of the chapter I shall summarize the theoretical approach to be adopted. That approach represents an attempt to restate in terms of recent work the essential features of the clonal selection approach which I developed in 1957–8.

The premises of clonal selection theory

Clonal selection theory in a modern guise must be expressed a little differently from the form used in 1958 but basically the premises of the theory are the same.

(a) There exist in the body populations of cells differentiated for immune function by their ability to produce antibody and to react in other ways to contact with specific antigen. These cells are referred to as 'immunocytes'. In the adult mammal they comprise a substantial proportion of the cells with the morphology of small lymphocytes as well as all plasma cells and a variety of immature and intermediate forms.

(b) Like the patterns which endow enzymic activity or antigenic individuality on other proteins, the specific pattern of antibody is determined by the genetic endowment of the cell which produces it.

(c) The range of immune reactivity of any immunocyte or clone of immunocytes is sharply limited by a process of phenotypic restriction. It may be subject to limited extension by subsequent somatic mutation.

(d) The origin of the diversity of immune pattern is to be sought at the genetic level. The important processes are probably (i) random choice for phenotypic expression of alternative gene combinations, and one or both of two types of somatic genetic change, (ii) 'scrambler' mechanisms of somatic recombination of the type recently suggested by Smithies and (iii) somatic mutation occurring within the relevant cistrons during the individual's life.

(e) Antigen acts essentially only as a signal or stimulus to such cells as are competent by the possession of antibody-like receptors to react to it.

Such a formulation is highly flexible in the sense that in any field of immunological investigation the precise form of theoretical interpretation can be modified to conform to the convenience of the situation. At the present time, for instance, there are a number of contentions opposed to aspects of my own interpretation of what is on record in the immunological literature. Some workers hold that it will soon be unequivocally demonstrated that transfer of capacity to produce immune pattern can occur from one cell to another. Others would base what most writers regard as the direct action of immunocytes on the adsorption of cytophilic antibody to immunologically neutral cells. Many immunologists are unconvinced that tolerance is wholly a matter of the *absence* of the corresponding immunocyte and would look for a more active process.

If any of these contentions are established, an extensive reorientation will become necessary but the central problem of accounting for the immune pattern in genetic terms will remain. At the present time the chief virtue of the clonal selection approach is that it provides a reasonable framework within which to interpret findings which involve both the population dynamics of lymphoid cells and specific immunological responses such as the production of antibody. This, in fact, is a concise statement of my present objective.

In this chapter I am concerned essentially with an orientating discussion of the biological principles germane to the development of selective theories of immunology. In writing this book, the greatest difficulty I have found is the utter impossibility of providing a logical sequence that will cover the subject matter of immunology in a single one-dimensional movement. Tolerance, for instance, can only be discussed in terms of interference with antibody production but the phenomena of tolerance are highly relevant to the nature of the differentiation of stem cell to immunocyte, which seems the logical point at which to start discussion of the whole immune process.

The solution I have adopted is, first, to assume some background of biological and immunological knowledge in the reader and to provide in this chapter a generalized summary of the approach that will be adopted. It is divided into two main topics which in one form or another cover most of the themes that need consideration:

1. Aspects of differentiation and somatic mutation which may be relevant to antibody diversity.
2. The origin and population dynamics of the lymphoid cells and the concept of the immunocyte.

The nature of antibody

There is no way of defining an antibody in any simple fashion. At the present time we regard as antibody any population of immunoglobulin molecules which has a specific capacity to unite preferentially with a definable chemical substance or configuration. The preferential capacity to combine with a given antigenic determinant is ascribed to the 'combining sites' of the antibody and its specificity is a manifestation of the 'immune pattern' of the antibody.

Before entering on any discussion of immune pattern, the concept of antigenic determinant needs to be clarified. It comes originally from Landsteiner's experiments with artificial antigens in which many molecules of some simple pattern, an arsanilic acid for instance, were chemically combined to a simple protein such as egg albumin. The antisera produced were first treated with the carrier protein to remove antibodies reacting with components other than the artificial hapten. Then, by appropriate precipitation tests with proteins carrying a series of related haptens plus inhibition tests in which the simple chemical blocked the capacity of the antibody to precipitate the full antigen, it became evident that the hapten was the only structure reacting with this population of antibodies. This conclusion has been confirmed and elaborated by refined experimentation in recent years. On current views any antigen (that is, a macromolecule or particle capable of reacting with antibody) can be regarded as a mosaic of configurations, of molecular twists and outlines, which are potentially antigenic determinants. Many of them, because they are identical or very similar to configurations in the animal injected, will be inert immunologically.

With this preliminary we can use the term immune pattern for the specific aspect by which antibodies of all types react with a given antigenic determinant. In man and most other mammals there are three major types of immunoglobulin which can function as antibody. The one present in highest concentration both in the total immunoglobulins of serum and in most standard antibodies is immunoglobulin G (Ig G or γ G). This form has been sufficiently studied at the chemical level to allow us to picture immune pattern on that molecule as the disposition of amino acid residues in two equivalent combining sites, one at each end of an elongate molecule. The molecule of a typical antibody is a highly complex structure. Strictly speaking, only myeloma proteins are available for the detailed study needed to define antibody protein structure. There is, however, no evidence whatever against the tacit assumption made by almost all immunochemists that an Ig G myeloma protein is a homogeneous population of a single type of antibody molecule produced by a clone of plasmacytes. There are indications that under special conditions large amounts of monoclonal antibody can be produced, but all that have so far been studied are heterogeneous. It cannot be wholly excluded that an antibody has some quality not expressed in a myeloma protein of equivalent type, but in this discussion it will be assumed that there is no such difference.

The Ig G antibody is a symmetrical molecule made up of two light chains each approximately of 22,000 mol. wt and two heavy chains of 50,000 mol. wt united by a relatively small number of disulphide bonds. Both chains are complex. The light chain of 214 residues is made up of two parts, each of precisely 107 residues. That including the N terminal group is rather highly variable from one Ig G myeloma protein to another, while the C terminal half is essentially identical except for the single amino acid change associated with the Inv a or Inv b antigenic character. The larger heavy chain is not so well investigated. The fact that a relatively large stable portion, now known as Fc, could be split off with pepsin without modifying antibody activity has been known for many years. The remaining Fd section has not yet been closely studied at the chemical level. It does, however, include a portion that varies in peptide structure from one myeloma to another, and it is the one section of the antibody molecule which all writers agree carries all or part of the combining site.

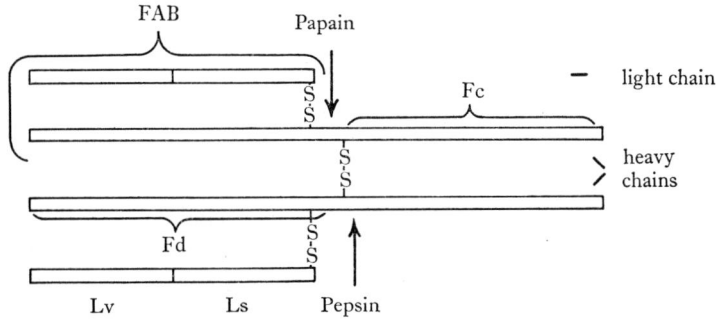

Fig. 5. The Porter diagram (modified) of Ig G structure, to indicate the various fractions and the site of action of papain and pepsin.

The highly variable character of the N terminal end of the light chain which is at least closely related to the combining site, plus the probability that the portion of the heavy chain which carries antibody specificity is also of variable constitution, points strongly but not absolutely to the currently popular view that these variations in amino acid sequence are in fact the basis of antibody specificity, of what we have called immune pattern. For reasons which may or may not stand up to future research, I have suggested that the variable portion of the heavy chain may be identical with the variable half of the light chain and therefore governed by the same cistron. A majority would probably regard the combining site as being derived from the mutual interaction of dissimilar segments on light and heavy chains. Irrespective of this diversity of opinion about the nature of the chains involved in the combining site, it seems probable that in general only a few residues (perhaps, as

Karush has suggested, about fifteen) are specially relevant to its specific character. Having regard to the very much greater extent of the 'variable' segment of the light chain (107 residues) than the length presumably involved in a combining site (7–10 residues), it must be kept in mind that the term 'combining site' has relevance only to the antigenic determinant being considered. If, as is suggested in a later diagram, the light and heavy chains may be closely related over a region of 20–30 residues, there could be possibilities of the same combining *region* carrying combining *sites* for two or more quite different antigenic determinants. If randomness of origin with determinate transmission of pattern is, as I believe, the essential character of antibody specificity, this would be bound to happen on occasion. Discussion of experimental results on the basis that any combining site is uniquely appropriate to a single antigenic determinant is as naïve as the belief that it was made to order to fit that determinant.

Irrespective of its relationship to the two chains, everything is consistent with the view originally due to Pauling that the combining site has a steric pattern and electronic configuration which make it unite more readily with the complementary configuration that we call an antigenic determinant than with any other molecular configuration. To be a little more precise, if we have a population of antibody molecules with identical combining sites so that we can speak of the population as a chemical species—antibody x—there will be a very limited class of chemical configurations which we can call collectively antigenic determinant X which will unite specifically with antibody x through the same combining site. Specific union can only be defined as firmer union than that shown by other substances tested. There is no absolute chemical equivalence between X and x. In one well-studied example, antibody to the glucose polymer dextran was shown to be able to react to some extent to the disaccharide maltose and successively more firmly up to the 5- or 7-hexose molecules.

We can also look at the relationship between antigenic determinant and combining site from the opposite side. In practice this will usually involve using a chemical hapten of known structure united to a natural protein or a synthetic polypeptide. Experiment has consistently shown that all available antibody populations—

those produced, for example, by immunizing rabbits with the artificial antigen—are highly heterogeneous.* In particular, there is still a wide variation in the avidity of union of different sections of the antibody population with the fully defined antigenic determinant. One must bear in mind that any soluble protein, notably

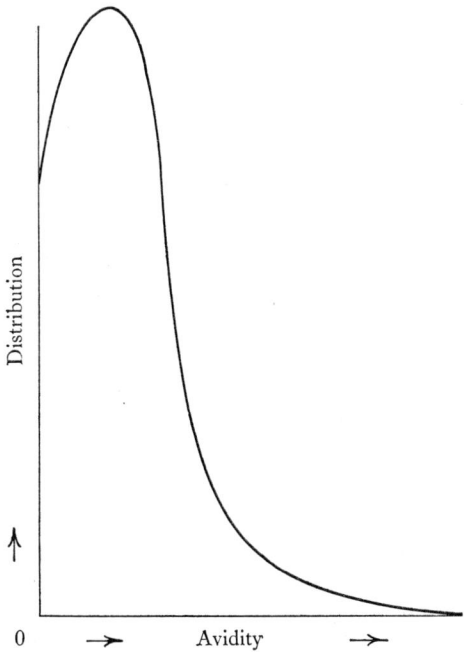

Fig. 6. To indicate the expected distribution of affinity of mixed immunoglobulins for any antigenic determinant. Only the small proportion of high avidity patterns to the right will be recognized as antibody.

serum albumin, has a capacity to adsorb a wide variety of simple chemical substances whose configurations are more or less equivalent to those groupings which can function as antigenic determinants. If it is correct to regard the emergence of new immune patterns as a random process, then for any given antigenic deter-

* The exceptions to this rule are those myeloma proteins which have a definable status as specific antibodies. The description by Eisen's group (1967) of a human myeloma protein active against antigens carrying dinitrophenyl as hapten is of special relevance.

minant there will be a fairly standard type of distribution, according to avidity, of the γ-globulin molecules present in a representative pool of serum from many members of the same species. The vast majority of immune patterns will have a negligible avidity of the same order as could be expected with any unspecialized protein. The distribution to be expected for higher degrees of avidity will be as shown in fig. 6. The highest possible degree of avidity will depend both on what arrangement of amino acid sequence and mutual disposition provides the strongest union and on how close to that optimal arrangement the initial pattern provided genetically can be brought by mutation or whatever other process is concerned in the 'generation of diversity'.

This character of the relationship between antigenic determinant and antibody is basic to any understanding of the concept of immunological pattern. The main objective of the present work is to seek an understanding of the nature of specificity and the 'soft edges' of specificity are an essential aspect of the problem.

The evidence is now overwhelming that the classical interpretation of protein synthesis as the transcription of information (coded pattern) in DNA to messenger RNA (m-RNA) and ribosomes where it is translated into an equivalent pattern of amino acids in a polypeptide chain is correct within its limitations. It is implicit in this that any protein that maintains its quality through successive cell generations is endowed with that quality by, in the last analysis, information held in the genome of the cell line concerned. There is nowadays no place for the 'instructive' theory that polypeptide chains are mechanically moulded into shape by contact with antigenic determinant. In one way or another there must be a genetic origin for the information that allows an antibody to be produced against a virus that may never previously have been met in the whole evolutionary history of the species.

The basis of diversity

The most evident fact about antibody is its heterogeneity. There are at least three different types of immunoglobulin which can carry immune reactivity in all mammalian species that have been studied. The range of immune pattern appears to be virtually unlimited. Antibody is produced predominantly by plasma cells

The theoretical approach

and if we agree that instructive theories are now untenable there are only two sources for that diversity of cells which is needed to account for the heterogeneity of antibody. One of these is differentiation, by which in some way a choice is made amongst the various potentialities developed over the course of evolution and stored in the genome. The second is by inheritable change within a somatic cell line, either by somatic mutation in the ordinary sense or by some type of intrachromosomal rearrangement or recombination. Whichever of these somatic mechanisms is concerned the effect will be the emergence of patterns which differ in random ways from the pattern of the zygote from which they derive.

Orthodox theory holds that every diploid cell in the body contains potentially all the information contained in the genome of the fertilized ovum. The process of differentiation consists of a programmed series of changes in the regions of information-containing DNA which are allowed to function. The essence of differentiation is that the changes are programmed under the control of the genome. The best criterion of differentiation is that it occurs uniformly in all individuals of a homozygous population in which environmental factors are held constant. Since all rabbits, homozygous or not, produce the three physically defined immunoglobulins A, G and M, we must accept the differences as resulting from differentiation in the cells that produce them.

Similarly, if it should be demonstrated that a stem cell from the bone-marrow is multipotent and, depending on the particular internal environmental niche in which it lodges, will develop into erythropoietic, granulopoietic or lymphopoietic cell lines, this would clearly also be the manifestation of a process of differentiation.

When, however, we come to look at specific immune pattern the picture is quite different. If we inject a series of animals of the same species with the same antigen and maintain all the conditions as uniform as possible, it is usual to find a proportion which fail to respond and a wide range of titre in those that do. This holds even in homozygous animals especially when a 'poor' antigen is used.

When an antiserum against a well-defined antigen like a hapten-protein complex is produced in a rabbit, detailed study of the antibody population will show a gross heterogeneity of the combining sites. The picture is not of something made to the pattern of the antigen but of a random population of diverse patterns whose only common feature is ability to react with the hapten.

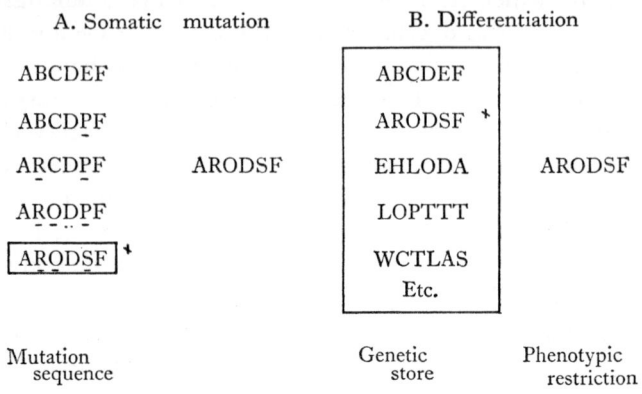

Fig. 7. Three origins for diversity: Schematic alternatives as to how the pattern ARODSF might arise in relation to a 'standard' pattern ABCDEF. A. Somatic mutation; B. differentiation; C. intergene recombination. Phenotypic restriction is operative in all.

From a quite different point of view the phenomena of tolerance necessarily imply that some random process is responsible for the production of cells carrying antibody patterns which, unless they are eliminated by the presence of circulating antigen, would be directed against antigens present in the body.

The theoretical approach

The essence of the situation is the *random* quality of the emergence of diversity and the evolutionary necessity that it should be random and that the random populations must be generated during the lifetime of the individual. If we use the conventional analogue of a protein pattern, a meaningful word in which letters represent amino acids, there are two basic ways by which a computer could be programmed to produce a random series of 10-letter words. One could provide in the memory all the 10,000 words that could conceivably be wanted and pick at random from these. Alternatively, starting with any 10-letter word, single-letter changes could be made at random, the result duplicated, other random single-letter changes made in each, and so on indefinitely. It is also obvious that the two processes could be combined in various ways. The problem at the immunological level is to discuss the pros and cons of 'randomized differentiation' or of 'accelerated somatic mutation' as the generators of diversity.

Diversification as a process of differentiation. Differentiation during embryonic and later development is basically a process of expression or inhibition of genetic potentialities in the fertilized ovum and the subsequent generations of descendant somatic cells. The complex diversity of function which we must postulate for antibody-producing cells is not unique in the vertebrate body. Primitive neurons seem almost to be programmed individually, each to move and direct its axon along an elaborately predetermined course. The control of pigmentation patterns in some organisms is almost equally elaborate. What is now known of the migration of pigment-controlling cells from the neural crest of the embryo does not make it any easier now than in Darwin's time to detail the process that gives the peacock its tail.

It must therefore be well within the capacity of evolution to devise a process by which genetic potentialities to cover every possible type of antigenic pattern could be present in the genome of the species. What is probably the most popular current interpretation of the heterogeneity of immunoglobulins and antibodies in one individual takes this point of view. Put perhaps oversimply, it is suggested that over the period of vertebrate evolution the primitive cistron responsible for the structure of a blood protein underwent repeated duplication, each new cistron then being susceptible to point mutation and, of course, selection for survival. Eventually, very large numbers of these mutated replicas of the original gene accumulated. Along with this process the rule was established that only a limited number could achieve expression in any one cell, the current mammalian rule being that two are used for the light chain, and four for the heavy chain of Ig G antibodies. There is no clue as to how many alternatives are maintained in the memory store, what the rules are for choice of this or that alternative and whether or not special rules apply to the cistrons whose product we recognize as variable segments in the myeloma proteins.

Many aspects of this approach must be accepted. It is almost inconceivable that the halves of the light chain do not represent the product of duplicated genes. The extensive range of antigenic types amongst immunoglobulins with determinants located on the heavy chain and in many cases precise genetic determination, demands a complex genetic situation that could well be based on duplicated cistrons.

Somatic mutation. It is an inevitable consequence of the evolution of a genetic system based on the replication of linear pattern in DNA that a proportion of errors should occur. In a very small proportion of the replicated chains there is a disturbance of the nucleotide sequence, and if the change has taken place within a structural gene the corresponding protein gene product will show an equivalent disturbance of amino acid sequence. At the level of germinal mutations the process is familiar in the changes observed in amino acid sequence in the variants of human haemoglobin, of insulin in different species, and of fibrinopeptides in the ungulates. The changes have in fact been used as one of the several independent methods of determining the triplet nucleotide code for amino acids.

There seems to be no reason for believing that error in replication is less likely to occur in somatic cells than in the germ cell line. On *a priori* grounds, one might believe that when a given segment of the genome in a somatic cell is regularly concerned with directing the synthesis of protein through the intermediary of messenger RNA, it would be *more* liable to accident than the corresponding region in a cell line concerned only with replication.

We will therefore assume that Orgel's figure of 10^{-8} per nucleotide per cell generation is of the right order of magnitude for point mutation, that is, for the simplest type of error in replication in somatic as well as for germinal cells. This does not rule out the likelihood that 'accidents' of one sort or another may also involve the genome of 'resting' cells which replicate only under emergency conditions.

There are in round figures 3×10^9 base pairs in the human diploid content of chromosomes or the likelihood of sixty errors at each replication of each cell. With perhaps 10^{12} cells replicating once a day or more frequently, there are almost hourly possibilities of every conceivable mutation occurring somewhere in the body. It becomes immediately evident that if large long-lived animals are to maintain functional and structural integrity, means of dealing with this flood of mutations must have evolved. Later on a case will be made for believing that the whole immunological process in vertebrates may have evolved to deal with this inherent weakness of living structure. For the present, all that need be emphasized is that if for any explanation of bodily function or disorder we have to call on somatic mutation there is a virtually unlimited reservoir of genetic accident available.

Any discussion of the significance of somatic mutation within the body must in principle take a similar form to the standard considerations of Darwinian evolution. Mutation gives rise to phenotypic change, any change will favour or prejudice chances of survival and any favourable mutation will eventually displace the former standard form of the species—or at the somatic level, of the cell clone concerned. If we confine ourselves to structural genes, the phenotypic result of point mutation or of grosser changes such as inversion or somatic recombination will be a modification of one or more points in the polypeptide sequence of a certain protein, enzyme, antibody or something else. Most changes will involve non-critical parts of the sequence, the gene product functions normally and the mutation in 10^{-6} or 10^{-8} of the cells of an organ or tissue will be unrecognizable. In another, probably large, proportion of mutant cells a vital region of a functional protein will be distorted and within a few cell generations the cell will become ineffective. In one way or another it will be eliminated and except perhaps for the transitory appearance in a stained section of a pyknotic nucleus, there will be no way of recognizing the occurrence of the mutation. A somatic mutation will in general only be recognizable if in one way or another the initial phenotypic effect can be magnified.

The effects of mutation are by definition inheritable and in broad terms no mutation will be recognized unless the mutant cell gives rise to a large number of descendant cells. There are three important ways by which this can happen. The mutation can occur in a cell at an early stage of embryonic development; it can give rise to a mutant that can proliferate faster and/or survive longer than its congeners; or it is so changed that it is stimulated to selective proliferation by some agent available in the internal environment. One example of each may be given:

(*a*) The first is exemplified in fleece mosaicism as described in Australian sheep by Fraser and Short. On rare occasions sheep-breeders find a lamb conspicuously different from its fellows by having patches of long loosely crimped wool contrasting sharply with the compact texture of the rest of the fleece. Search for such exceptional lambs amongst a sheep population, probably effectively ten million animals, provided a group of 30. Amongst these, one animal had approximately 50 per cent of its skin surface covered with the abnormal long wool, two had 20–25 per cent, and as the proportion of skin area diminished so the number of animals showing that proportion increased. The interpretation by the investigators was that the mutation in question could occur at any stage of development. If it involved one of the two cells from the first division of the fertilized ovum, half the fleece would be involved, at the next division the likelihood of the mutation would be doubled but the proportion of fleece affected would be halved, and similarly for the further stages of segmentation.

(*b*) Proliferative advantage from mutation is probably responsible for every spontaneous appearance of a malignant tumour as well as for all the increase in invasiveness (progression) observable either in the original host or on transfer to suitable animal recipients. An example of non-malignant change may be taken from experiments using Till and McCulloch's method of clonal growth of haemopoietic cells in the spleen of lethally irradiated mice. If cells from bone-marrow or foetal liver are injected intravenously into such a mouse, white 'colonies' of multiplying donor cells are easily visible in the spleen 10 days later. A suspension of cells from such colonies can be similarly injected into another irradiated mouse and the passage sequence carried on. With adult cells the passage series eventually fails but, on two occasions, passage of foetal liver cells gave at second or third passage a few larger colonies. At the next passage the spleens were fully colonized by cells of uniform primitive type resembling lymphoma cells. Passage could be continued indefinitely. The two strains differed in significant properties and it was evident that they were two independent mutants which had a strong proliferative advantage compared to normal cells in the depleted splenic environment. Neither had any malignant characters and they differed completely from malignant lymphoma cells by being unable to colonize the spleen of normal mice.

(c) It is the essence of the clonal selection approach that what determines the immunological specificity of a lymphoid cell clone is the pattern of a particular segment of the genome and that differences between such patterns have arisen by a randomly acting genetic process. A significant part or almost the whole of this process seems likely to result from somatic mutation. This cannot be established directly, but it is possible to show experimentally that when such cells have arisen they are specifically stimulated to proliferate by the corresponding antigen. Jerne's technique of producing discrete plaques of haemolysis each centred on a cell producing and liberating antibody against sheep red cells provides a way of directly counting antibody-producing cells. It can readily be shown both *in vivo* and *in vitro* that secondary stimulation with sheep red cells will stimulate a sharp proliferation of effective cells. A dozen different types of less direct evidence have led to the same conclusion.

There is a strong body of opinion which holds that the normal process of ageing represents essentially the accumulation of somatic mutations throughout the body and secondary results that may arise from the increasing loss of efficiency of various organs. In the opinion of Curtis, the most important aspect is genetic change in cells such as those in the liver which are normally replaced only at very long intervals or following emergency damage. In thinking of mutation in the ordinary sense it is convenient to consider mutation rate in terms of error per replication but even in bacteria it is known that mutation may occur in resting organisms. If the quality of cells in the mouse liver is tested by provoking mitosis during regeneration after damage by carbon tetrachloride, it is found that there is a steady accumulation of abnormalities of mitosis with age and there is other indirect evidence from functional anomalies in liver tumours that mutations are frequent. In view of the intense and varied biochemical functions of the liver we can be certain that there is a constant process of transcription from DNA to m-RNA. Although the precise physical nature of the transcription process is unknown it undoubtedly involves partial uncoiling of DNA and separation of the two strands, possibly with breaking and repair of the transcribing strand. Error and accident could well be frequent enough in these processes of activation, transcription and repression to account for the observed frequency of mutation.

Wherever there is a potentially harmful bodily function, there will usually accompany it some form of homeostatic mechanism to minimize the likelihood of damage. One of the most interesting recent developments in bacterial genetics is the description of a mechanism, apparently involving three enzymes, by which it is possible to excise and repair short segments of DNA within which incompatible chemical changes have occurred. It is not known whether this can also occur in vertebrate somatic cells but the possibility is worth bearing in mind that if any region of the genome should for evolutionary reasons benefit by having a high rate of mutation, such a mechanism for excision and repair could be intimately concerned. An abnormally high local concentration of such enzymes could conceivably be adapted to make small excisions and inversions much more frequent in certain sections of the genome than elsewhere. If somatic mutation is the essential origin of differences in combining site pattern, this local mutation rate must necessarily be higher than in other regions of the genome. There is a rather distant analogy to this in the highly mutable 'hot spots' of Benzer in the phage genome.

The balance of probability. At the cytological and serological level there seems to be no means by which one can differentiate between

The theoretical approach

the two hypotheses: (*a*) that diversity of immune pattern depends wholly on a strictly random selection from a polycistronic mechanism within which germinal mutations accumulated over the period of vertebrate evolution are stored and (*b*) that superimposed on a complex genetic control of the various segments of the immunoglobulins there is a local process of accelerated somatic mutation or some more extensive but still random chromosomal rearrangement which involves the cistron(s) responsible for the segments that give rise to the combining site of antibody. On either alternative it is axiomatic that there is a strict process of phenotypic restriction by which the segments selected remain constant throughout the clone of descendant immunocytes. This would leave open the possibility of further somatic mutation within the immunocyte clone.

It is obvious that both alternatives may be broadly correct, and that either accelerated somatic mutation or the currently popular suggestion of intrachromosomal interaction of genes with recombination could greatly reduce the number of duplicated cistrons required to give the observed diversity of pattern.

If any decision is possible with available techniques it will have to be on a basis of analyses of amino acid sequences and, unless some other material than myeloma proteins becomes accessible, success seems to be extremely unlikely. Even the study of the variable chains in, say, 100 myeloma proteins produced in a strictly homozygous subline of BALB/C mice might not provide enough material for a definite decision.

In all subsequent discussion when the term 'somatic mutation' is used in relation to diversity in specific immune pattern it can be read as equivalent to any type of random inheritable change differentiating one line of immunocytes from another. Perhaps the next major development in experimental immunology will be the provision of a technical approach by which the present dilemma of interpretation can be resolved.

The role of the lymphocyte

The immunological significance of the lymphocyte was probably the most active topic of immunological research in the period 1960–5. Before 1960 it is fair to say that the function of the lymphocyte was unknown, although many felt that it must be primarily immunological, and at one period there had been strong claims that it was the antibody-producing cell. In 1958 I wrote that the only cellular basis for a clonal selection theory must be the lymphoid cells comprising in a single series both lymphocytes and plasma cells. This, however, was based on general considerations, mainly that there was no other available system of cells, rather than on direct experimental evidence.

Three converging lines of experimental approach have led to the recognition of the lymphocyte as of central importance.

The thoracic duct lymph in the rat contains an almost pure suspension of lymphocytes, most of them small lymphocytes. From a study of the effects of depletion of the lymphocyte population by prolonged drainage of the thoracic duct Gowans was led to a broad series of investigations in which various modifications of this technique were used. These showed that depletion of lymphocytes could prevent a primary antibody response, that this incapacity could be remedied by infusion of small lymphocytes, and that under appropriate conditions of antigenic stimulation a proportion of labelled small lymphocytes developed into large pyroninophilic cells capable of mitosis.

The thymus in the young animal is a very active site of lymphocytic multiplication and for a long time it has been known that lymphatic leukaemia in certain strains of mice was initiated in the thymus and could largely be prevented by thymectomy. In extending work of this sort J. F. A. P. Miller examined the results of removing the thymus surgically on the first day of life. With appropriate strains, an important series of observations could be made. First the mice developed normally for some weeks and then suffered a chronic fatal disease with wasting and loss of lymphoid tissue. During the period of apparent health, homografts and even heterografts of skin were not rejected and there was failure to produce antibody in response to several common antigens. Lymphocyte levels were low but there was often a normal level of γ-globulin in the serum, and plasma cells were common in lymphoid tissue. None of these findings were completely regular, even in Miller's hands, and with their extension to other strains and species a rather confused situation developed that has not yet been fully explained. At the present time it is clear that the thymus in the young animal is a very active centre for lymphopoiesis and that it produces humoral agents intimately concerned with the differentiation of lymphocytes and with the functioning of the immune system. There is strong evidence that a large proportion of lymphocytes produced in the thymus do not reach peripheral lymphoid tissues and almost equally valid evidence that the lines of immunocytes which develop are derived from progenitors differentiated in the thymus. Irregularities in the experimental results have been ascribed to racial variations in the time and rate of liberation of lymphocytes in the prenatal period and to the type of microorganismal infestation that develops after birth.

The third approach derives from the use of phytohaemagglutinin to induce mitosis in lymphocytes, as mentioned earlier in relation to delayed hypersensitivity. Under appropriate conditions, the small lymphocytes enlarge to form pyroninophilic DNA-synthesizing cells which subsequently divide. This behaviour fell so neatly into line with Gowans's findings *in vivo* that there was a violent 'gold rush' of clinical investigators to the new field.

The small lymphocyte can best be regarded as a highly mobile carrier of genetic information with no more executive capacity than is needed to stimulate it to take the form of a functioning cell. There is a growing consensus of opinion that the circulating lymphocytes represent a morphologically uniform population of cells with a wide range of functional potentialities. In bone-marrow there are numerous cells morphologically resembling small lymphocytes which have no immunological function. On rather slender positive evidence these are widely regarded as stem cells from which any of the mobile mesenchymal cell types, monocyte, granulocyte and immunocyte, as well as the red cell series, can develop. The line to be taken is ascribed to the action of appropriate hormones present in high concentration in particular areas of differentiation. If this is true, it becomes illegitimate to equate the lymphocyte morphology with any particular functional capacity. There may be excellent evidence that macrophages are derived through circulating monocytes from small lymphocytes in the bone-marrow. This does not mean that small lymphocytes of established immune function can give rise to peritoneal macrophages. Again, everything suggests that immune lymphocytes can pass through a pyroninophil blast intermediary to initiate a clone of plasma cells—a bone-marrow lymphocyte is almost certainly incapable of this. If we omit the bone-marrow and the other haematopoietic regions for the time being, lymphocytes arise by mitosis and proliferation in the thymus, and in peripheral lymphoid tissue in spleen, lymph nodes, Peyer's patches and elsewhere. In the young mammal the thymus is the most active centre of lymphocyte production and for reasons which will need later discussion it can be regarded as the standard site for the differentiation of stem cells to lymphoid cells of immune function which henceforward will be referred to as *immunocytes*. In addition there is a growing opinion that similar primary differentiation to immunocytes can also take place in other lymphoid tissue sites along the gastrointestinal tract. It is becoming common to differentiate between thymus-dependent cells, differentiated in the thymus, and those not so dependent. With some residual uncertainty the functions of delayed hypersensitivity and homograft immunity are ascribed to thymus-dependent cells, while antibody production in general is not thymus dependent. From what is known of the bursa of Fabricius in fowls it can be taken that the process of differentiation in the still largely hypothetical 'gut-associated lymphoid tissue' has the same general character as in the thymus.

Based largely on evidence from grafting infant thymus from mice whose cells are acceptable by, but karyotypically distinguishable from those of the host, it is now accepted that there is a rapid turnover of cells in the thymus. The view that differentiation to immunocyte takes place in the thymus is becoming increasingly popular and, if this is accepted, the existence of what I have called the 'censorship function' of the thymus seems to be unavoidable.

As a prelude to the discussion of this function of the thymus in relation to tolerance, the following outline of cellular changes in the normal thymus of a young mammal may be offered.

Stem cells from the bone-marrow reach the thymic cortex via the blood. Here, they settle in close relation to the reticulo-epithelial cells and under the influence of the local hormonal environment become actively mitosing large lymphocytes. The descendants are medium and small lymphocytes and at a certain point the proliferative potential of the clone is exhausted. The small lymphocytes produced remain for 3–4 days in the thymus and then either die *in situ* or pass to the circulation, probably via the local lymphatics. There is much histological evidence of cell destruction in the form of pyknotic nuclear fragments, and calculations based on the intensity of mitosis in the thymus suggest that 90–99 per cent of the cells produced may be destroyed.

A small proportion of the cells leaving the thymus can be experimentally identified in peripheral lymphoid tissue. If the view is correct that the function of the thymus is to differentiate stem cells to immunocytes, these cells go to swell the reservoirs of immunocytes available to be called on when any antigen with which they are capable of reacting reaches the tissue. Peripheral production of lymphocytes takes place in germinal centres and the rather inconclusive evidence is consistent with the view that a germinal centre is a clone of cells developing from a single stimulated immunocyte. Germinal centres always arise in lymphoid tissue, but opinion at present is against the view that most of the adjacent small lymphocytes are derivatives of the germinal centre they surround. Details are still lacking but there is convincing evidence that newly produced small lymphocytes are rapidly distributed throughout the lymphoid tissues of the body with the notable exception of the thymus. In every primary lymph follicle there must be thousands of different immune patterns represented by the cells which compose it. This becomes of great importance when we are concerned with following the path by which antigen stimulates the cells which will produce antibody.

Always with the reservation that it is not possible to equate small lymphocyte morphology with immunocyte function, it still remains highly probable that the peripheral lymphocytes observed in spleen lymph nodes and aggregations along the gut are in fact immunocytes of various types. There are three features of these cells which are of great immunological importance.

The first is their characteristic mode of entry and exit into lymphoid tissue. Entry is from the bloodstream by passage through the cytoplasm of swollen endothelial cells of capillaries or venules. These swollen cells are characteristic of lymphoid tissue and appear to have a specific stickiness or other form of attraction for circulating lymphocytes. The traffic is apparently strictly one-way, from capillary lumen into the substance of the lymphoid tissue. Movement *from* a lymph node is solely via the efferent lymphatics.

The second point of importance in this preliminary discussion is the relationship of the plasma cell to the lymphocyte. This is still controversial and some immunologists would keep the two cell types quite distinct, deriving the plasma cell from perithelial cells around small blood vessels. On the other hand, a majority now take the view that a small lymphocyte antigenically stimulated to a pyroninophil blast can be directed either to multiply as lymphocytes or, in an appropriate environment, to initiate a clone of plasma cells. If, as seems likely, the non-thymic origin of plasma cells becomes firmly established, it will depend on the site of differentiation how the activated cell will develop.

The third concerns the fate of lymphocytes and plasma cells. Both may be very long lived. After a single exposure of a rat in the early stage of antibody production to a large dose of tritiated thymidine, labelled small lymphocytes and mature plasma cells can be seen for at least six months. The great majority of both types are much shorter lived and only a very small proportion of small lymphocytes undergo activation to blast cells. Small lymphocytes are extremely susceptible to cytotoxic agents including at least one physiological substance, cortisol, and reasons will be given later for regarding this vulnerability as a way of making available the amino acids and nucleotides of their substance to local or general metabolic pools as needed. Plasma cells are more resistant to such agents but tend to disappear rapidly after an antigenic stimulus ceases to act. There is no evidence that mature plasma cells ever develop capacity to de-differentiate to blast form and renew mitotic activity.

Tolerance in relation to immunocyte origins

Without being aware of its significance, experimental embryologists who found that a piece of skin or a limb bud could be transferred from one species of amphibian embryo to another were demonstrating immunological tolerance many years ago. Quite extensive grafting of chick embryos was done in 1937–40 by Willier's group but the importance of the difference between embryo and adult was not recognized. Within the conventional field of immunology the first important findings were Owen's discovery that bovine dizygotic twins regularly showed two blood groups and that the presence of two distinct types of red blood cell usually persisted for life in both twins. In 1949 Burnet and Fenner discussed Owen's results along with those of Traub, who found that congenital infection of mice with the virus of lymphocytic choriomeningitis gave rise to a long-lasting asymptomatic infection. They regarded both as evidence of toleration by the embryo of what would in the adult be rejected as foreign, and introduced the concept that the differentiation of self from not-self was the central problem of immunology. It was predicted that appropriate injections of antigens in the embryo would give rise to subsequent tolerance of that antigen. Eventually the prediction was abundantly fulfilled but, as is the way of simple biological concepts, new experimental and clinical phenomena make it impossible now to present any unitary picture of immune tolerance.

Although it is relatively simple to produce tolerance by neonatal injection of a variety of soluble proteins, serum albumin for example, there are many antigens such as fibrinogen, bacterial flagella and bacteriophage where only partial degrees of tolerance can be produced in some species, and none at all in others. In most cases homograft tolerance can be produced but it is much rarer to be able to induce acceptance of a heterograft. There are now many ways by which degrees of tolerance or, better, unresponsiveness, can be produced in adult animals by, as it were, flooding the animal with a soluble foreign protein, by X-irradiation or by the use of immunosuppressive drugs and even (with a properly chosen antigen and a suitable mouse strain) by the injection of a very small dose of antigen.

The original concept of tolerance was that an essential part of the process of embryonic development was the establishment of a taboo on immune response to any of the normally circulating components of the body. In most respects this seems to be a self-evident necessity but it is a tradition of immunological experimentation to press far beyond the bounds of the normal and there has been no serious difficulty in showing that, with intense immunological stimulation, antibodies against almost any natural component of the body can be produced. This, however, no more proves that there is no normal homeostatic process preventing such responses than the appearance of hyperpyrexia in malaria indicates that there is no physiological control of body temperature.

The early work on tolerance was concerned with the situation in which a foreign antigen persists in the body either in the form of an alien cell chimera or a tolerated virus infection. Such conditions could readily be tested by grafting appropriate skin or examining for the continuing presence of the virus. Even in these fields, however, there were indications of partial tolerance, a condition that is much more frequently observed when attempts are made to establish tolerance to soluble antigens.

If a neonatal animal is given a series of relatively large injections of a soluble antigen it is usual for no antibody to be produced, and for this unresponsiveness to a challenge by the same antigen to persist for a variable period. The results of such experiments vary greatly from one individual to another, and if several different methods are used for measuring antibodies reactive with the antigen it is rare to find an example of tolerance that will embrace them all.

It is now clear that there are a great many conditions when an animal will fail to respond, or respond poorly, to an antigenic stimulus which in a majority of 'normal' control animals will produce easily demonstrable immune responses. No single interpretation can be valid and there are several ways of looking at even 'classical' neonatal tolerance.

(a) In the thymus or in any other site of primary differentiation, it is believed that a stem cell becomes an immunocyte because it has been stimulated to produce a receptor equivalent, at least, to the combining site of antibody in the sense that it can react with an appropriate antigenic determinant. This immune pattern of the receptor is of random origin and as likely to react with a body component as with a foreign antigen. It is a necessary part of any clonal selection theory that whenever a cell differentiates as an immunocyte carrying a pattern complementary to any antigenic determinant present in the thymic environment, contact with that antigen will initiate a destructive or inhibitory reaction which will prevent the development of the cell as an immunocyte. In the absence of cells which can react to produce antibody there can be no production of antibody.

Within the thymus there is very active cell proliferation and destruction so that one can confidently assume that in addition to potential antigens in plasma and intercellular fluids, all the vast number of potential antigenic determinants within any unspecialized cell will be available in the thymic environment. If the basic hypothesis of destruction by antigen–receptor contact in the thymus is correct, there will be a sufficiency of 'self' antigens there to ensure that a very large proportion of newly differentiated immunocytes should be destroyed by this process.

(b) For some substances to be antigenic, particularly in young animals, it may be necessary for them to be coated with γ-globulin (natural antibody). Otherwise they will not be taken up by phagocytic cells in such a way that they can be presented to immunocytes in an effectively antigenic form. Since normal antibody is presumably produced by immunocytes which have passed the thymic 'censorship' and have been unspecifically stimulated, this is essentially only an operational variant of (a).

(c) The immune response to any antigen is always complex and will normally include production of antibody in the form of all three types of immunoglobulin and the appearance of a variety of immunocytes. The relative intensity of each component will vary greatly from one situation to another and there are circumstances where one type of antibody can mask some other type of immune response against the same antigen. Antibody itself has a well-marked feedback capacity to prevent the initiation of any more production of antibody by the same antigen, and this phenomenon can be responsible for some examples of partial unresponsiveness. Experimental allergic encephalomyelitis in rats can be prevented by immune serum; enhancement of transmissible mouse cancer by antiserum is well known. When tolerance to a certain soluble antigen is measured by one method, for example the nonimmune curve of removal of labelled antigen from the circulation, it is quite common to find discrepancies in two directions. An apparently tolerant mouse may show antibody detectable by some other method, and a rabbit which has apparently 'broken tolerance' may fail to produce any precipitating antibody. The possibility almost diametrically opposite to (*b*) that, on occasion, tolerance may be mediated by antibody, must always be kept in mind.

(*d*) If unresponsiveness is due basically to the absence of cells which can respond to antigen, it could result either from destruction of such cells by antigenic contact or from the descendants of a stimulated cell all being forced into an irreversible phase of differentiation. Most immunologists regard the mature plasma cell as an end cell no longer capable of replication or of differentiation into a cell which can replicate. If all the available immunocytes capable of reacting with antigen X are irreversibly committed to plasma cell formation, a state of unresponsiveness must develop until new cells of the required pattern emerge as a result of mutation and differentiation.

Some writers have suggested that there is no such thing as tolerance on the grounds that by sufficiently strenuous treatment an animal can be made to produce antibody against any of its components and even to die of autoimmune disease. This is an illegitimate argument unless we assume that tolerance must be all or nothing. Partial tolerance is easily demonstrated and the effect of large doses of antigen given with Freund's complete adjuvant is merely the end of a continuous spectrum.

My own view would be that (*a*) is the predominant mechanism by which tolerance, including natural tolerance to body components, is mediated and that in experimental studies it may often function by way of the mechanism described in (*b*). The other two approaches are particularly important in relation to partial tolerance.

It must be emphasized here as elsewhere in immunology that tolerance is a soft-edged phenomenon and always partial. When we say that a given antigenic determinant reacts specifically with a combining site on a receptor, this can mean only that the union is a reversible one of such affinity that it can be manifested in some experimentally demonstrable fashion. The affinity level necessary will vary with the reaction being used. This is of special relevance in studying the phenomenon of loss of tolerance when the antigen in question is withheld for long periods.

If tolerance or unresponsiveness is due to the temporary absence for any cause of cells with which the antigenic determinant can react significantly and if there is a constant flow of new mutant patterns finding expression in the thymus, it is self-evident that in the absence of the antigen there will be an opportunity for new reactive immunocytes to emerge. The likelihood of their doing so will diminish with thymectomy and with age. For a time, at least, the clones concerned will probably be directed against only one antigenic determinant of the antigen or represent low avidity patterns with only partial reactivity for the antigen.

SUMMARY

This outline should give a broad indication of the theoretical approach to be adopted. It is essentially Darwinian natural selection applied at the cellular level to clones instead of at the level of the organism and the species. This general concept can be summarized as follows.

The specific immune pattern presented by the combining site of an antibody molecule or the receptor of an immunologically competent cell is genetically derived. It is still uncertain whether the pattern of the combining site is the responsibility of a single cistron or whether, like the immunoglobulin molecule as a whole, it arises from the convergence of several streams of genetic information. Whatever the source of genetic control, the pattern arises by a random process operationally equivalent to somatic mutation. Associated with the random determination of the immune pattern a strict phenotypic restriction must become operative which limits the cell to the production of one type of immunoglobulin and one pattern of combining site.

It is a function of the thymus and any other sites of primary differentiation to eliminate any newly differentiated immunocytes reacting with sufficient avidity with any antigens that are accessible in the organ.

Immunocytes that pass this censorship colonize lymphoid tissue and are ancestral to the general lymphocyte–plasma cell population of the body.

Any such immunocyte carrying an immune pattern complementary to an antigenic determinant present in the body, for example as part of a bacterial invader, will be liable to proliferate and so give rise to a clone of cells with similar potentiality. Once any newborn mammal has had an opportunity to experience the impact of antigens from the environment, the lymphoid system can be pictured as an intermingled population of cell lines or clones, those present in largest number being reactive against commonly experienced foreign antigens. The number of distinct clones probably increases to a plateau at adult life but the relative populations of each clone will be highly variable, a reflection at all times of the recent antigenic experience of the individual. The element of a Darwinian situation are all present. The numbers of essentially autonomous genetic elements, the lymphoid cells, are large, perhaps around 10^{12} in man, giving adequate opportunity for mutation, and the selective advantage of an accidentally appropriate pattern is enormous and extremely rapidly expressed.

3 The thymus in relation to the origin and differentiation of lymphoid cells

THE FUNCTION OF THE LYMPHOCYTE AS A MOBILE INFORMATION CARRIER

The small lymphocyte is probably the commonest mobile nucleated cell of the body. Its origin and functional differentiation must always remain the central problem of immunology viewed from the cytological aspect. An immediate difficulty arises in the rapidly developing view that under the name 'lymphocyte' or 'small lymphocyte' we may be lumping together many different types of cell. In particular, the lymphocytes commonly seen in the bone-marrow may have different potentialities from those in the circulation, lymph nodes and spleen, and these again from those in the thymus. Other workers, however, while accepting these observable differences, see no reason why genetically similar cells should not show different behaviour as a result of their sojourn in different internal environments.

All body cells, apart from haploid germ cells, are assumed to contain the full complement of genetic information present in the fertilized ovum from which they developed. The problems of defining the limits of a certain morphological type of cell and tracing its line of origin by progressive differentiation are probably insoluble by any single experimental approach. The lymphocyte is particularly difficult to define as its morphology is undistinctive. It is known that some small lymphocytes may become large pyroninophil cells capable of mitosis, and there is strong evidence that either directly or by way of these active cells, even macrophages, plasma cells, mast cells and fibroblasts may be derived from cells with the morphology of small lymphocytes. If this is true it suggests the need for adopting an attitude to the small lymphocyte that marks it off from all other cell types. We shall adopt the hypothesis that a lymphocyte is a mobile repository of genetic information without any executive organization of the cytoplasm beyond that necessary for its free mobility through tissues, plus receptors of some sort which can mediate the capacity of environmental stimuli to mobilize the particular store of information required. If we include all populations of small lymphocytes defined simply on a morphological basis, they presumably include cells whose genome is at various stages of differentiation not necessarily always directed toward immunological function.

In any emergency situation one can see the value of having always available large numbers of cells, morphologically small lymphocytes but representing perhaps many thousand clones each of which has a differentiated potentiality, which can be called into action by appropriate stimulation. If only 1 in 1,000 cells are of the needed potentiality the number can be rapidly raised to 10 per cent by a series of six or seven binary divisions of the stimulated cell within a few days. It would be reasonable, too, that to provide the special building blocks needed for the rapid expansion of a badly needed clone, lymphocytes not needed should be broken down at random. This would present the trophic function of lymphocytes referred to or hypothecated by numerous writers and provide an evolutionary rationale for the abnormal vulnerability of lymphocytes to irradiation, corticosteroids and cytotoxic drugs.

THE ROLE OF THE THYMUS

From this operational outlook by which the lymphocyte is regarded simply as a mobile store of genetic information with no immediate executive responsibility, it is not necessary to assume that all lymphocytes arise from a common source at some stage in embryonic development. In recent years, however, it has become clear that the thymus plays an important part in the development and functioning of lymphocytic populations in both mammals and birds. There is strong evidence that in the placental mammals that have been studied in any detail the embryonic thymus is the source of the first lymphocytes, and through late embryonic life, and at least until adolescence, is an important centre for the control of lymphocytic activity. There is no good evidence against the speculation that all lymphocytes could be traced back to origin in the epithelial cells of the thymus primordium but, equally, there is nothing to counter the assumption that primitive blood-forming cells at any stage of development could also take on the appearance of lymphocytes. The evolutionary approach suggests that thymus, lymphocytes, γ-globulin and capacity for immune response appeared together in the higher cyclostomes.

Embryologically the epithelial cells of the early thymus seem to take on lymphocytic character under the stimulus of adjacent mesenchymal cells at a time when there are no other lymphocytes in the body. Failure of the thymus to develop may be associated with almost complete absence of lymphoid tissue and virtually no circulating lymphocytes, but these cases seem to vary considerably from one to another and some show only moderate reduction of blood lymphocytes. Removal of the thymus on the first day of life in certain strains of mice gives rise to a situation of generally impaired immunological effectiveness. J. F. A. P. Miller's first accounts suggested that virtually total loss of immune responses was the rule if thymectomy was complete. The results with other strains of mice and other species have been in the same general direction but less striking. It appears that in mice and placental mammals generally there is active production of lymphocytes from the thymus before birth and neonatal thymectomy has no special virtue in itself. It merely cuts off a process at a variable time after its initiation.

Opinion is still fluid in regard to the relative importance of the thymus as a source of lymphocytes or as an endocrine organ producing hormone(s) controlling immunological function. Any general statement must therefore involve an arbitrary choice between alternatives at certain points and will eventually be found to be unduly simplified. With these reservations we can use experimental, comparative and clinical sources of information to summarize the function of the thymus as follows:

(*a*) The thymus is the primary centre for differentiation of immunocytes and provides the progenitors of the various clones of lymphoid cells which eventually colonize the peripheral lymphoid tissues. The actual proportion of the cells produced in the thymus which find it possible to do this is probably very small in adult life but considerably higher in prenatal and neonatal periods.

(*b*) For the first few days of life the colonizing lymphocytes and

The thymus

the clones to which they give rise need the persistence of a humoral agent produced by the non-lymphocytic tissues of the thymus if they are to remain indefinitely viable.

(c) In the neonatally thymectomized mouse there is a gross deficiency in the types of lymphocyte available and there are patchy deficiencies in the types of immune responses that can be initiated. In general the capacity to reject homografts or to display delayed hypersensitivity reactions is depressed more than the ability to produce conventional antibodies.

THE STRUCTURE OF THE THYMUS

In a young animal, a 4- to 8-week-old mouse or a child of ten for example, the thymus is still large and very actively producing lymphocytes. Yet its removal at this stage appears to have practically no effect in impairing immunological responses. The only way to demonstrate impaired function is to expose the animal to some severe stress such as near-lethal X-irradiation. Under such circumstances the full recovery of immune function is more rapid in the presence of a thymus than in its absence.

A great deal of attention has been paid to the dynamics of the lymphoid cells which make up the main mass of the thymus in the young animal. The basic finding is that there is a rapid turnover of cells which, apart from proliferation, destruction and liberation into the general circulation, involves a relatively slow but continuous entry of new stem cells from extra-thymic sources. When two mutually compatible mouse strains, one of which carries a recognizable marker chromosome, are available, parabiosis experiments can be used to provide an almost physiological process of lymphocytic interchange. Under these circumstances it was possible to show that after five weeks with a common blood circulation the two partners had almost reached an equilibrium in lymph nodes and spleen, and even in the thymus 12 per cent of the mitoses were of the partner's type. Grafts of neonatal thymus undergo atrophy and depletion before redeveloping normal histological structure. The conditions are therefore more or less unphysiological but the findings are consistent that within three weeks the mitoses seen in the graft are wholly of host type.

To provide a structural basis for envisaging the cellular interchange we may adopt the interpretation that has been derived from electron microscope studies by Clark (1963). In fig. 8 it is modified slightly to include the macrophages ('PAS cells') which are believed to have an important functional role. In Clark's view, the thymus is an epithelial organ densely honeycombed with packets of proliferating lymphocytes in the cortex, and with the medulla irregularly infiltrated with lymphocytes and other cells mostly associated with blood vessels. An individual packet is shown in the

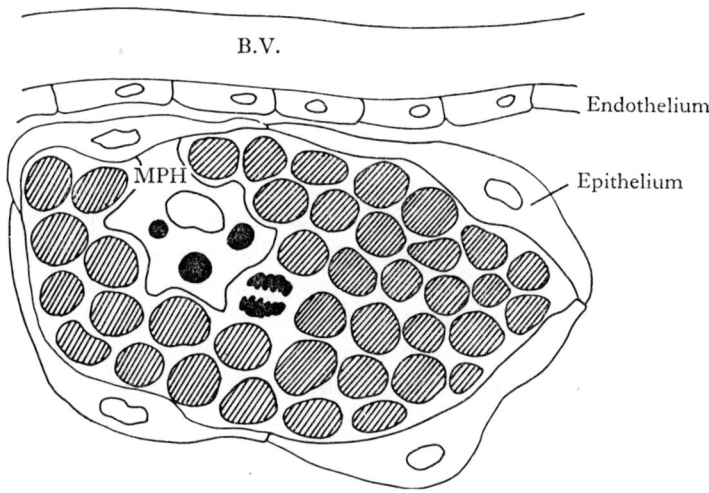

Fig. 8. The unit of cortical cells in the thymus (Clark packet). B.V. = blood vessel; MPH = macrophage.

diagram. Essentially it is a nest of actively multiplying lymphocytes plus one (or occasionally more) macrophage usually recognizable by its content of phagocytosed nuclear debris. The packet is completely enclosed in a tenuous capsule of epithelial cells with a minimal amount of supporting tissue, including collagen and elastic fibres.

The great majority of the thymic cells are lymphocytes; large, medium and small. In the cortex their close-packed distribution in Clark packets provides a different texture from the randomly distributed lymphocytes in primary follicles of lymph node or spleen.

In smears or impression preparations the cells are typical lymphocytes. If collections of thymic lymphocytes are compared with those of the thoracic duct or with circulating lymphocytes there are certain differences, usually rather subtle ones that do not necessarily hold for other strains or species. In mice there are at least two antigens which can differentiate thymic lymphocytes from the great majority of peripheral lymphocytes. These are shown by cytotoxic tests and may, in part, depend on the susceptibility of thymic cells to damage. Absorption experiments, however, indicate that a real, if labile, antigen is concerned.

Whenever thymic cells, i.e. cells from the cortex, medulla and connective and perivascular tissues of the organ, are compared with cells from lymph node or spleen in any aspect of immune function they are much less effective, sometimes appearing inert. At the risk of error it seems reasonable to accept the evidence as indicating that lymphocytes in the cortex with their active but controlled multiplication (*a*) have a serologically differentiable surface antigen not found in peripheral lymphocytes, (*b*) have no power to produce antibody *in situ* or *in vitro*, (*c*) produce no immediate graft-versus-host reaction and (*d*) when opportunities are provided for thymic cells to pass to spleen and lymph nodes, immune competence to react with antigen may become demonstrable.

Changes in cell numbers and types within the thymus
In the course of ageing and under stress a variety of structural changes can be observed in the thymus. It is well known in human pathology that at autopsy after any illness lasting more than a day or two there is thymic atrophy, most marked in the cortex. The picture can be simulated in experimental mice by administration of a milligram of hydrocortisone, moderate local or general irradiation, a large but sublethal dose of almost any cytotoxic agent and any severe, acute or subacute infection. Any of these will, in the mouse, result first in the necrosis of many cortical cells with pyknosis and active phagocytosis of nuclear debris, followed by the progressive depletion of the lymphocytes in the cortex. Within a day or two the cortex may be almost empty of lymphocytes. It appears greatly shrunken and composed of epithelial cells, macrophages, occasional plasma cells, and structural elements associated

with the blood vessels. After removal of the stress the cortex refills with lymphocytes.

In ageing there is a general diminution of thymic weight with a relative expansion of medullary area in relation to cortex. In man both cortex and medulla are also progressively replaced by fat; and in old individuals, although an atrophic thymus can be found at autopsy, section shows only shreds of thymic medullary tissue.

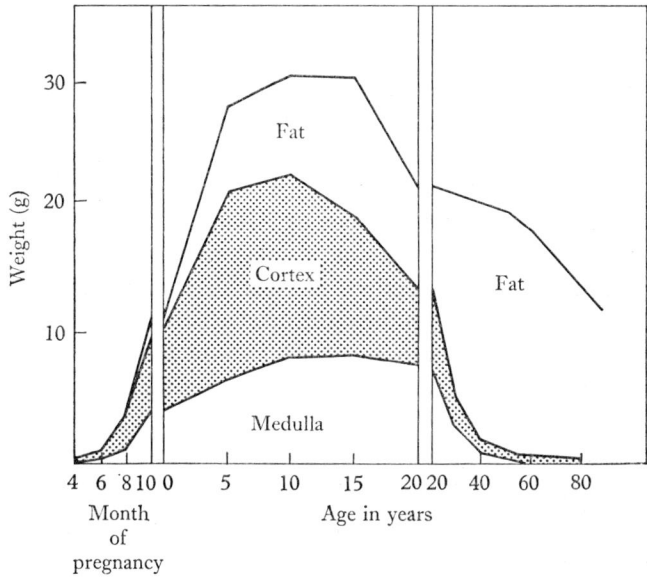

Fig. 9. Changes with age in the weight and composition of the human thymus. Redrawn from J. A. Hammar (1936), *Die normalmorphologische Thymusforschung im letzten Vierteljahre*. Leipzig: Barth.

In mice one finds a variety of appearances in older mice including cellular accumulations in the medulla. In the autoimmune strain NZB and its hybrids with which I have had much experience, there is an almost regular development of germinal centres in the medulla and a variety of secondary changes. In these strains both mast cells and plasma cells are common and I have seen a number of sections in which large areas of cortex have been converted *en masse* to mast cells and in the hybrid (NZB × NZW) F_1 areas of cortex almost wholly replaced by pyroninophil cells. The impression is overwhelming in both conditions that lymphocytes in the cortical packets have been transformed directly either to mast cells or pyroninophil cells closely resembling immature plasma cells.

These are essentially pathological conditions but they point toward an unsuspected lability of differentiation of thymocytes that may be relevant to the theme that their differentiation to immunocytes is the main function of the thymus.

The significance of the thymus in the perinatal period

Congenital failure of the thymus to develop in man or its removal surgically in the immediate neonatal period in mice, both produce striking effects which are not seen as a result of thymectomy later, even if this is only a week after birth. The discovery of the effect of neonatal thymectomy in mice by Miller in 1960–1 was almost wholly responsible for current interest in thymic function. As shown in the previous section, the fact that later removal of the thymus has little effect on the apparent well-being of a mouse does not mean that the thymus functions only in the perinatal period. The main virtue of neonatal thymectomy is that the effects produced are gross and can be readily demonstrated within a few weeks or months. Few investigators like to wait for a year or more before the result of an experimental manipulation becomes apparent.

The effect of neonatal thymectomy varies greatly with the species of animal used and in the mouse (the species most commonly studied) with the strain. There is no visible effect of neonatal thymectomy in the dog and very little in the rabbit. The effect in the rat is clearly demonstrable but there is only a partial and quantitative depression of immune function. Only in certain strains of mice and in that immunological curiosity, the golden hamster, is the effect of neonatal thymectomy of the classical type described by Miller in his first papers. Initially then, we may consider the nature and significance of the classical result.

In the strains C3H and (AK × T6) F_1 neonatal thymectomy has no effect on the growth of the infant mouse for several weeks. Until then it gains weight normally and looks healthy and, if it is raised in germ-free conditions, may remain healthy indefinitely. Reared conventionally, a wasting disease whose nature is still controversial, sets in, and the mice die at around three months of age. This, however, allows a reasonable period over which tests of immunological capacity can be carried out. Restricting ourselves to this period, it is found that the mice show a level of circulating lymphocytes about half the normal value and lymphoid tissue reduced to about the same extent. Plasma cells are present in the intestinal tissues and in lymph nodes and spleen. There are variable changes in the serum proteins but usually all the immunoglobulins can be detected.

Of immunological deficiences the most outstanding is the capacity to accept homografts of skin and even heterografts of rat skin. Antibody-producing capacity is reduced but when a number of antigens are used there is an almost random-appearing mixture of ability and inability to produce individual antibodies.

The capacity of various manipulations to restore immune competence to neonatally thymectomized animals has been extensively studied. Amongst the effective procedures are early grafting of neonatal syngeneic or allogeneic thymic tissue, and repeated injections of syngeneic thymic cells or of relatively large amounts of syngeneic spleen cells. Thymic tissue implanted in Millipore chambers intraperitoneally is also effective. Injection of syngeneic bone-marrow cells or foetal liver does not protect nor does a 'successful' graft of rat thymus. Most workers have failed to show significant effects of cell-free thymic extracts but this may merely reflect inadequate dosage.

Perhaps the most significant findings are (a) the failure of bone-marrow cells to return immune capacity either in the neonatally thymectomized mouse or in the older mouse subjected successively to thymectomy and lethal X-irradiation (although in the latter case bone-marrow can 'rescue' the animal and, with thymic tissue in Millipore chambers, reconfer immune capacity) and (b) the ability of adult syngeneic spleen cells in adequate dose to return immune capacity. In terms of our general hypothesis these are compatible with the views: (i) That bone-marrow contains cells which can give rise to immunocytes but only in the presence of a thymus or an adequate concentration of thymic hormone. In their absence bone-marrow cells are immunologically inert. (ii) If an adequate number of compatible adult lymphoid cells are provided, the neonatally thymectomized animal can remain immunologically competent at least for a considerable period.

The comparative anatomy of the thymus
More is known about the function of the thymus in the mouse than in any other mammal and there is enough to suggest that apart from some differences in the timing of its development the situation in other placental mammals, including man, is functionally similar. There are, however, anatomical and embryological differences. In most mammals the thymus develops from the third branchial pouch and in the course of development migrates into the thorax. In the guinea-pig the organ remains in the neck. Many marsupials have two sets of thymuses, a pair of cervical thymuses derived from the third branchial pouch and a thoracic thymus from the fourth and fifth pouches. All have a microscopic structure similar to that of placental mammals, and there is evidence from the American opossum that their function is broadly similar.

Entry of cells into the thymus in the postnatal period
It is now certain that among the circulating cells of the blood are some from which may be derived lymphocytes, plasma cells, erythrocytes, macrophages and granulocytes and, in all probability, vascular endothelium and fibroblasts. It is the simplest of a number of as yet unverifiable alternative hypotheses to believe that the 'stem cells' concerned may initially be capable of differentiation in any of these directions and that the actual route along which they are differentiated is determined by their sojourn in an appropriate internal environment for an adequate period. There is relatively firm evidence that such stem cells arise from the bone-marrow (and perhaps any other sites of haemopoietic activity).

Evidence from parabiosis indicates a continuous changeover of the proliferating cortical lymphocytes in the thymus. Our current hypothesis is that any stem cell, that is, a relatively undifferentiated cell, which can enter the structural units of the thymic cortex is there subject to differentiation to an immunocyte. This is a term which it is convenient to use for any cell, lymphocyte, plasma cell or other, which has specific immune reactivity of any sort. In our usage it will imply a good deal of interchangeability between different morphological or functional characters within a single clone of immunocytes (fig. 10).

Autoradiographic studies using tritiated thymidine, plus more old-fashioned methods using counts of mitotic rates under a variety of conditions, have given a reasonably consistent picture of the cell dynamics of the mouse thymus. There is nothing substantial to suggest that the behaviour of the thymus in the mouse is in any way exceptional amongst mammals. There is a very high level of proliferative activity amongst the large and medium lymphocytes; 70–80 per cent being labelled by a single intravenous injection when fixed an hour later. A proportion of all mitoses involve differentiation toward the standard form of the small lymphocyte,

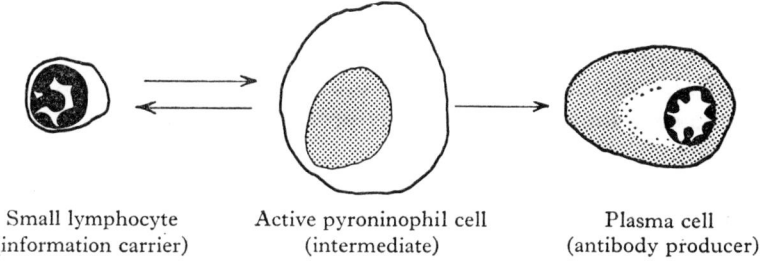

Small lymphocyte (information carrier)   Active pyroninophil cell (intermediate)   Plasma cell (antibody producer)

Fig. 10. The immunocyte concept.

and at a certain point two small lymphocytes are produced by division of a medium lymphocyte and do not multiply further in the thymus. On the average, such small lymphocytes spend 3–4 days in the thymus from their time of birth. Then they disappear. It is still an unsolved problem as to what happens to the great majority of cells produced by mitosis in the thymus. A proportion undoubtedly die *in situ* as judged by the constant presence of pyknotic debris in macrophages. A common belief is that large numbers leave the thymus as small lymphocytes but, for some reason, the great majority are autolysed and disappear as individual entities soon after entering the circulation. However, even if the output of cells which develop into viable clones is something less than 1 per cent, this might well be adequate for any immunological function, such as the provision of new immune patterns, which may be dependent on the thymus.

The thymus

In discussing the basis of immunity it is impossible to start at one point and progress logically to a complete synthesis. In addition to the incompleteness and sometimes the contradictions of the experimental evidence, each set of phenomena is influenced by a variety of factors that it would be more convenient to discuss in some other setting. The significance of the entry of perhaps 5 per cent of new clones per day to the thymic cortex is one of these difficulties. It can only be discussed adequately in terms of immune pattern and the origin of diversity within immune pattern (see chapter 6). Here then, in the context of thymic function, we can simply accept the existence of specific immune pattern as something based on genetic information and phenotypically expressed only when the cell has been enabled to synthesize protein carrying immune pattern. The first function of that protein is to serve as one or more cell receptors, the essential feature of clonal selection theory being that the receptor has broadly the same pattern as that of the combining site of antibody produced by other cells of the clone.

The picture of thymic function which has been rapidly developing, viz., that it is the most important and perhaps the only source of new immune pattern, seems to require two distinct capacities of the thymus—that it should be the sole site at which stem cells can become immunocytes and that it should release into the general circulation only immunocytes which are not reactive against body components. This requires some preliminary discussion of the process of differentiation in general and of the thesis that in immunocytes new patterns arise by somatic mutation or some operationally equivalent process.

On modern genetic theory, every cell of the body carries the whole of the genetic information present in the diploid complement of chromosomes as soon as fertilization is complete. The cistron or cistrons concerned in determining immune pattern are present in every cell and, more particularly, in every stem cell capable of entering the circulation. If the region concerned is subject to normal mutability or has developed an increased mutability as an evolutionary requirement, the stem cells, by the time of birth, will have accumulated a wide range of potential patterns. In the absence of appropriate differentiation, however, the patterns will never be expressed. It matters not in the least that a skin cell or an epithelial cell in the small intestine is potentially an ancestor of an auto-immune forbidden clone. If it is not differentiated to an immunocyte it can do no harm.

The nature of differentiation is still unknown but it is reasonably clear that *adjacent cells* play a very important part. In the thymus, entering cells are intimately associated with the reticulo-epithelial cells that seem to endow the thymus with its individual character as an organ. They almost certainly provide the differentiating environment. The stem cell enters a Clark packet, proliferates and, by hypothesis, the 'immune cistron' is de-repressed. Synthetic

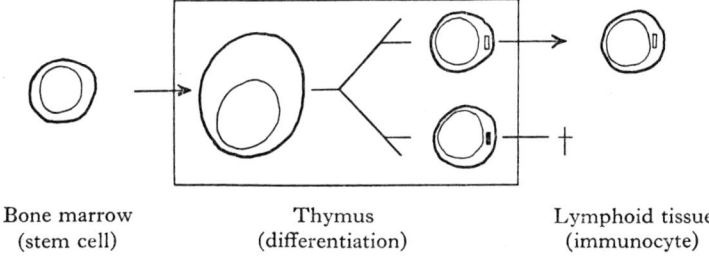

| Bone marrow | Thymus | Lymphoid tissue |
| (stem cell) | (differentiation) | (immunocyte) |

Fig. 11. To illustrate the role of the thymus in differentiation and 'censorship'. With differentiation, immune pattern emerges and the cell becomes reactive to contact with antigen. Open rectangle = 'non-self' pattern; black rectangle = 'self' pattern.

activity for the product, in the first instance as receptor rather than as antibody, is initiated. By the time the terminal small lymphocytes are produced, the receptors must be functional.

At this point the second postulated function of the thymus comes into play. When a newly emergent receptor can react specifically with any antigenic determinants present in the thymic environment, the cell carrying it must be destroyed. Depending on a number of possible factors, destruction may take place as soon as the receptor is present at all, perhaps in the large or medium lymphocyte phase, or it may be delayed until the 'sensitized' cell is liberated into the circulation. Whatever the details, the essential feature claimed for this hypothesis is that the only newly differentiated cells which can give rise to normal clones of immunocytes are those which fail to react with accessible body components.

The thymus

This postulated double function of the thymus is virtually the only way in which the facts can be interpreted within the framework of clonal selection theory. A point which has not so far been mentioned in this context is that in the thymus a cell being made ready for one defined type of differentiation is likely to be temporarily highly labile and easily influenced by abnormal stimuli to develop along an aberrant line of differentiation. This is the most likely interpretation of the very wide range of morphological cell types to be seen when thymic lesions develop in the 'autoimmune' mouse strain NZB and its hybrids. In addition to occasional massive change to pyroninophilic cells approaching plasma cells in character, or to mast cells, a variety of other cell types may be present in affected areas. Some may have come via the circulation but, even so, the form they take in the thymus must be determined largely by the nature of the environment provided.

The existence of a thymic agent active on lymphocytic function has been known since Metcalf's work in 1956 and it is probable that this plays an important part in the various actions that have been ascribed to the internal environment of the thymus. In appropriate experimental situations it can be shown that the presence of thymic tissues in Millipore chambers implanted in the peritoneal cavity can restore capacity to reject homografts both to neonatally thymectomized animals and to animals thymectomized at a later stage and then subjected to a lethal irradiation dose with 'rescue' by bone-marrow cells. This is perhaps a little at variance with the special importance ascribed to the actual thymic environment, since it indicates a capacity of thymic agents to allow manifestation of immunocytic capacity in other environments than the thymus. It does, however, strengthen the claim that the internal thymic environment may have a potent effect on cells differentiating within it.

In summary then, the function of the thymus in postnatal life is to serve as a source of new immune patterns to ensure an adequate supply of 'information' to deal with any significantly likely emergency. This is done by making use of all the genetic information relevant to immune pattern that has been developed in the cell genome either during the course of vertebrate evolution or as a result of somatic mutation or equivalent processes during the life of the individual. This information will be accumulated in the first instance within the stem cells of the haematopoietic system. Each cell must carry a number of alternative potentialities as to the type of immunoglobulin it will produce and each, depending on its line of somatic descent, will have accumulated changes due to somatic mutation. The nature and extent of the potentialities in each stem cell must be deferred for later discussion but the materialization of one potentiality only is the essence of differentiation. Those stem cells which enter the thymus are constrained to differentiate to immunocytes, that is, by expressing one potentiality to produce receptor protein or antibody of immune quality. Once such receptors are in existence the cell becomes susceptible to positive or negative stimulation by the antigenic determinants which are sterically complementary to the immune pattern. In the thymic environment such contact results in death of the cell either within the thymus or soon after its liberation to the circulation. As will be discussed later, this provides the essential basis for natural immune tolerance of body components.

The function of thymus and bursa in birds

The avian thymus is unlike any seen in mammals, being composed of a string of ovoid lobules running along each side of the neck. In the chicken there are usually seven lobules, each in a young bird of 10–12 weeks being about 6–10 mm in longest diameter. Embryologically the epithelial thymus first shows the appearance of lymphocytes at ten days' incubation. It persists through life but with a seasonal cycle of partial atrophy with relative medullary enlargement followed, after the breeding season, by a redevelopment of cortical tissue and increase in weight.

Another organ whose function is in many ways parallel to that of the thymus is the bursa of Fabricius, which develops as an epithelial sac budding from the dorsal region of the cloaca. From and after the fifteenth day of hatching, lymphocytes appear; probably by the entry of stem cells from the blood, although direct conversion of cells in the epithelial nodules to lymphocytes is perhaps not wholly excluded. In one way or another a multilobular lymphoid organ develops. It reaches a maximum size of 1·5 to 2 g and atrophies at sexual maturity. This atrophy is presumably a

The thymus

response to hormonal stimulation and, following this clue, an important means of inhibiting the development of the bursa has been developed in the form of treatment of the embryo with testosterone or related androgens.

Either by hormonal treatment in the embryo or by surgical bursectomy immediately after hatching, chickens lose completely or almost completely their capacity to produce antibody against any of the standard types of antigen. This can occur without any significant reduction in the immunoglobulin content of serum.

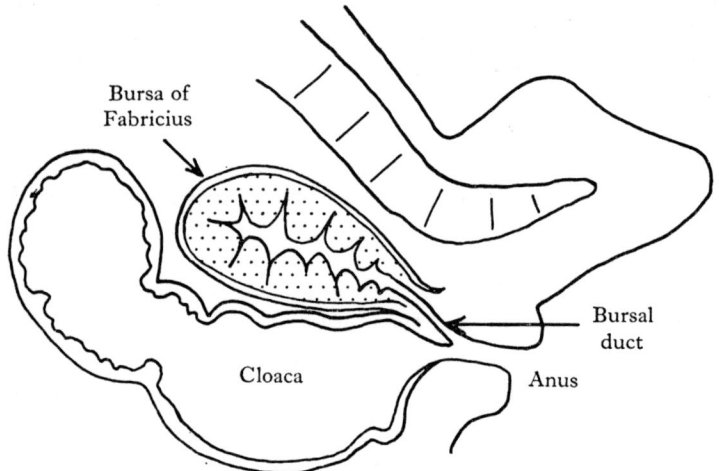

Fig. 12. The relationship of the bursa of Fabricius to the cloaca in the chicken.

Bursectomized animals with intact thymuses show no difference in the time of rejection of homografts or in the capacity to produce graft-versus-host reactions in appropriate recipients. There is some difference of opinion in regard to sensitization by tuberculin, but there is acceptable evidence that bursectomized chickens incapable of producing antibody can respond to treatment with CNS tissue plus adjuvant by the development of 'allergic' encephalomyelitis.

Neonatal thymectomy is difficult to carry out successfully in chickens but all reports consistently show a prolongation of the time of skin homograft rejection. Other features reported are a diminution in the number of circulating lymphocytes and *no* diminution in the capacity to produce graft-versus-host reactions on the chorioallantois.

There is an unfortunate lack of information on many aspects of bursal and thymic function in chickens and one would feel that an intensive study of this system is urgently needed. If, as appears superficially to be the case, we have the mammalian thymic function divided between two avian organs, there must be great scope for the further analysis of that function. The bursa is *not* an antibody-producing organ and, in a bird immunized with sheep red cells, contains no cells capable of producing antibody plaques by Jerne and Nordin's technique. The fate is not known of the lymphocytes produced so abundantly in the bursa. There is, however, evidence that (as in the mouse thymus) multiplying clones are constantly reinforced by new stem cells from perhaps thymus or bone-marrow.

Two groups have provided evidence that soluble products from bursal cells in diffusion chambers can regenerate immune capacity to some extent in bursectomized chickens. There is evidence that plasma cells are absent or very rare in the spleens of bursectomized chickens but there appears to be no consistent diminution in the concentration of immunoglobulins in serum.

Without a great deal more information no satisfactory interpretation of the avian thymus–bursa relationship is possible. I have suggested as a hypothesis with heuristic potentialities—and under the influence of a related hypothesis due to Good—that the thymus is responsible, as in mammals, for the differentiation and 'censorship' of immunocytes but that if they are to give rise to proliferating cells of antibody-producing type they must be exposed to a hormone produced by 'gut-associated lymphoid tissue'. This exposure could occur by the entry into the bursa of cells partially differentiated in the thymus or by contact with bursal hormone at a distance. Present opinion, however, is swinging rather rapidly to the view that the bursa and its mammalian analogues receive stem cells direct from the bone-marrow and differentiate them to potential antibody-producing immunocytes. Any further elaboration of this hypothesis can be left until p. 92, where it can be brought into relation with some of the features of human immunopathology.

4 The immunocyte: its definition, recognition and distribution

At the cellular level the central problems of immunology concern the differentiation, genealogy and interconvertibility of the various types of mobile nucleated cells present in the circulation, wandering through tissues or accumulated in bone-marrow, thymus or the peripheral lymphoid organs. These include the granulocytes (polymorphonuclear leucocytes, eosinophils and basophils) and the rather enigmatic tissue mast cell. The cells of the lymphoid series from blast through medium to small lymphocyte and the related plasmablast to mature plasma cell series, contain what, following Dameshek, we shall call 'immunocytes', but it should be emphasized at once that it is not possible to equate morphology with immune function. Finally, there are the cells of the reticulo-endothelial system primarily defined on their phagocytic capacity but differing very considerably from one site to another.

No immunologist has any doubt that the process of antibody formation and all the other basic activities of the immune response take place within cells of these groups. The problem is to co-ordinate what is known at the morphological level, including the sequence of progenitors and the range of differentiation, with the immunological behaviour of tissues, discrete cell populations or single cells.

THE EXPERIMENTAL DEMONSTRATION OF IMMUNE FUNCTION IN CELL POPULATIONS

There are a number of possible approaches, most of which will be mentioned only briefly as now having little more than historical interest.

Surgical removal of spleen or thymus has only minor effects on the immune reactivity of an animal. Rather more has been learned by using the technique of shielding a particular part of the body or a single organ when an animal is heavily X-irradiated using a dose sufficient to annul all immunological response to an antigen given in the next day or two. The most interesting finding was that, in the rabbit, shielding the appendix which has much lymphoid tissue and many plasma cells allows almost full retention of antibody-producing capacity. In a sense this is taken to indicate not that antibody is mostly synthesized in the appendix but that there are mobile cells in the appendix which within a few hours can effectively restock the various lymphoid organs depleted of their lymphocytes by the irradiation. An operationally equivalent procedure would be to obtain from a syngeneic animal an adequate number of living lymphocytes and use them to restore immune capacity to an animal rendered immunologically inert by whole-body irradiation. There are many variants of this approach. Nearly all require that the recipient must not actively reject the transferred cells and that it should be incapable of producing the antibody under study. Both ends can be attained by recent X-irradiation or the use of embryonic or neonatal animals.

The principal difficulty in all such experiments is that any suspension of cells from an animal, whether from spleen, bone-marrow, blood leucocytes or thoracic duct, is a heterogeneous population. Usually the most that can be said is that from a mixture of cells of which the differential count in a stained smear is such and such, a certain immune response is obtained with doses of cells equal to or greater than x, x being usually of the order of some millions of cells.

For many years now, it has been known that suspensions of cells from any organ of a primed animal that contained relatively large numbers of lymphocytes, plasma cells and macrophages could give rise to antibody production under such experimental conditions. The role of the plasma cell as a major producer of antibody has been universally accepted since 1948 and modern work has been largely directed toward establishing the immunological role of the lymphocyte.

From all points of view the most suitable source of lymphocytes is the thoracic duct, and recent opinion in this field has been greatly influenced by Gowans's exploitation of the opportunities so provided. Most thoracic duct cells are small lymphocytes but there is always a proportion of large and medium lymphocytes some of which may be indistinguishable from plasmablasts. By suitable manipulation almost all the large cells can be eliminated and by administration of such material Gowans and collaborators have shown that immune capacity may be lost and regained under the following circumstances:

(*a*) Chronic drainage of the thoracic duct in rats produces severe depletion of lymphocytes, and such animals can neither produce antibody against a standard antigen such as sheep red cells, nor reject a skin homograft which differs by only minor histocompatibility factors.

(*b*) Such depleted animals can be restored to normal immunological capacity by the administration of thoracic duct cells from a compatible donor.

(*c*) Rats rendered tolerant to skin homografts lose their tolerance when given syngeneic normal thoracic duct cells.

(*d*) Thoracic duct cells from a donor immunized with tetanus toxoid conferred on a syngeneic recipient the ability to give a secondary-type response to challenge with the same antigen.

(*e*) Using suitable pure strains of rats differing by major histocompatibility factors, injection of thoracic duct cells into an allogeneic recipient produces a severe graft-versus-host reaction. In the course of this a proportion of small lymphocytes in the inoculum are converted to large pyroninophil cells capable of mitosis.

These findings are consistent with what has been obtained by the use of less suitable material in the form of cell suspensions from spleen and lymph nodes. No one now has any serious doubt that within any large population of lymphocytes taken from an animal of defined immunological status there are subpopulations of lymphocytes capable of transferring capacity to react in fashions corresponding to the immunological ability of the donor. This does not of course mean any more than that small lymphocytes can carry specific immunological information. It does not allow identification of individual capacity in any given cell or provide a measure of the proportion of the lymphocyte population with specific activity. For this, methods applicable to single cells are necessary.

THE FUNCTIONAL RECOGNITION OF INDIVIDUAL IMMUNOCYTES

An immunocyte is a cell that can react with a specific antigen in some recognizable fashion, and a number of ways have been devised by which the specific immunological reactivity of single cells can be demonstrated. The most direct is to use a sensitive test to measure the production of antibody by an isolated cell. Another method is to observe under the microscope whether visible antigenic particles adhere to the surface of a given cell. Immunofluorescent methods are more generally applicable to detect either immunoglobulin or, by the 'sandwich' method, specific antibody. Finally the recognition of immunoglobulin by using ferritin-labelled antiglobulin can be used to identify immunocytes in electron micrographs of tissue or cell sections.

The role of the plasma cell

Since Astrid Fagraeus's work in 1948 there has been little doubt that the plasma cell is the predominant producer of antibody and in this section it will be convenient to sketch the confirmation of this opinion by the use of modern methods.

In ordinary histological sections or smears, plasma cells are easily recognized by their round nuclei with lumps of chromatin giving a clock-face appearance and fairly abundant basophil cytoplasm. The basophilia is due to large amounts of RNA and sections made for electron microscopy show that this RNA is part of the characteristic mechanism of protein-synthesizing and -secreting cells, the endoplasmic reticulum. In plasma cells, as in the cells of the pancreas or any other protein-secreting gland, there is a dense accumulation of close-packed flattened vesicles, smooth on the inside, roughened on the outside, with enormous numbers of ribosomes. The ribosomes represent the site of protein synthesis and it has now been clearly demonstrated by the use of an antigen (ferritin) which can be seen in electron micrographs, that antibody accumulates within the vesicles. It is reasonable to believe that this accumulated immunoglobulin is liberated either continuously or intermittently into the surrounding fluid. This has not yet been experimentally established and the possibility exists that what is seen within the vesicles is a stored reserve rather than antibody at an intermediate stage of a continuous process of synthesis and secretion.

A more general approach is by the use of fluorescent antibody. By appropriate chemical manipulation it is possible to attach a highly fluorescent dye (e.g. fluorescein) to an antibody molecule without damaging its power to combine with antigen. The combination can thus be used as a specific stain for antigen if we wish to find, for instance, where a certain antigen is located in a section of lymph node in an immunized animal. If the animal was inoculated 24 hours previously it will be found that the reticulo-endothelial cells (macrophages) will be stained and fluoresce brilliantly under appropriate illumination. Neither lymphocytes nor plasma cells are stained by this method.

To use the method to detect immunoglobulin in or on a cell and, by implication, so to identify it as an immunocyte, the immunoglobulin is regarded as an antigen. The best technique if human cells are to be studied is to produce in rabbits specific antisera against human A, G and M immunoglobulins and prepare specific fluorescein-coupled antibodies. Further refinements can be introduced by preparing specific sera against one or other type of light chain (see chapter 5). In this way it has been found that all three immunoglobulins may be produced by plasma cells, mature and immature.

The sandwich technique makes it possible to show that plasma cells in an immunized animal contain specific antibody. A section usually made from frozen tissue is first treated with *antigen* and washed. Antigen is thereby attached to antibody if this is present in the cell and a considerable proportion of antigenic determinant groups will be left on the surface available for binding to fluorescent antibody and specific for the antigen being studied.

Finally, there are two direct methods by which single cells can be shown to produce functional antibody. Both will be discussed at more length in subsequent chapters.

The first is to separate a single cell from the local lymph node of an immunized animal, wash it and allow it to secrete antibody into a tiny volume of fluid. The antibody can then be detected if a sufficiently sensitive test is available. One method, developed by

Nossal and Lederberg, is to immunize rats with the flagellar antigen of a *Salmonella* strain. Flagellar antibody attaches to and entangles the flagella responsible for the motility of bacteria. If a washed lymphoid cell from a rat immunized with flagellar antigen of *Salmonella adelaide* is left in a microdroplet of saline for an hour and then five or ten motile bacteria of the right strain introduced, we have a sensitive system for the detection of antibody. If the cell is producing antibody, the bacteria will be immobilized within a minute or two. If it is not, the bacteria will swim around actively for an indefinite period. With this method, virtually all the cells which produce antibody are plasma cells or early members of the plasma cell line.

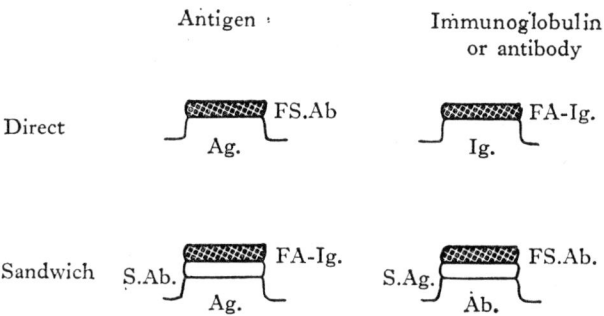

Fig. 13. Detection of antigen, immunoglobulin and antibody by fluorescent antibody. FA-Ig. fluorescent antiglobulin; FS. Ab. fluorescent specific antibody; S. Ab. specific antibody; S. Ag. specific antigen.

Antibody against certain bacteriophages can be detected in very small amount and a basically similar method has been to take the fluid secreted into a microdrop by a single cell and test this for phage-neutralizing power.

Another method involving individual cells uses a different principle. If the antibody being studied is one that can damage red cells and produce haemolysis, it is possible to incorporate cells being tested for their production of this antibody and an excess of 'target' red cells in a thin agar layer. A cell-secreting antibody will then be surrounded by red cells to which the antibody becomes attached. Such cells are vulnerable to haemolysis by fresh guinea-pig serum (complement) and after such treatment one sees scattered over the uniform layer of red cells small circular holes (plaques) which are colourless and almost transparent. Under the microscope a single cell will be found in the centre of each plaque; obviously the source from which the antibody was derived. Again it is found that some of the cells are plasma cells, but most of them are large and medium lymphocytes or immature plasma cells, presumably capable of further proliferation.

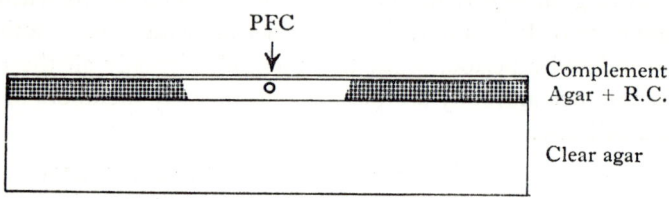

Fig. 14. The principle of antibody plaques by the Jerne–Nordin method. The upper layer contains a mixture of splenic cells and red cells (antigen). After incubation the plaques are 'developed' by complement.

By all these methods, plasma cells can be identified as antibody or immunoglobulin producers but it is recorded in almost all the relevant papers that occasionally or frequently positive results were obtained from cells morphologically not plasma cells. Some had the appearance of small lymphocytes, and some have been shown to contain only weakly developed endoplasmic reticulum.

Immune function in individual lymphocytes

Basically similar methods have been used and in fact many of the positive findings have been in the course of experiments in which plasma cells gave the most frequent and conspicuous positive appearances.

It is perhaps significant that positive findings are more common in conditions associated with typical delayed hypersensitivity reactions or with conditions such as homograft immunity and graft-versus-host reactions which are more analogous to delayed hypersensitivity than to antibody production, i.e. in 'thymus-dependent' conditions.

The only impressive results by the use of the sandwich technique are those of Raffel's group in guinea-pigs sensitized respectively

Plates 1, 2, 3. Phases of the immunocyte. Electron micrographs at a magnification around 15,000× of cells from rat lymph nodes. (Provided by Mr A. Abbot of the Walter and Eliza Hall Institute.)

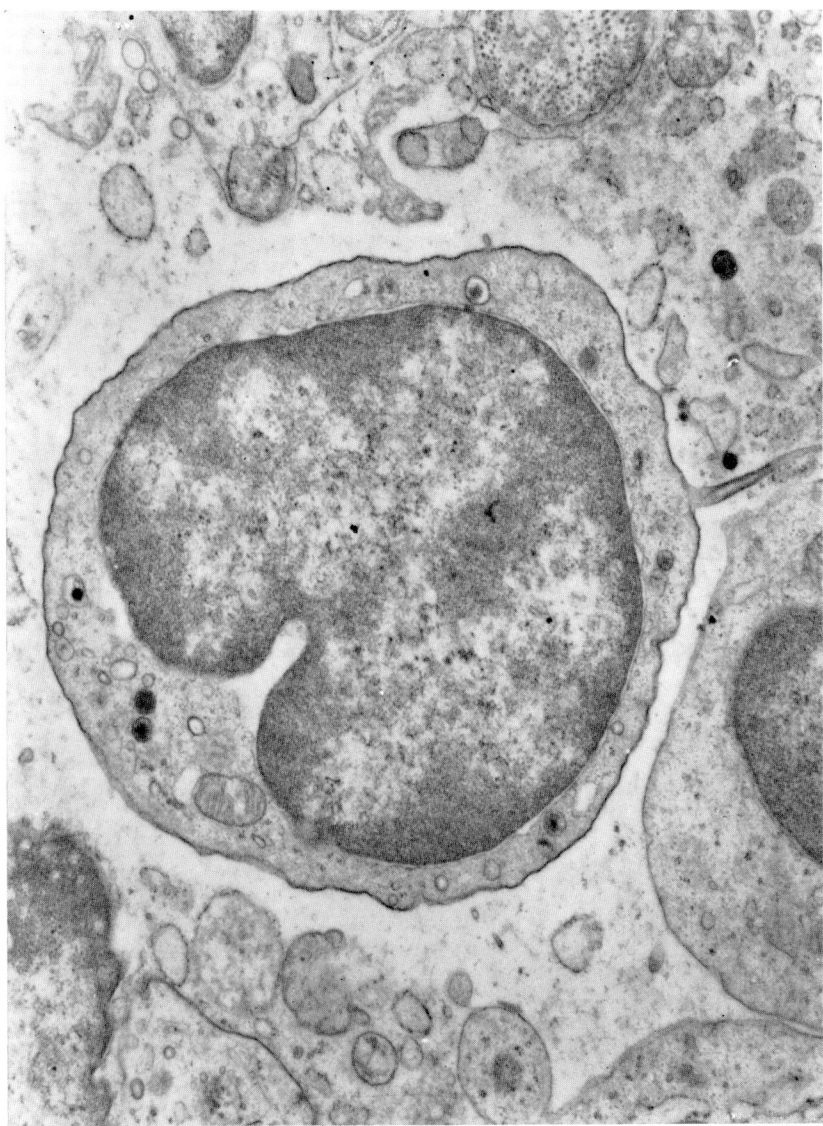

1. *Small lymphocyte.* The standard carrier of cellular information. Note the high nuclear–cytoplasmic ratio, the relative emptiness of the cytoplasm showing only one mitochondrion in this section, and the density of the nucleus without a clearly-visible nucleolus.

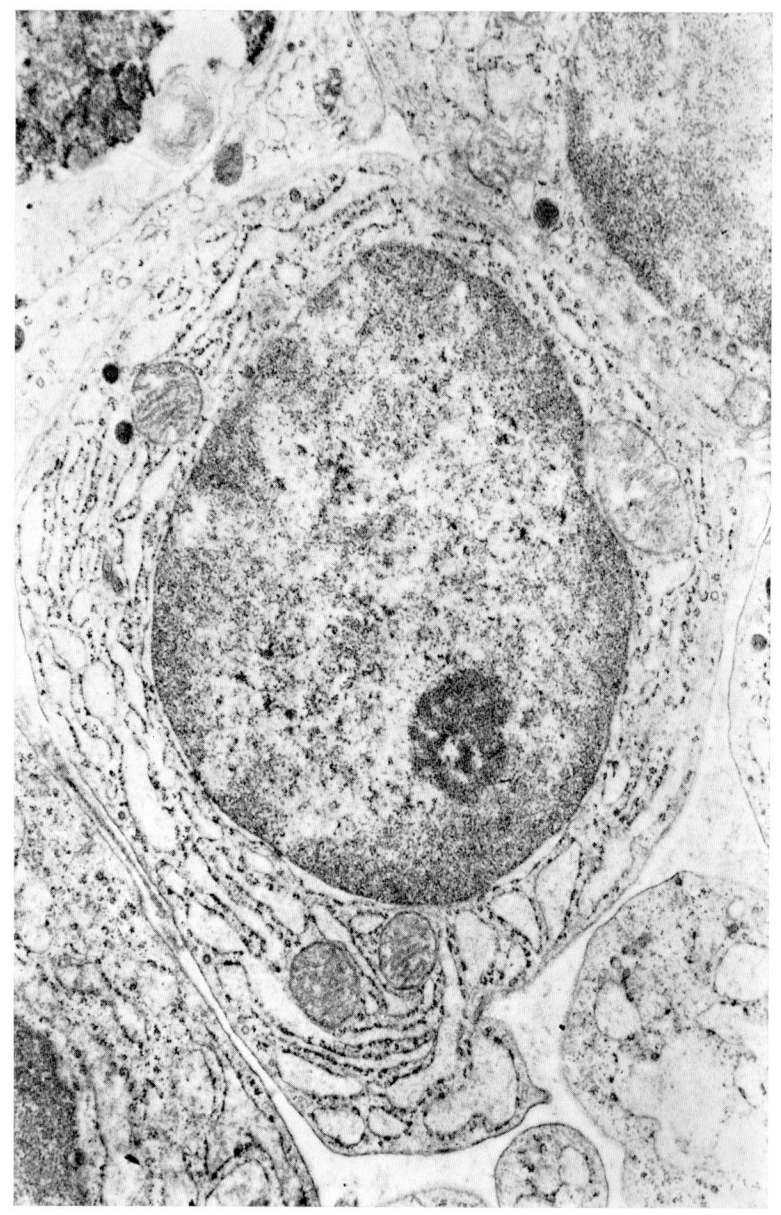

2. *Immature plasma cell.* The most significant producer of antibody. Note the large nucleus with conspicuous nucleolus, well-marked endoplasmic reticulum with ribosomes, and three mitochondria.

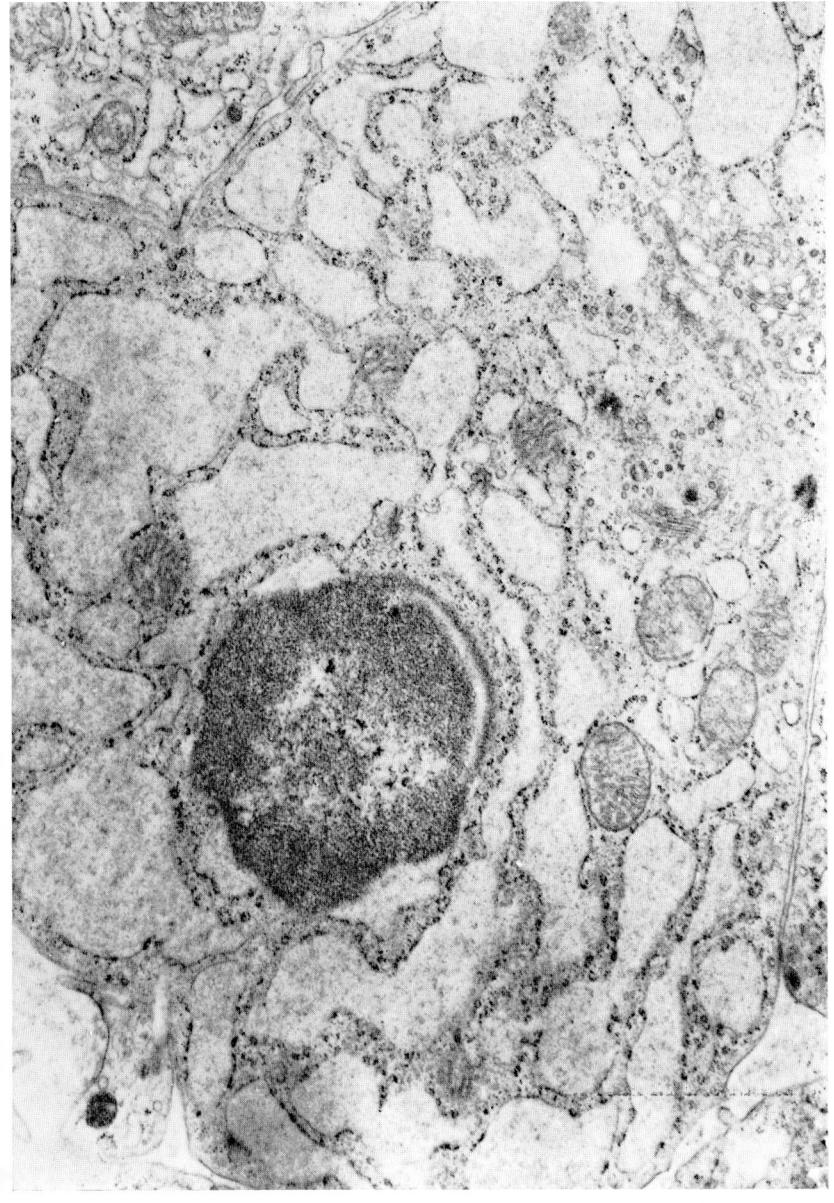

3. *Mature plasma cell.* The end stage of the antibody-producing cell. Note that the nucleus is small and beginning to show pyknotic degeneration. The endoplasmic reticulum is extensive and vacuolated and there are numerous mitochondria.

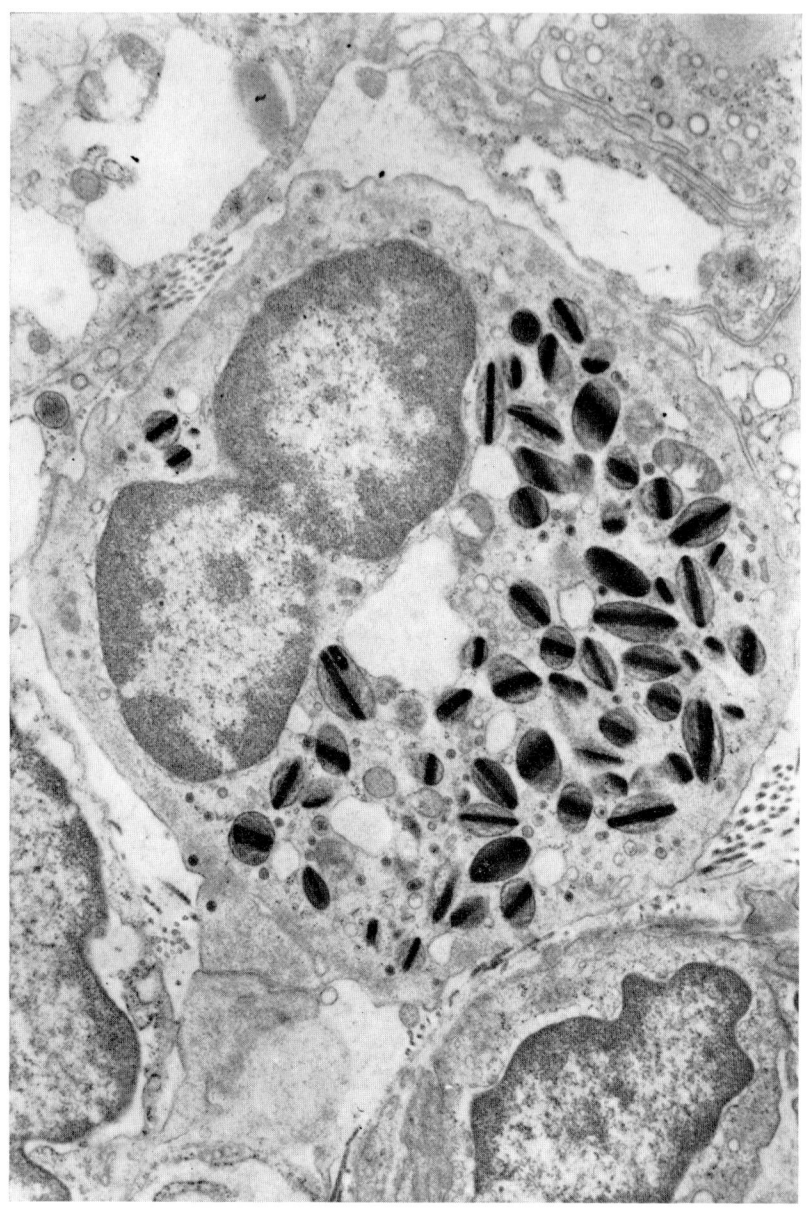

4. Eosinophil granulocyte (rat), characteristically reactive to antigen–antibody complexes. Note the bilobed nucleus and the characteristic granules with crystalloid inclusions. (Provided by Mr A. Abbot.)

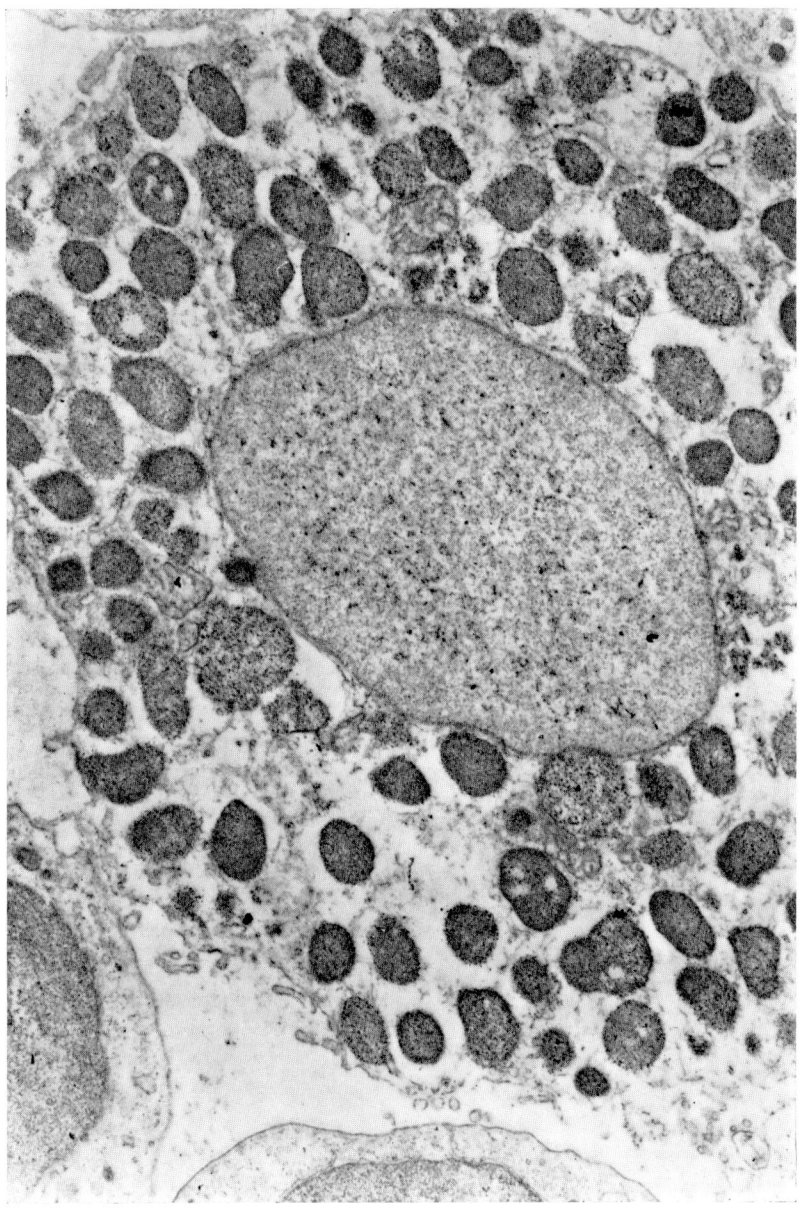

5. Mast cell (rat) responsive to stimulation by liberation of histamine, serotonin and heparin. Note the large rather variable granules responsible for the characteristic metachromatic staining and which contain the pharmacologically active agents. (Provided by Mr A. Abbot.)

Plates 6 and 7. *The relationship of macrophages to the uptake of antigen.* Electron-micrographs of lymph node sections from rats given heavily labelled flagellar antigen. By a combination of autoradiographic and electron microscopic techniques the location of antigen is shown by the dense black deposits of metallic silver. (Electron micrographs provided by Professor G. J. V. Nossal, Dr Judith Mitchell and Mr A. Abbot.)

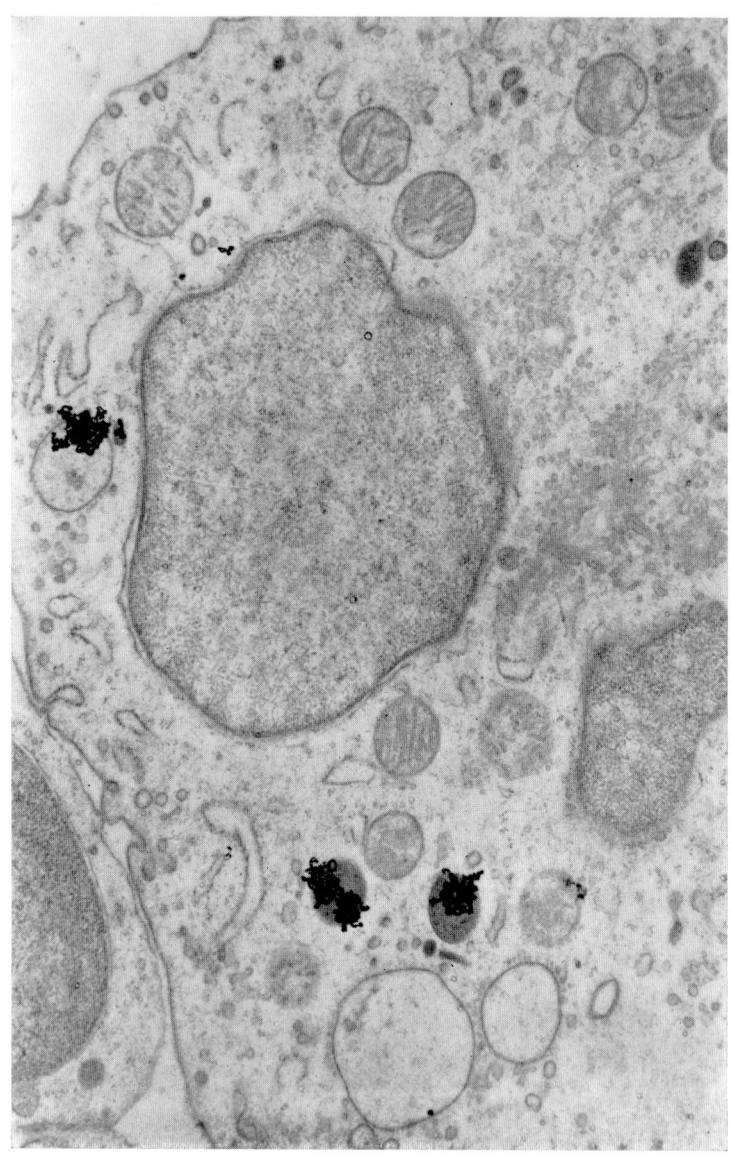

6. Medullary macrophage showing concentration of antigen in lysosomes (phagosomes). None is present on the surface membrane of the cell.

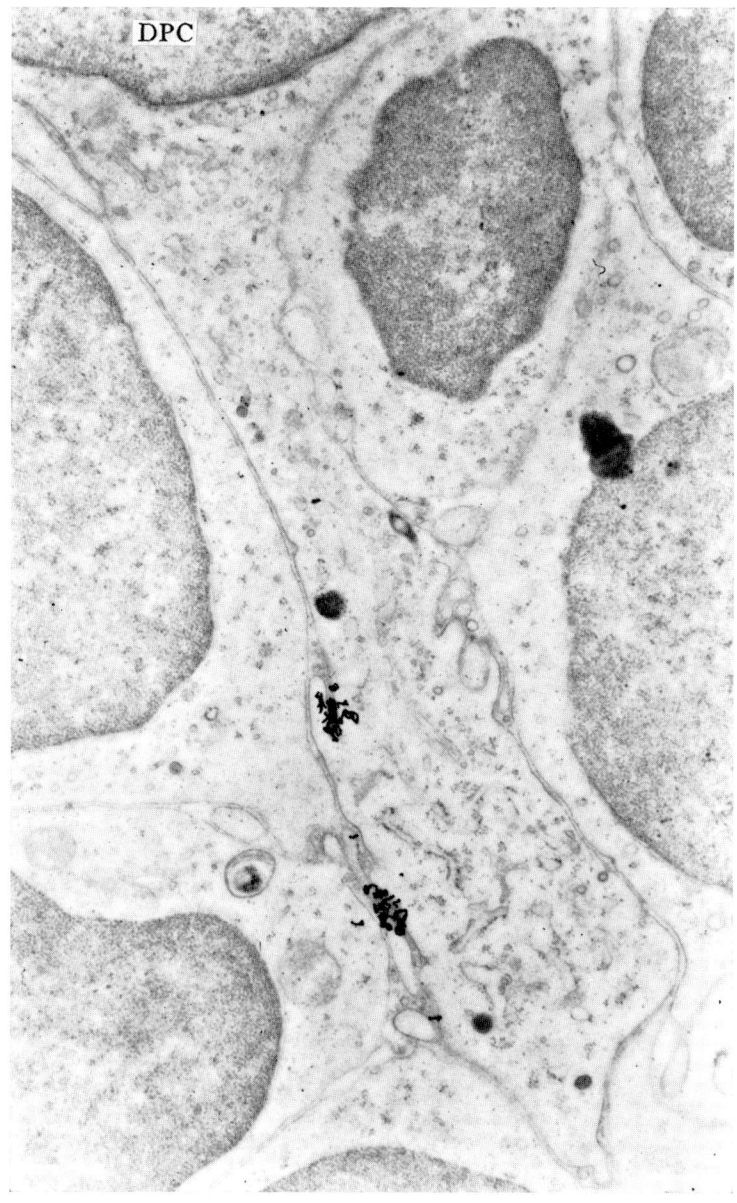

7. Localization of antigen on the cell membrane of the dendritic phagocytic cell. DPC = the nucleus of the phagocytic cell involved; the other nuclei are those of small lymphocytes.

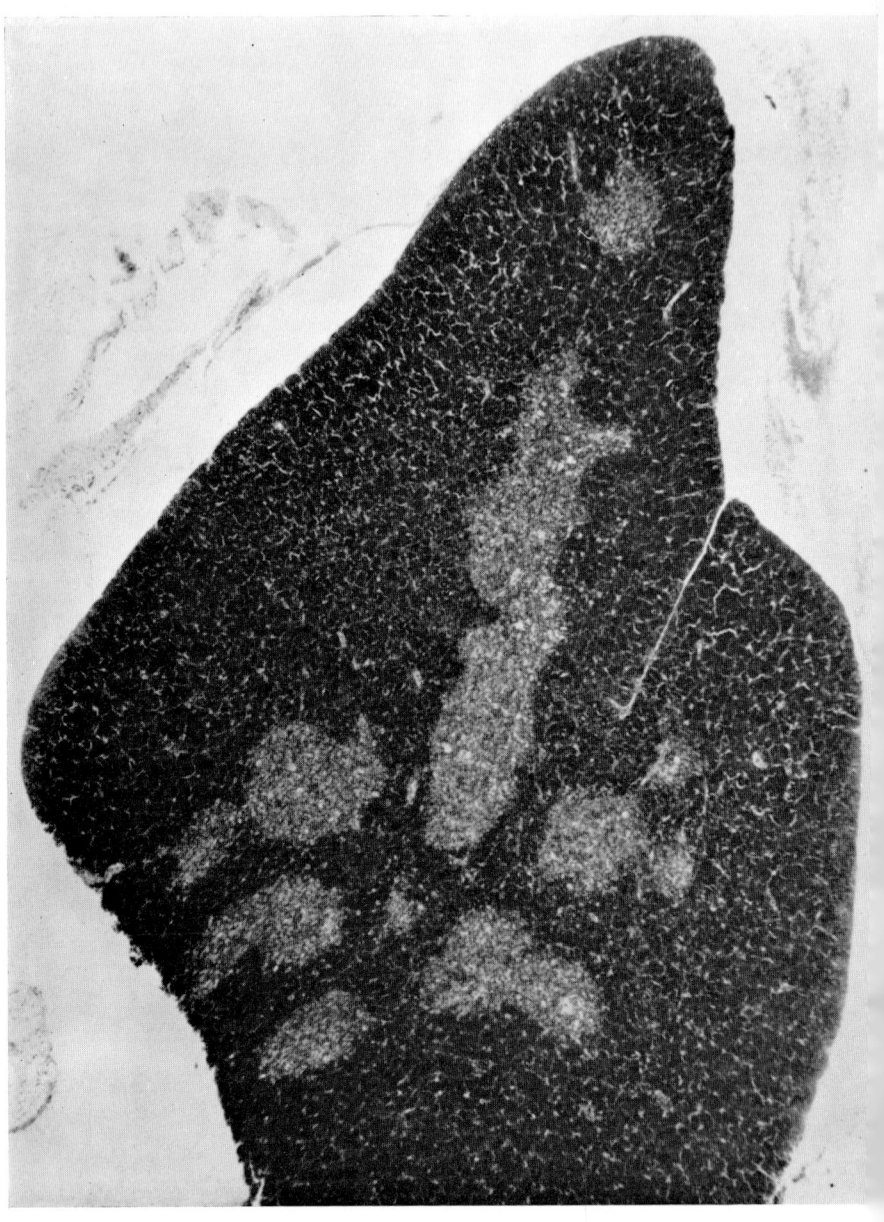

8. Section of thymus from a young mouse to show the sharp demarcation of cortex (dark with close-packed nuclei) and medulla.

by tuberculous infection and by the injection of encephalitogenic protein. Animals showing positive tuberculin reactions or typical experimental allergic encephalomyelitis gave lymphocyte populations of which '6–20 per cent' or '5–10 per cent' of small lymphocytes showed specific fluorescence when treated with antigen and fluorescent antibody. There are other less fully established reports that tuberculoproteins are more readily taken up by lymphocytes from sensitive individuals than from normals.

Basically similar studies have been made in which the tuberculoprotein (PPD) was conjugated with fluorescein and used to determine the percentage of reactive lymphocytes. In positive tuberculin reactions the percentage reacting ranged from 1·5 to 9 per cent; in negative reactors ten of eleven showed less than 1 per cent.

Evidence for the presence of immunoglobulins in or on lymphocytes is more extensive. Using immunofluorescence techniques to study human cells, van Furth found that cells, mostly medium lymphocytes, could be found in thoracic duct lymph, giving active fluorescence for M, G or A immunoglobulins; small lymphocytes both in the thoracic duct lymph and in the blood showed weak staining for M only. In all situations, medium lymphocytes showed more marked fluorescence and included some positive for A and G. In line with much other evidence indicating that the 'small lymphocytes' of bone-marrow may be a distinct cell type, these showed no evidence of any immunoglobulin. Equally interesting was the finding that cells in foetal thymus showed no fluorescence at a time when spleen cells showed M or G immunoglobulins. The general impression from these results is that many large and medium lymphocytes are, in fact, cells in the process of becoming plasma cells rather than small lymphocytes. The latter cells produce either M immunoglobulin or none at all.

The other field of interest for the individual characterization of lymphocytes is stimulation of human small lymphocytes to blast formation and mitosis *in vitro*. It is too early to generalize, but what has been published seems to establish that a proportion of small lymphocytes can be stimulated by specific agents as well as by a variety of nonspecific ones such as phytohaemagglutinin. Among confirmed examples are the regular occurrence of blast transformation in lymphocyte populations from tuberculin-positive individuals when the cells are treated with tuberculoprotein; transformation is also seen regularly when lymphocytes from two different individuals are mixed. There are also accounts of individual cases of severe drug reaction to 'Dilantin' and of infantile eczema with specific response to the appropriate antigen. In experimental animals the only well-documented account is of stimulation by allotypic antiglobulin serum which is not relevant here (see p. 168).

TABLE 1. *Presence of immunoglobulins G, A and M in cells*

	Plasma cells	Small lymphocytes
Thymus	G A	—
Spleen	G A M	M
Lymph node	G A M	M
Thoracic duct	G A M	M
Bone-marrow	G A M	—

— no immunoglobulin detected.
Based on R. van Furth (1964). Doctoral thesis, Leiden.

It is rather striking that so far there are no reports of equivalent reactions in immunized animals and no recent confirmation of claims that any type of immunization not associated with the production of delayed hypersensitivity in human beings will produce appropriately reactive lymphocytes. As a tentative conclusion we may state:

(*a*) that many large and medium lymphocytes are cells of the plasmacyte series and can produce one or other of M, G or A immunoglobulins;

(*b*) that the only immunoglobulin produced by small lymphocytes is M—most produce none;

(*c*) that small lymphocytes associated with delayed-hypersensitivity-type reactions may have an exceptional type of surface reactivity for the sensitizing antigen;

(*d*) that the bone-marrow population of cells with the morphology of small lymphocytes is not part of the immunocyte group.

COMMITMENT OF IMMUNOCYTES

In the second half of this chapter the aim is to describe the population dynamics of lymphoid cells, their movements, sites of proliferation, morphological and functional modification and final disposal. At this stage we assume that each immunocyte, that is, every descendant of a lymphoid cell differentiated to immune function in the thymus or elsewhere, carries receptor sites of specific character capable of reacting with a restricted range of antigenic pattern and often only with a single group of closely related determinant patterns. This is more fully discussed in chapter 8. It will also be accepted that, in mammals, cells carrying new immune patterns first emerge from the thymus, retaining, however, the qualification that future research may require the recognition of other primary sources of new cells possibly analogous to the bursa of Fabricius in chickens.

In the previous chapter it was concluded that immunocytes are differentiated in the thymus and there subjected to a scrutiny for immune patterns capable of reacting with antigenic determinants of accessible body components. Only a minor proportion of the lymphocytes produced in the thymus give rise to continuing clones after leaving it. Many are destroyed in the organ itself, others may enter the circulation and for one reason or another prove non-viable. Nevertheless, the mass of direct and circumstantial evidence points to the conclusion that all the immunocytes in the body are descended from cells which have been differentiated in the thymus and have passed thence to the circulation.

Most deductions as to what happens when differentiated cells leave the thymus must be made from indirect evidence. Such deductions give rise to a fairly well-established picture, many details of which are subject to change with the accumulation of future information. With this qualification, what happens seems to be as follows.

About three days, on the average, after their last mitosis, small lymphocytes leave the thymus and enter the blood circulation either directly or indirectly. A majority of these are lost, perhaps as a result of stimulation received in the thymus. Of those which can be traced, most lodge in lymphoid tissue. Indirect but persuasive evidence indicates that most of those that lodge in lymph nodes are to be found in the paracortical areas rather than in lymph follicles. If we slightly anticipate later discussion, these small (and medium) lymphocytes of immediate thymic origin bring immune patterns whose origin is unrelated to the immunological experience of the body. They are uncommitted or progenitor immunocytes, each with its characteristic immune pattern awaiting stimulation, and they represent the only way in which fresh supplies of 'new' immune patterns can arise. Everything suggests that these newly produced cells are vulnerable. In all probability any high concentration of antigen will be lethal, perhaps not so much in virtue of the amount but of the sequence of specific stimuli. There is good evidence for the existence of a thymic hormone necessary for the viability of cells recently released from the thymus. In the absence of continued production of some humoral product by thymic epithelial tissue the new cells cannot mature to the level at which they can manifest any of the demonstrable functions of immunocytes. Once cells have passed this vulnerable stage there is no evidence that thymic hormone is necessary. Economy of hypothesis is to assume that thymic epithelium secretes a single protein hormone which, in addition to the well-documented effect of mediating the survival of newly liberated cells, is also concerned in stimulating proliferation and differentiation of cells entering the thymus and in facilitating the elimination of 'self-reactive' cells. The additions, however, are at the present time wholly speculative.

Contact of an uncommitted cell with an antigenic determinant capable of union with its specific receptors can have, of course, other effects than the destruction of the cell. There is rather uncoordinated evidence that (a) the cell may be induced directly to synthesize and liberate Ig M antibody and (b) it is de-differentiated to a blast-type cell from which a relatively small descendant clone of 'committed immunocytes'—morphologically lymphocytes—is derived. The conditions that determine whether destruction or some type of positive immune reaction follows contact with specific determinant are largely unknown, and what is known is better left to chapter 8.

Here, our concern is with the fact that after preliminary contact with a given antigen an animal gives a much more active immune response. In cellular terms it now has a population of committed immunocytes. In a sense the uncommitted immunocyte is a hypothetical entity needed to account indirectly for many observational and experimental facts. Committed immunocytes are the lymphocytes which can be demonstrated to respond specifically to antigen.

The change from the uncommitted to the committed immunocyte can be most readily and probably correctly pictured as involving an increase in the number of specific immune receptors (which may now be in the form of Ig M antibody molecules) and in their accessibility to antigen in the environment.

THE STRUCTURE OF PERIPHERAL LYMPHOID TISSUE

For many years it has been clear that spleen and lymph nodes are the tissues most directly concerned with immune processes. For technical reasons, most recent experimental work on cellular immunology has been concerned with the cells of accessible lymph nodes, either popliteal or auricular, and it will be convenient to base general discussion of the function of lymphoid tissue on this work. In all probability the lymphoid tissue of the spleen and the extensive accumulations of lymphoid tissues along the alimentary tract, from tonsils downward, play a basically similar role.

Lymph node structure

The essential features of a peripheral lymph node are shown in fig. 15. The afferent lymph carrying any antigenic material from its catchment area enters at the periphery and is distributed over the lateral sinus, from which it percolates through more or less definite channels into the cortex and eventually is collected into the lymph sinuses associated with the medullary cords and brought to the efferent lymph vessels at the hilus. Lying immediately beneath the lateral sinus is the cortical tissue with a number of areas of more closely packed small lymphocytes, the primary lymph follicles. Within these, secondary follicles or germinal centres develop under antigenic stimulation. Toward the hilum of the node the medullary cords, more or less closely packed, represent essentially small blood vessels surrounded by a sheath of tissue infiltrated by lymphoid cells and delimited by the lymphatic endothelium lining the channels which come together to form the efferent lymph vessels. Between the cortex and medulla is the paracortical lymphoid tissue which is not clearly demarcated into primary follicles and is labile in amount and distribution according to the degree of stimulation of the node. In general, small lymphocytes predominate in the primary follicles and the paracortical areas; the germinal centres characteristically contain large lymphocytes and variable numbers of medium lymphocytes and lightly

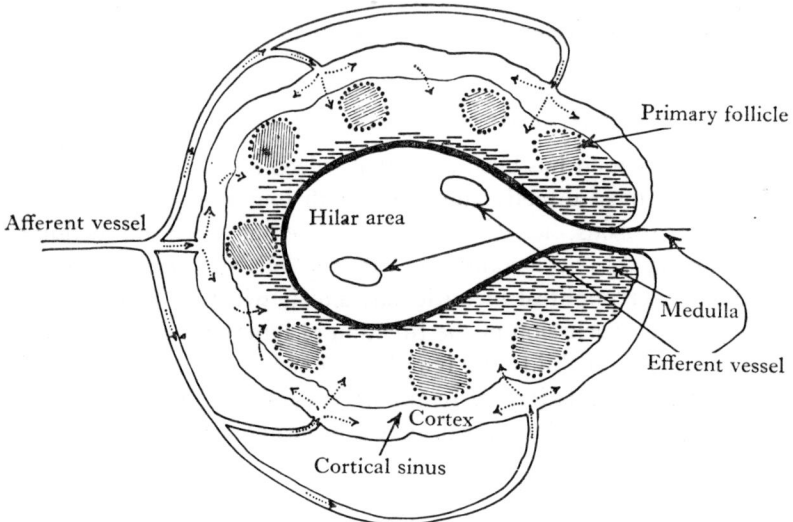

Fig. 15. Schematic diagram of a popliteal lymph node from a young rat. From G. J. V. Nossal, G. L. Ada and C. M. Austin (1964). Antigens in immunity. IV. Aust. J. exp. Biol. med. Sci. **42**, 311.

pyroninophilic cells. In active lymph nodes the main concentration of plasma cells is in the medullary cords but there are also many pyroninophilic cells in the paracortical area. Phagocytic cells of the reticulo-endothelial system are numerous and are most conspicuous in the wall of the peripheral sinus and of the lymph channels in the medulla. In addition there are the dendritic cells which form an inconspicuous reticulum through the cortex and which appear to play a major role in presenting antigen to cells of the lymphoid series.

The distribution and character of the blood vessels have an important bearing on the immunological function of the lymph node. In a typical rat lymph node the arterial supply enters at the hilum, and primary arteriolar branches, each within a medullary cord, run directly to the cortex where they divide into capillaries. These are relatively inconspicuous compared with the smallest venules, which show many areas of cuboidal endothelium and are tortuous and numerous. They leave the cortex via the medullary cords and at the hilum join to form the draining venous trunk. The medullary cords are most clearly seen in an oedematous lymph node. They are surrounded by lymphatic endothelium, on the lymph sinus side of which are numerous macrophages (littoral cells). There is a single unbranching central arteriole or venule with venules about ten times as frequent as arterioles. Patches of cuboidal endothelium may be present at any part of the venule but it is more frequent near the cortex.

The generally accepted view of the embryology of lymph nodes is that they arise by the accumulation of lymphocytes around appropriate regions of the developing network of lymph channels. Lymphocytes and lymph nodes do not appear until the time that the thymus contains lymphocytic cells, and the view that all or most primitive lymphocytes arise from the thymus, and by colonization and proliferation give rise to the peripheral lymphoid accumulations, is widely but by no means universally held.

The immune function of the lymph node

In the developed lymph node the most important functional feature is the extensive entry of small lymphocytes from the blood and equivalent discharge of cells by the efferent lymphatic. In the popliteal lymph node of the sheep this may correspond to a complete turnover of cells once every seventy hours. Entry from the blood is across the relatively thick-walled postcapillary venules which are characteristic of all lymphoid tissue. Lymphocytes are highly mobile cells and they have been noted to have a special tendency to enter the cytoplasm of certain types of epithelial cell in tissue culture and of intestinal epithelium *in situ*. On the other hand those who have studied the movement of leucocytes microscopically in rabbit ear chambers or preparations of mesentery

The immunocyte

have never recorded the passage of a small lymphocyte through the capillary wall. Polymorphonuclear leucocytes, eosinophils and monocytes pass readily at the junctions between two endothelial cells.

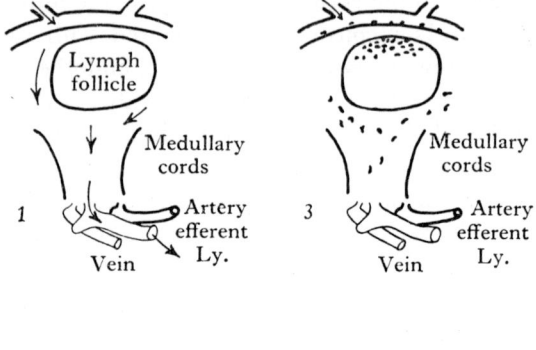

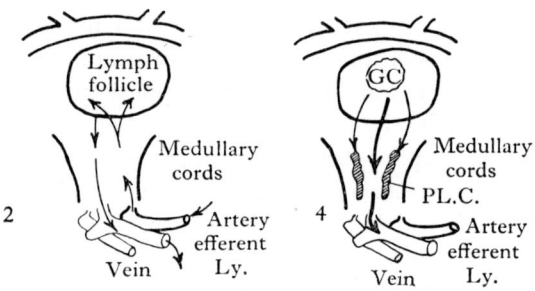

Fig. 16. Movement in a peripheral lymph node. A series of simplified diagrams to indicate: 1. The flow of lymph; 2. The movement of lymphocytes entering by the blood, leaving by the efferent lymph trunks; 3. Distribution of antigen reaching the node by afferent lymphatics; 4. Probable movement of proliferating immunocytes. Pl. C. = plasma cells; GC = germinal centre; Ly = lymphatic.

The capacity of small lymphocytes to leave the bloodstream via the postcapillary venules of lymphoid tissue in large numbers has been adequately established. It must follow that the cuboidal endothelium of the venules concerned must differ significantly and adaptively from normal capillary and venular endothelium. The patchy distribution of the cuboidal character suggests that a local, rather than a genetically determined process may be concerned.

There are interesting implications of the simplest formulation of such a process—that in any accumulation of lymphocytes and antigen-retaining reticulum there will be a continuing liberation of an agent with the effect of making venular endothelium 'attractive' or 'sticky' for lymphocytes passing through in the blood. 'Permeability factors' can be extracted from lymph node cells and it is possible that such extracts contain the hypothetical agent responsible for maintaining the cuboidal state of the venular endothelium in lymphoid tissue.

Such a hypothesis might be of value in interpreting the process by which lymph nodes and other lymphoid accumulations develop. If, whenever for any reason a group of lymphocytes come together, the adjacent postcapillary venule develops this specific permeability for small lymphocytes, a 'gravitational' process will give rise to an increasing aggregation around which presumably the characteristic architecture and vascular supply of the lymph node will develop.

The afferent lymphatics are so disposed as to bring to the node any antigenic material appearing in their field of drainage as well as any lymphocytes or other mobile cells present in the tissue fluids. They embouch into the peripheral sinus and so bring antigen into close relationship to the cortical aspect of the primary lymph follicles. The functional anatomy of the lymph follicle can best be elaborated by following the fate of a labelled antigen, such as the *Salmonella* flagellin of Nossal's group injected into a footpad of the rat. There are many phagocytic cells lining the various lymph paths and sinuses in the draining popliteal node and a large amount of antigen is taken up by these. From the immunological angle these seem to be unimportant compared with the dendritic phagocytes that are inconspicuously interspersed amongst the lymphocytes of the primary follicles. When lymph nodes are examined at daily and weekly intervals, after such an injection the dense accumulations of labelled antigen seen at 24 hours soon vanish from most of the sites. A proportion of macrophages in the medullary and paracortical areas remain heavily loaded for weeks and with even a very small dose of antigen there is prolonged persistence in the dendritic reticulum cells of the primary follicles. With the appearance of germinal centres the labelled area is distorted to form a long-lasting cap on the cortical side of the germinal centre.

Our hypothesis is that these reticulum cells are important repositories for antigen—perhaps sites where its physical character is modified. In the living follicle we are almost compelled to think of the lymphocytes as individually mobile so that a continual sequence of cells can come into contact with extensions of the cytoplasm of the dendritic antigen-containing cells. Quite rapidly, any lymphocyte in the follicle capable of reacting with the antigen present will have an opportunity to do so, and it is probably legitimate to regard any such population as a random sample of the whole complement of lymphocytes (or immunocytes) in the body.

Functionally speaking, the most important feature of a lymph node is the mobility of the cell population it contains. In the lymph leaving the popliteal node of a large animal, such as the sheep, are large numbers of lymphocytes which can be shown by appropriate labelling experiments not to be produced in the node. Approximate calculation suggests that about 10 per cent of the lymphocytes entering the node in the blood pass through vessel walls into the node, while an equivalent number leave by the efferent lymphatics. Similarly, if such a node is subjected to heavy (2,000 r) local irradiation to destroy all its contained lymphocytes and the situation examined 24–48 hours later, it is found that the cell content of efferent lymph is virtually unaltered, as is the capacity of the node to produce antibody on appropriate stimulation.

Evidence from a wide variety of experimental procedures shows that the lymphoid cell population of every primary lymph follicle in the body is constantly changing. Cells enter from the blood and for the most part leave the node by the efferent lymphatics, eventually to return to the blood circulation by one of the main lymphatic trunks. It follows that every accumulation of lymphocytes in the body that is not under immediate antigenic stimulation will contain representatives of virtually every clone of immunocytes that has been produced. This high degree of mobility is of great importance for anyone interpreting results of immunological experiments on individual lymphoid regions *in vivo*, whether they are lymph nodes, Peyer's patches or focal accumulations produced experimentally.

Antigenic stimulation from, say, a foot-pad injection, has two main morphological effects on the lymph node: (*a*) an increase in the numbers of plasma cells largely in the medullary cords and

(b) the appearance of germinal centres (secondary follicles). At an appropriate time, antibody is detectable in the efferent lymph or in extracts of the node. There is still uncertainty about the cellular interpretation of these changes. One feels, however, that there is significant evidence in favour of one interpretation and none yet available to disprove it. According to this interpretation, an immunocyte activated by contact with the corresponding antigen lodges in lymphoid tissue in one of two situations: (a) in the substance of a lymph follicle or (b) in a medullary cord. In the lymph follicle, which may be in the same or in a lymph node distant from that in which the cell was stimulated by antigen, the activated cell proliferates to give rise to a clone of large and medium lymphocytes which remain in contact until the stage of small lymphocytes is reached, so giving rise to a germinal centre. All the progeny will, apart from incidental mutation, be of the same immune pattern as the initiating immunocyte. Everything indicates that a high proportion of newly formed small lymphocytes pass rapidly into the circulation. Certainly few of those present around the germinal centre are derivatives of it.

A proportion of lymphocytes undergoing mitosis can be seen in regions of the lymph node other than the germinal centres, and the relative contribution made by germinal centres to new cell production in the node is not clear. If one accepts the demonstration that medium lymphocytes synthesizing DNA are present in the circulation, it seems likely that some of these have been produced in germinal centres and also that on lodgment in a lymph follicle they may continue to divide for a generation or two. It is not impossible, therefore, that outside the thymus all production of small lymphocytes takes place in germinal centres. One senses, however, a growing opinion that lymphocytes associated with delayed hypersensitivity are *not* produced in germinal centres.

The origin of the numerous plasma cells in the medullary cords is controversial. It may be still too early to discard the old view that they arise from perivascular reticulum cells, but the whole present trend is to regard them as derivatives by direct descent from activated immunocytes. Our own experience in examining lymph nodes of mice and rats seems to be consistent with the view that at least a substantial proportion of plasmablasts arise in germinal centres and move through the paracortical region to the medullary cords. During this process, proliferation and maturation occur. The possibility that stimulated immunocytes in the circulation may pass through the endothelium of the capillaries or venules in medullary cords and there develop as plasma cells is by no means excluded.

There are some important aspects of plasma cell physiology still to be elucidated. One of the most important medical problems in the immunological field is the nature of agammaglobulinaemia where lymphocytes are normal and appear capable of a number of immunological functions. Plasma cells, however, do not appear in response to antigenic stimulation, antibodies are not demonstrable and only very small amounts of immunoglobulins. A rather similar picture is seen in bursectomized chickens and the best current hypothesis is probably that in both instances a hormonal factor is missing that is needed to allow the initiation by an activated lymphocyte of a plasma cell clone. What evidence there is points to the hormone being derived from associations of lymphoid cells with epithelium of entodermal origin.

The other important problem concerns the regions in which plasmablasts multiply and mature plasma cells accumulate. In the normal animal, plasma cells are conspicuous in the medulla of lymph nodes and in the red pulp of the spleen where most are found immediately adjacent to Malpighian bodies. In pathological situations (autoimmune disease) they are characteristically found at the periphery of lymphoid cell accumulations. In lupoid hepatitis in man they may outline the periphery of the liver lobules. All these findings suggest that plasma cells develop and function preferentially where there is an adequate supply of oxygen and nutrients via the blood. The requirements for lymphocytic multiplication in germinal centres, thymic cortex or fortuitous accumulations seem to be less critical.

MOVEMENT OF LYMPHOCYTES

Every cubic millimetre of normal mammalian blood contains a few thousand lymphocytes, mainly small lymphocytes, and this number remains approximately constant. Appropriate studies with labelled cells, however, indicate an average stay of only a few hours in the circulation. The population is being constantly changed and one of the major problems in cell dynamics for the future is the means by which homeostatic control of the numbers of circulating lymphocytes and other leucocytes is mediated. A closely related problem may well be the homeostasis of immunoglobulin levels in the plasma. Both must be postulated as background conditions in considering other aspects of the population dynamics of immunocytes.

In discussing the population dynamics of lymphocytes it is first necessary to repeat what has already been said about the heterogeneity of small lymphocytes. Everything points to the small lymphocyte as the common morphological form of a cell that is functionally inactive but has potentialities of function that may be needed elsewhere in the body. From bone-marrow one can obtain populations of small lymphocytes capable of 'rescuing' lethally irradiated mice. Small lymphocytes from thoracic duct lymph are inert in this respect. In any discussion of the immunological function of small lymphocytes it must be understood that all statements made should be construed as referring to 'a significant proportion of the cell population under study', not to morphological small lymphocytes as a whole, or even to what may often be a majority of the cells in the experimental population.

It is now certain that many small lymphocytes are immunologically competent in the sense that they can be shown to react specifically with antigens and/or contain demonstrable immunoglobulin in or associated with cytoplasm. On the now almost axiomatic assumption that many different functional or potentially functional types are included under the morphological guise of the small lymphocyte, it becomes necessary to stress that any discussion of any particular category of these cells must consist rather largely of hypotheses designed to offer indirect experimental approaches for their verification or disproof. With the general acceptance of a clonal selection approach as background one such hypothesis is as follows.

Small numbers of viable small lymphocytes leave the thymus and settle for longer or shorter periods in lymph follicles or elsewhere in lymphoid tissues. These are differentiated immunocytes in the sense that contact with a certain antigenic determinant can be recognized by its capacity to initiate functional changes of one sort or another in the cell. In view of the capacity for nonspecific stimuli like phytohaemagglutinin to induce mitosis in lymphocytes, we can probably assume with reasonable certainty that there are also generalized physiological stimuli other than antigen which can stimulate activity of more or less equivalent character. The characteristic feature of the response to an *antigenic* stimulus capable of inducing antibody production is the appearance of germinal centres and plasma cell accumulation in the lymph nodes draining the area involved.

The situation can be represented by the entry of antigen A via the afferent lymphatics to a lymph node where the cortical areas contain, amongst thousands of other types of lymphocytes, a few representatives of clones carrying receptors (or fixed antibody) a, which can unite with antigenic determinant A. Contact of such a cell with A may be either direct or by cell-to-cell contact with a dendritic macrophage which has taken up antigen A. The result will depend on many factors of which the concentration encountered of the antigen and the local internal environment where the stimulated cell lodges may be the most important. The *significant* response may well be one in which the primary immunocyte takes on the character of a large pyroninophilic cell, synthesizes small amounts of Ig M-type antibody and replicates to produce eventually a clone of small lymphocytes, perhaps in the process giving rise to a germinal centre. The result will be the development of a clone of 'committed' immunocytes which will be rapidly distributed to all lymphoid accumulations. These committed immunocytes are probably those which can be implicated in the following phenomena:

(*a*) They carry small amounts of Ig M in the cytoplasm.

(*b*) On stimulation by antigen they liberate M-type antibody and undergo mitosis.

(*c*) In suitable internal environments some of the descendants follow the plasma cell sequence, synthesizing and liberating first M-type and later G-type antibody.

(*d*) Other descendants take the form of small lymphocytes—memory cells—which persist as carriers of immunological memory.

In general the more intense the antigenic stimulus the larger the population of specific immunocytes that will develop.

In some such fashion the overall population of lymphocytes in the body will come to be made up of an immense variety of clones, with the number of representatives of each being a rough measure of the frequency and intensity of exposure to the antigen concerned.

Large numbers of lymphocytes are present in normal tissues other than lymphoid tissues, and there are accumulations in regions subject to any of a wide variety of subacute or chronic pathological processes. It is probable that lymphocytes pass more readily through the postcapillary venules of lymphoid tissues than through any other type of vascular endothelium, but the total of lymphocytes wandering through the general tissues of the body must be very large. This holds especially for the submucosal tissues of the intestinal tract.

On almost any conceivable formulation of the life history of the lymphocyte only a very small proportion of small lymphocytes will give rise to descendant clones. The vast majority are end-cells and their eventual fate requires discussion.

One of the corollaries of the concept that the body's lymphocyte population maintains a vast number of clones with differing immune patterns, from which a relatively small number of individual cells are 'chosen' by antigen for selective proliferation, is that large random populations could, if necessary, be sacrificed to provide building blocks for the synthesis of nucleic acid and protein by the proliferating clones. It has already been suggested that this may take place on a large scale in the thymus. The small lymphocyte is notoriously the most vulnerable cell of the body to the destructive action of X-irradiation, corticosteroids and cytotoxic drugs. Everything points to this vulnerability as having an important evolutionary role. In clonal selection theory it is important that a cell capable of reacting with an antigen should under certain circumstances be susceptible to destruction by contact with that antigen. This is the basis of tolerance and immune unresponsiveness. It is equally likely and reasonable that when active immunologically stimulated proliferation of immunocytes is taking place in the body, many other lymphocytes are being broken down to return their components to the metabolic pool. It is universal to find pyknotic fragments of lymphocytic nuclei wherever lymphocytic proliferation is taking place. The evidence in regard to the disintegration of lymphocytes *in vivo* is still fragmentary and no quantitative data are available. Until methods to obtain the facts have been worked out it will be impossible to estimate the relative proportions of lymphocytes which (*a*) give rise to descendant cells, (*b*) are disintegrated *in vivo* or (*c*) are released into the external environment on mucous membranes or in secretions. There is no doubt that large numbers of lymphocytes are shed into the alimentary canal.

SUMMARY

The picture of the lymphocyte and lymphatic tissue that has emerged with the application of modern methods is very different from what it was only a decade ago. It is an altogether more dynamic concept and presents some lessons that are still incompletely learnt. It is evident that histologists have always been inclined to interpret appearances in tissues as being derived from other cells which are either present or have been present in the same tissue. This holds to a less extent but still significantly for autoradiographic and other methods of 'functional' histology.

It seems now that we must picture all accumulations of small lymphocytes as transitory populations always changing in two important respects. Within the tissue itself the constituent lymphocytes are presumably moving in random fashion and constantly changing their situation both in relation to other lymphocytes and to the cells more firmly attached to the collagen and reticulin fibrils that give form to the structure. Within that framework the lymphocytes can be pictured almost as the proverbial 'bag of worms'. The actual cells making up the local population are also changing at a rate which has been estimated for the popliteal lymph node of the sheep as corresponding to a complete turnover every seventy hours. Cells are constantly leaving by the afferent lymph vessels while others are entering from the blood. As far as lymphocytes are concerned, the whole lymphoid tissues of the body, with the important exception of the thymus, form a single compartment with essentially random, but also randomly restricted, movement throughout the whole system.

Summary

Although cells of the lymphocytic series are highly mobile, the cells which are associated with them are much less so. The individuality of a lymph node is preserved by the cells which are not lymphocytes, and everything points to the importance of some of these cells in taking up and retaining antigen. This is a point to be discussed in more detail in relation to the cellular aspects of antibody production but it is essential to an understanding of the circulation of the immunocytes.

If antigenic molecules are held by cells fixed to the sponge-like matrix of the peripheral lymphoid organs, the combination of short-range mobility and progressive replacement from elsewhere seems ideally suited to ensure that every lymphocyte that can react with an antigenic determinant which has entered the body will have an opportunity to do so.

5 The nature of antibody

As soon as methods for the demonstration and titration of antibodies had been established, efforts were begun to identify chemically the constituent of serum responsible. It was evident that antibody had the general characteristics of protein and that it was predominantly present in the globulin fractions as defined by contemporary methods of salt precipitation. By the 1930s it was established that antibody was globulin, resembling any other serum globulin in its chemical and physical characteristics except for a specific capacity to combine with the corresponding antigen.

The modern phase of immunochemistry can be dated from Tiselius's work on the electrophoresis of serum proteins by which he defined α-, β- and γ-globulins. Separation of these fractions indicated that nearly all antibody was contained in the most slowly moving fraction, the γ-globulin. For many years γ-globulin was generally used as the appropriate chemical designation for antibody, although from an early stage it was well known that, while standard rabbit antibodies had a molecular weight around 160,000, the intensively studied equine antibodies to pneumococcal polysaccharide antigens were approximately 10^6 mol. wt.

THE IMMUNOGLOBULINS

With the progressive development of more refined chemical, physical and immunological methods for studying soluble proteins, it has become clear that there are several types of globulin which can carry the specific reactivity of antibodies. It is now conventional to refer to these as immunoglobulins, of which the three types commonly recognized in mammalian (including human) sera are Ig G, Ig M and Ig A.

It is certain that these are not the only physical types of immunoglobulin even in healthy animals. There are already indications that in mice and guinea-pigs there are two varieties of G, and a fourth type, D, has been described in man. Another type, Ig E, which may be pathological, has been recently demarcated. Immunoglobulins are usually studied in the form of antibodies obtained from normal individuals, but a great deal of information has also been obtained from immunoglobulins produced in pathological excess by patients with multiple myelomatosis and some related conditions. Rightly or wrongly, many deductions about the nature of antibody have been based on findings with such myeloma proteins and from this angle they will need to be discussed at some length in this chapter.

TABLE 2. *Human immunoglobulins and related abnormal proteins*

Normal (Concentration, mg/ml)	Pathological	Molecular weight
Ig G 0·8–1·5	Ig G (My. pr.)	150,000
Ig A 0·06–0·2	Ig A (My. pr.)	150,000 and multiples
Ig M 0·04–0·12	Ig M (My. pr.)	900,000 ±
Ig D trace	Ig D (My. pr.)	150,000 ±
Light chain (K or L)	Bence Jones protein	22,000
Heavy chain (Ig G)	—	50,000

My. pr. = Myeloma protein.

The primary differences between immunoglobulins by which the three types are defined are as follows:

(*a*) Molecular weight around 160,000 for G and A, and around 1 million for M, with corresponding sedimentation coefficients of 7 (6·6)S and 19S. Ig A is prone to aggregation and it is common to find a fraction with a sedimentation coefficient S_{9-11} which may represent a dimer.

(*b*) Specific *antigenic* characters differentiating A, G and M which allow their recognition either by gel-diffusion reactions in agar or by immunofluorescence methods.

(*c*) A characteristic distribution of electrophoretic mobility within each molecular type giving easily recognized lines in the patterns obtained by immunoelectrophoresis.

The biological characteristics of the three types of antibody will need to be discussed at length in relation to many facets of immunology, but for preliminary orientation the differences may be summarized as follows.

Antibodies of Ig M structure are the first to appear on immunization with almost all types of antigen and make up most 'normal' antibodies. In the later stages the titre of M antibodies is reduced and their place taken by antibodies of G type. When bacterial polysaccharides are used as antigen, M-type antibodies persist and their normal replacement by type G is not easily demonstrable. This is probably mainly due to the relative ineffectiveness of Ig G antibodies as compared with Ig M in producing some of the commonly used antigen–antibody reactions. Where direct comparison is possible, M antibodies attach more firmly to antigenic particles and against red cells as antigens are, molecule for molecule, many times more effective as haemolysins.

The classical antibody produced by deliberate immunization with protein antigens is of G type and almost all the refined chemical work to be mentioned later has been done with such antibodies. It is probable that biologically speaking they are less important than M and A types. G antibody is less readily attached to tissue cells than A and readily passes the human placenta into the foetus.

Ig A-type antibodies are found in all mammals and one subclass of these probably represents the antibody or reagin found in hay fever patients. The two important biological characters of Ig A antibodies are the ease with which they attach to body cells and, perhaps closely related to this, their special function of being concentrated in and secreted by glandular epithelium (in mammary, parotid and probably other glands).

Secondary differences at the chemical level include the failure of A antibodies to precipitate with antigen, perhaps, as suggested by Karush, because their two combining sites are too close together to allow lattice formation with antigen. M immunoglobulins contain a much higher content, 12·2 per cent of carbohydrate, than A with 10·5 per cent, or G with 2·8 per cent. It is an important point of similarity that all antibodies of M, G and A types may have in common the antigenic characters based on 'light' chains and the specific character of the combining site.

THE HETEROGENEITY OF ANTIBODIES

Even within each of the immunoglobulins, antibodies are highly heterogeneous and with every refinement of physical, chemical and immunological technique for separating and characterizing soluble proteins the number of subpopulations of antibody molecules that can be separated increases. To anyone interested in a clonal approach to immunology this is the most important quality of antibody. Its significance has been greatly increased as a result of studies on myeloma proteins obtained from patients with multiple myelomatosis. Essentially this is a conditioned malignancy of relatively highly differentiated plasma cells. By what is perhaps in some sense a circular chain of reasoning, most of these myeloma proteins are believed to arise by the proliferation of a single mutant cell to form a uniform clone of thousands of millions of cells. Hundreds of myeloma proteins of human origin and considerable numbers of similar proteins from plasmacytomas of mice have now been studied in detail. The results can be simply, but I believe legitimately, summarized by saying that each myeloma protein provides an example of what a single antibody-producing cell can produce. Normal serum contains immunoglobulins in a heterogeneous mixture produced by thousands or millions of distinguishable clones of globulin-producing cells.

The great experimental advantage of myeloma proteins is the ease with which they can be isolated and purified from a patient's serum. Each patient provides an individual protein. A few are quite anomalous but 90 per cent of them can be identified as physically and antigenically typical A, G or M immunoglobulins. Within each Ig group, however, are individual differences and the results suggest strongly that *any* type of immature plasma cell can undergo this particular type of inheritable change. In addition there are anomalous conditions which produce proteins of the same general quality but not equivalent to any of the normal forms. These include the 'heavy chain' proteins and the Bence Jones proteins, both of which may be present as an abnormal component of the blood plasma. In addition, a large proportion of typical myeloma patients excrete large amounts of Bence Jones protein in the urine. This is now known to be composed of the light chains characteristic of the complete myeloma protein and, as such, having the same antigenic quality and amino acid composition. Urinary Bence Jones protein is therefore a convenient source of material for chemical studies of light chain.

The monoclonal character of a typical myeloma protein is evidenced by its uniformity. Instead of a broad zone on electrophoresis there is a single sharp spike; antigenically it reacts only with one of specific A, G, M or D antisera and, unlike any purified normal immunoglobulin, only one of the two alternative κ or λ antigens of the light chains is represented. While these chapters were being written it was reported that at least three myeloma proteins (Ig G) had a definite antibody specificity and were therefore true monoclonal antibodies with a specific combining site. This should lead to an important set of new advances. Already on the basis of the evidence from myeloma proteins it can be confidently assumed that any given clone of immunocytes will produce *physically* and *antigenically* uniform populations of antibody molecules. Most immunologists will probably soon be driven to agree that the immune pattern of all *antibody* produced by the clone will also be homogeneous.

Recognition of the heterogeneity of immune pattern in an antiserum produced against a single (but always complex) antigen goes back to the early days of bacterial serology. If a rabbit was immunized against bacterium B, an antiserum was produced which not only agglutinated B but also a wide range of more or less closely related cultures, A and C for example. If, now, the antiserum was repeatedly treated with A bacteria to remove all antibody capable of reacting with A, it would still react relatively strongly with B and probably with C. After washing the A bacteria, antibody might be eluted from them by a suitable technique. In such negative and positive manipulations it was possible to fractionate the antiserum into different subpopulations of antibody molecules to almost any degree of elaboration. Even when a single artificial hapten was used as antigenic determinant, cross-testing with haptens of related molecular structure revealed antibody molecules with different degrees of avidity for the homologous antigenic determinant and of cross-reactivity with related antigens.

A few myeloma proteins of Ig M type react as rheumatoid factors, i.e. as if they were antibodies against partially denatured γ-globulin. There are many difficulties in interpreting the meaning of this result and, at the experimental level, rheumatoid factor is an unsatisfactory type of antibody for detailed study. Nevertheless, the existence of one type of myeloma protein with antibody character resulted in a concerted effort to detect a myeloma protein that would react with a chemically definable antigenic determinant. Now that several of these have been found, it will be of immense interest to determine the range of cross-reactivity of a 'pure' antibody, something that has not yet been possible and which is vital for the understanding of many phenomena relevant to the nature and origin of immune pattern.

THE CHEMICAL STRUCTURE OF IMMUNOGLOBULIN G

The Porter diagram

In view of the heterogeneity of antibodies it has become necessary to concentrate chemical studies on examples of antibody which can be obtained in considerable amount and be readily purified. Most work has been done on G-type antibodies prepared in rabbits with artificial antigens carrying a suitable haptenic group as antigenic determinant. In man, chemical work has tended to be concentrated on G myeloma proteins or Ig G from normal individuals studied without regard to specific immune pattern, but there have been some important studies on specific antibodies.

In general, the approach has been to dissociate the immunoglobulin molecule into relatively large polypeptide chains and to ascertain the distribution on such fractions of the various functional qualities of antibody or immunoglobulin. It is now accepted that the 'Porter diagram', shown in slightly modified form in fig. 5, is a satisfactory schema for representing the structure of human or rabbit Ig G as deduced from such studies. The first methods to be used involved the use of proteolytic enzymes. In a commercial process developed in 1936 the fragment Fc was split off by pepsin leaving an active complex of two light chains and the Fd portions of the heavy chains. The modern approach was opened by Porter's use of papain with cysteine which produced essentially two fragments from each molecule, one containing a single antibody site and named Fab, and the other, the Fc fragment, which is part of the heavy chain. These procedures of limited proteolytic enzyme action have been supplemented by the development of methods to reduce S–S bonds by cysteine or mercaptoethanol and separate the chains by suitable manipulations while they were maintained under conditions preventing reunion.

The Porter diagram indicates that Ig G is built up of four polypeptide chains, two light of mol. wt 20,000 ± and two heavy of mol. wt 50,000 ±, united by disulphide bonds. There is a reasonable likelihood that the heavy chain may be composed of a large segment (Fc) and a smaller one (Fd) carrying the piece which plays the major part in forming the specific combining site. There is a real possibility that both the light and heavy chains are made up of more than one genetically distinct polypeptide chain. For the present, however, there is no decisive evidence that more than two genetic loci for light and heavy chains respectively are concerned. In addition, a relatively small oligosaccharide molecule is attached to an aspartic acid residue in the heavy chain (Fc segment). The carbohydrate contains 3 galactose, 5 mannose, 2 fucose, 10 acetylglucosamine and 1 sialic acid units.

Antigenic qualities

If we confine ourselves for the time being to human immunoglobulins, the first functional quality to be discussed is the distribution of antigenic determinants. These can be studied by producing antibodies against purified immunoglobulins or fractions thereof, either in a distant species such as the rabbit, or in the more closely related rhesus monkey. Even more illuminating results can be obtained by making use of the antibodies found under pathological conditions in humans which react against one or other determinant of their own immunoglobulins; the 'rheumatoid factors' represent the most important source.

Such serological studies of human immunoglobulins, in the first instance with rabbit antisera, nowadays almost always made against a single myeloma protein or its fractions, have shown that:

(*a*) The heavy chains characteristic of immunoglobulins A, G and M are serologically distinct.

(*b*) Light chains of Ig G can be divided into two serologically distinct types, K and L.

(c) A and M immunoglobulins also have the same K and L types of light chain.

(d) All human beings have both K and L light chains which are present in a ratio of $\pm 2\text{K}:1\text{L}$.

(e) A single plasma cell produces K or L but not both, while nearly all myeloma proteins are either wholly L-type or wholly K-type.

(f) The specificity of the combining site (that is, the immune pattern of the antibody) is uninfluenced by these antigenic characters. Any standard human antiserum will show antibody activity in immunoglobulins A, G and M of both K and L types.

(g) Using antisera made in rhesus monkeys, at least four subgroups can be recognized in the heavy chains from Ig G.

The findings from human antisera are complex and involve two systems. The Gm antigens (a+), (b+), (f+) are found in various combinations in individuals, (a+b+f+) being common and (a−b−) combinations being never seen. Again, myeloma proteins have only one antigen or none and studies of plasma cells by fluorescent technique show Gm(a+) or Gm(b+), but never both. The Gm determinants are located on the heavy chain, (a+) and (b+) on the Fc fragment, (f+) apparently close to the disulphide bond holding light and heavy chains together.

The Inv antigens are on the light chains. Inv a is found on K myeloma chains but never on L, while Inv b may be on both. Myelomas Inv(a−b−) are found, although normal globulin of this character is not known to occur. These points are important in relation to phenotypic restriction—an important topic in chapter 6.

Electrophoretic qualities

The immunoglobulins A, G and M are most clearly delineated by the use of Grabar's technique of immunoelectrophoresis. Ig G shows a particularly long arc which in itself is a clear indication of the heterogeneity of net charge within the population. More detailed information can be gained by using one of the modifications of starch-gel electrophoresis. When light chain molecules are separated from normal Ig G and examined by this method, a complex pattern of bands emerges which appears to indicate that ten levels of net positive or negative charge are possible for any mammalian species, the distribution in any given species being concentrated over three to five adjacent levels. Heavy chain shows a broader band with no sign that it could be resolved into a series of separate lines.

The regularity of the spacing of the light chains indicates that with the relatively small chains of a constant molecular weight around 20,000, each step represents one unit difference of net electric charge, the replacement of a neutral by a basic amino acid or vice versa. It indicates equally that the light chains present in an individual serum have a high degree of heterogeneity in addition to Inv a and b, and K or L characters.

This heterogeneity is not seen in myeloma proteins. Each shows a single heavy band at a position corresponding to one of the components of the light chain population in normal immunoglobulin. In most preparations there is a weak adjacent band which may represent an artefact arising in the course of preparation, or evidence of a secondary mutation within the plasmacytoma cell clone.

Amino acid sequences of light chains

It has become almost an article of faith with immunologists that the differences between the myeloma proteins of two individuals are formally equivalent to the differences between the antibodies produced by distinct clones of immunocytes in the same individual. This may be wrong: myeloma proteins have not yet all been shown to carry a specific combining site. In several places in this book the question is raised of the possibility of the combining site being a distinct peptide unit with its own genetic determination. However unlikely this is it has not been excluded, and it could be that some myeloma proteins differ from antibodies in failing to possess any such unit. I believe, however, that more than one myeloma immunoglobulin has already been shown to have a typical combining site and it is on this assumption that the argument will be continued.

The light chains of a human immunoglobulin have a molecular weight of $\pm 22{,}000$, corresponding to 214 amino acid residues. Perhaps the most interesting biological discovery of the last year

The chemical structure of immunoglobulin G

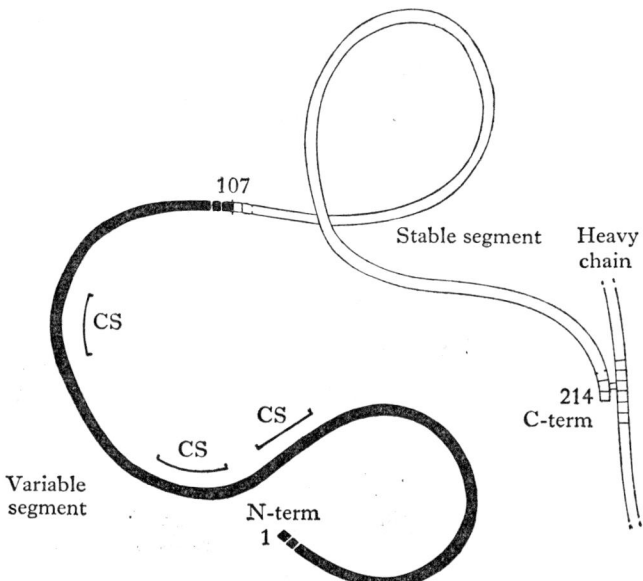

Fig. 17. The light chain of a human immunoglobulin drawn approximately to scale to show the 'variable' and 'stable' segments and the attachment to heavy chain. CS = approximate size of a combining site.

```
1                                                                         25
Asp Ile Glu Met Thr Glu Ser Pro Ser Ser Leu Ser Ala Ser Val Gly Asp Arg Val Thr Ile Thr Gly Gys Glu Ala
Glu     Val Leu                 Thr         Leu         Pro         Glu             Ala Ser Leu Ser          Arg Ser
                                Thr         Pro Val     Leu                         Ile Ala
                                Asp
                                Leu
                                Gly
```

Fig. 18. The first 25 amino acid residues in human K light chains to show variant and invariant positions. From Smithies's (1967) data.

White = invariant; hatched = showing one of two alternate amino acids; dotted = with one change in addition to any showing the alternate choice; black = hyper-variable. 1st row—full amino acid sequence; 2nd row—alternates; 3rd row—irregular changes.

or two has concerned the amino acid sequences of some selected K-type light chains from myeloma proteins. A comparison of three type K Bence Jones proteins shows that the chain is divided into two equal parts in which amino acid residues 1–107, numbered from the N terminal end, show great variation from one protein to the other, while the C terminal half, 108–214, is common to all three except for some single amino acid replacements of which the most interesting is associated with the change in no. 191 from leucine to valine. This corresponds to change in serological character from Inv a to Inv b.

In the N terminal end there are numerous differences but the length of the variable segment is 107 residues in all and there are a number of common features. The commonest type of difference is replacement of a single amino acid by another but there are short sequences of quite different character. To the present, no regularity in or convincing interpretation of the changes from one protein to another has been recognized. The differences suggest that, subject to the maintenance of certain invariant features of which one is the length of the segment, a completely random set of changes in the genome has been laid down at some phase and stabilized during the whole period of active proliferation. What bearing this may have on the nature and specificity of the combining site can be deferred to the next chapter.

Although the definitive work has been done on human material, workers with mouse myeloma and rabbit antibodies have obtained presumptive evidence that this division of the light chains into variable and constant halves holds also in these species. There is already a strong indication that the variable half may have an important role in relation to the combining site.

The combining site

Physico-chemical studies have established the existence on the classical Ig G antibody of two identical and symmetrical combining sites to which the corresponding antigenic determinant can attach. From the ease with which a combining site can be blocked by relatively small hapten molecules it is deduced that the specific area involved is quite small, perhaps involving no more than ten to twenty amino acid residues. It is certain that the site is wholly a configuration of amino acid residues with a very strong likelihood that residues on both light and heavy chains are concerned.

The bivalence of Ig G antibody has been fully established by chemical methods (equilibrium dialysis and fluorescence quenching), by the immunological properties of fragments and reconstituted preparations, and directly by electron microscopy. The evidence that both combining sites on a given Ig G antibody molecule are identical is incomplete since all natural antibodies are heterogeneous. Most immunologists accept the likelihood that there is at least a very close approach to symmetry of the two sites. There is no evidence of the existence of hetero-ligating antibody with two different specificities although by appropriate recombination of half-molecules from different sources it can be shown that such hybrid molecules can be readily recognized. Fractionation of an anti-dextran by specific adsorptions gave results which on the whole were in accord with uniformity of the two combining sites but did not exclude a certain degree of disparity. It seems to be legitimate, until experimental evidence to the contrary is put on record, to accept the symmetrical character of the Ig G antibody and to expect no difference in the specificity and avidity of the two combining sites.

The size of the combining site has been studied in detail by Kabat and collaborators for human antibodies against the simple polysaccharide, dextran. It is possible to prepare a complete series of homologous oligosaccharides in the form of chains of glucose units from isomaltose (2) up to a 7-unit chain. These have a measurable blocking power in inhibiting precipitation of dextran which at first increases with increasing size. With most human antisera there was no improvement in inhibition beyond the hexasaccharide. This is therefore considered to have a configuration approximately complementary to that of the combining site and of about the same size. There is a widespread convention to think of the combining site as having the quality of a cavity into which the antigenic determinant fits, but I do not know of any documented discussion of the point. One can hardly doubt, however, that there is some special quality which allows only two small areas on a large protein molecule to serve as combining sites. The only hint available is that tyrosine appears to be present consistently in the combining site, perhaps indicating that two tyrosine residues in some special configuration is the important feature.

Opinion has varied from time to time as to the relative importance of heavy and light chains in their contribution to the specificity of the combining site. Separated chains are never as active as the original or the reconstituted molecule but in most experiments the heavy chain has been more active than the light one.

A more direct approach has been to use reagents which can modify the site by combining with certain amino acids. By using the reagent on antibody in which the combining site is protected by attachment of specific hapten and comparing this with the effect on unprotected antibody, an indication of the importance of a particular amino acid can be gained. Iodination, for instance, gives results indicating that tyrosine is significantly involved in most combining sites but to a much more important extent in some antibodies than in others. A modification of this experiment, in which the two isotopes ^{131}I and ^{125}I are used, allows a recognition of the peptides concerned in the combining site in the sense of being protected from iodination in the presence of hapten. The results obtained by Pressman's group suggest that the light chain carries the significant tyrosine residues and by implication plays the greater part in forming the combining site.

An elaboration of the same general approach due to Doolittle and Singer is to use the technique of affinity labelling. In this the hapten, dinitrophenyl, is presented to the antibody in the form of a compound, *m*-nitrobenzene-diazonium-fluoborate, which forms azo-links with tyrosine residues in the combining sites. If the reagent is suitably labelled with tritium, the tyrosine residue concerned can be recognized in peptide maps of the various fragments of the antibody. In this way it was shown that the tyrosine was present in both light and heavy chains. The peptide involved has an average size of 25 ± units and a generally hydrophobic character. It is heterogeneous and in all these respects there is a striking similarity between the peptides from heavy and light chains. The heterogeneity points very strongly to the 'variable' segments of both heavy and light chains being involved.

One cannot resist trying to draw the modern findings on the fine structure of Ig G antibody into a speculative statement based on a suggestion I made at Canberra in December 1964. This is that there is a 'specific chain' involved directly in the structure of the combining site and that this chain appears four times in the immunoglobulin molecule as a portion of the Fd segment of the heavy chains and the variable segment of the light chains. On this view the combining site is made up of two adjacent identical sequences, one on the heavy chain, the other on the light, and the special quality of the combining site may well be due to this duplication of a potential adsorbing pattern. This hypothesis has the important advantage of requiring only one section of the genome to be subject to the 'randomization' process responsible for the heterogeneity needed to give an adequate number of immune patterns.

If it is established that the variable portions of light and heavy chains are quite different, as Putnam believes is the case, a more cumbersome picture must be accepted. One would have to assume that the interaction of two genetically distinct variable chains would result in certain regions being held together by appropriate short-range forces to produce a duplex in which the two sets of amino acid residues have only a general resemblance to each other. This is still needed to account for the Singer–Doolittle results. Provided the interchain forces are definite and regular enough to ensure that the product of all cells of the clone has the same combining site structure, no serious change in the argument is necessary. This modification does, however, make the emergence of the final pattern of the combining site an even more random process than we have envisaged.

Versatility of the combining site

At this point it may be worth while to examine briefly the implications of the almost universally adopted picture of a small combining site made up of a few, perhaps twenty, amino acid residues. It is easy enough to say that a sequence of even ten amino acids can be arranged in 20^{10} or 10^{13} different ways, but this is meaningless without some indication of the evolutionary background by which adsorptive specificity arose. This involves a brief comment on the nature of enzyme action.

The extraordinary number and range of activity of the enzymes which can be extracted and isolated from tissues and micro-organisms must mean that there are as many molecular groupings which can serve as substrates for enzyme action or competitive inhibitors as there are potential antigenic determinants. All enzymes are wholly or predominantly protein and it is becoming clear that the active site is often (or always) a relatively short segment of polypeptide. In egg-white lysozyme, for instance, the site of attachment of competitive inhibitors has been accurately located. Generally, the active site seems likely to be considerably smaller than the combining site of an antibody.

It is clear that by suitable disposition of amino acids in sequence, active sites can be produced which are capable not only of allowing specific adsorption of almost any conceivable biological substrate but also, by joint action of the sequence, able to facilitate the molecular and electronic rearrangements that take place in the substrate. Enzymes are more fundamental than antibodies and no one would dispute that proteins have evolved primarily because of their unique suitability as biological catalysts. The same requirement has been presumably responsible for the 'choice' by evolutionary processes of the standard twenty amino acids. The first necessity for enzymic action is a capacity for specific adsorption, and protein has unique potentialities in this respect. Clearly, the same quality has been exploited in the evolution of specific immune pattern.

Qualities of the Fc segment

The Fc fragment of the Ig G heavy chain is of standard structure except for the changes corresponding to the Gm allotypes (in man). Its function seems to be to attach antibody to cells and to determine the passage of Ig G antibody through cellular membranes such as the foetal rabbit yolk-sac or the intestinal wall of newborn rats or mice. There is good evidence that the fixation of antibody which confers passive anaphylactic sensitization to reactive tissues is via some portion of the Fc fragment. Since in both these functions homologous antibody is significantly more effective than heterologous, it is necessary to postulate some specific relationship between an animal's immunoglobulins and something which can be regarded as a receptor on a wide variety of cells.

In seeking a general biological significance for this function one naturally looks at the basic function of immunoglobulins to serve as opsonins. It is probably significant that γ-globulin is the only common autologous protein that is readily taken up by macrophages, including the dendritic phagocytic cells of lymph follicles. The suggestion would be that the structure of some part of the Fc region is adapted to unite to some surface component common to a variety of body cells including macrophages and a variety of epithelial and connective tissue cells. It is highly probable that cytophilic antibody represents a fraction of immunoglobulin in which the Fc component is more accessible than normal. Since the carbohydrate unit of Ig G is associated with Fc, the possibility must be kept in mind that the carbohydrate may be wholly or partly responsible for this type of union.

There is also evidence that the catabolism of Ig G, including the three 7S immunoglobulins $\gamma 1$, $\gamma 2a$ and $\gamma 2b$ in mice, is regulated by the concentration of these immunoglobulins in the plasma and that the responsible component is the Fc fragment. Brambell (1966) has offered a general hypothesis that all these functions depend on the uptake of Ig G molecules by pinocytosis with destruction of any proteins not capable of making specific union with receptors in the wall of the phagolysosome. The hypothesis has an *ad hoc* quality since it is difficult to see how union of a protein determinant to a vacuole wall receptor could protect the protein against a high concentration of protease in the vacuole or how it is subsequently released into the plasma or some other fluid.

Recapitulation of the structure of G-type antibody

Obviously the more we know about the chemical structure of antibody the better position we are in to understand the process of its production. It is the basic contention of this book that at every stage in the development of science there is need to choose the current interpretation which allows the clearest understanding and the best practical use of the facts as they have been determined. If that interpretation can be put in the form of a hypothesis which can, in principle, be disproved by experimental approaches, it will also help to speed further advance in understanding.

In the case of G-type antibody the picture that emerges in 1967 is as follows.

The antibody molecule is a complex structure of polypeptide chains based on the combination of two light and two heavy chains.

The genetic control of the various functionally distinct sections is still a matter for speculation and will remain so until the structure of the combining site and its relation to the light and heavy chains is clarified. We are almost compelled to accept as significant the resemblance in the length and location of cysteine residues between the variable and stable segments of the light chain. There is also the hypothesis, much less adequately based, that a segment of the heavy chain has a variable structure equivalent to that of the variable half of the light chain. It would simplify the situation, and be in general concordance with such processes as the evolution of the haemoglobins, to consider the immunoglobulin molecule as having evolved by the duplication and independent mutation of a single primitive cistron coding for 100–110 amino acids. The light chain would correspond to two and the heavy chain to four of the basic units and there is nothing to indicate how many of these duplicated and independently modified cistrons there are in the genome.

The structure of the oligosaccharide must have a complex set of genetic determinants but appears at present not to be directly relevant to the problem of immune specificity.

The molecule is symmetrical. Both combining sites have the same specificity and avidity, both light chains are of the same antigenic character, and what evidence there is suggests that the two heavy chains must also be identical. This symmetry has the implication that, having regard to the diploid character of somatic cells and the several loci concerned, *a high degree of phenotypic restriction must be operative*. If n is the number of loci concerned and if there were no necessity for molecular symmetry, there should be 2^n patterns of globulin producible by any diploid cell instead of the one symmetrical pattern which is observed.

The combining site is produced by the juxtaposition of portions of the 'variable' segments attached to the light and heavy chains. The precise character of the site will depend mainly on the amino acid sequence of the variable chains but will also be influenced by factors such as the net charge on the whole light chains and the accuracy with which the two variable chains are mutually arranged. Here, a certain degree of accident may be involved, but otherwise it appears that in a given cell or clone all the details of the antibody globulin produced are genetically determined and the principle of phenotypic restriction operates. For any change to occur, an appropriate *genetic* change must first take place either by somatic mutation or by some alternative process with a similar overall result.

The classical instructive theory of antibody production has few points of contact with what interests us today, but it should not be dismissed without adequate reason. Broadly, it assumes that physically similar antibodies of different specificity differ only according to their secondary and tertiary folding and the subsequent formation of intramolecular disulphide and hydrogen bonds. It should follow, therefore, that when these bonds are broken and a wholly random secondary folding induced in strong urea or guanidine solutions, it ought not to be possible to restore immune specificity. Two well-substantiated claims to have successfully restored a large fraction of specific combining power by careful return to normal environments have been published, and there appears to be a growing consensus of opinion that the final configuration taken by any protein depends far more on the linear sequence of amino acid residues in its polypeptide chain(s) than on any other factors.

In some sense the picture we have adopted is derived from the preconception of a selective approach to antibody formation. It is still remotely possible that an antigenic determinant introduced into the nucleus of a globulin-synthesizing cell might in some at present inconceivable fashion lead to the replacement of an existent segment of DNA by one producing a pattern complementary to that of the antigenic determinant to which it was exposed. Any less cumbersome alternative way of accepting an 'instructive' approach to antibody formation hardly seems possible in the present state of knowledge.

THE STRUCTURE OF A- AND M-TYPE ANTIBODIES

Far less work has been done on the structure of the other types of immunoglobulin for quite simple technical reasons. Antibodies of type A do not precipitate with antigen so that it is virtually impossible to obtain specifically purified antibody for chemical studies. In one example of antibody of this type, where conditions for study were unusually favourable and defined chemical haptens were the antigenic determinants concerned, results were interpreted as corresponding to a molecule with two combining sites close together so that the molecule could not function as a bridge holding two antigen molecules together. This is an attractive picture which may well apply to all A antibodies for, in addition to accounting for failure of precipitation, it offers a reason for the readiness with which such antibody attaches to body cells. In G antibody, attachment to complement and to body components generally is by the Fc segment of the heavy chains, and the configuration of the A molecule may leave this region of the molecule more accessible for contact with a cell surface. The much larger carbohydrate content may also be significant in this respect.

The large M-type antibodies are approximately five times the size of A or G immunoglobulins and on reduction of S–S bonds give rise to 7S components. It is reasonable therefore to think of them essentially as pentamers of molecules resembling A with a considerable addition of polysaccharide. Where direct comparison is possible, as in haemolytic reactions, M antibody is much more active than G, perhaps to be related to the greater number of combining sites which can be brought to bear on a given surface. In most discussions, M-type antibodies are referred to as 19S and are recognized in practice by the fact that simple treatment with 2-mercaptoethanol destroys their specific reactivity. The correlation between 19S sedimentation and susceptibility to inactivation by 2-mercaptoethanol holds for adult mammalian sera but not necessarily for immunoglobulins from other classes of vertebrate.

Electron micrographs of G and M antibodies have been published but not of A-type antibody. The possibility has, however, been suggested that A antibody is bivalent but with the two combining sites very close together. It is also known that larger forms can be found of A antibody with a sedimentation constant around 11 S which may be dimers or trimers. I have found it useful to picture the physical form of the three immunoglobulins as shown in fig. 19. This provides a simple way of visualizing such phenomena as lattice formation by M and G but not A-type antibodies, the much greater complement-fixing power of M, and the special capacity of A to attach to tissues. The possibility that the pentamer of A shown as M may have five rather than ten accessible combining sites has been suggested.

The problem presented by the change from M to G antibodies in the early stages of the primary response will be discussed later, but here it should be noted that when a small hapten is used the avidity of the combining sites of G and M antibody present around the times of the change is similar. Although the character of the heavy chains differs in the three types, everything suggests that the portions which give rise to the combining sites are the same in each.

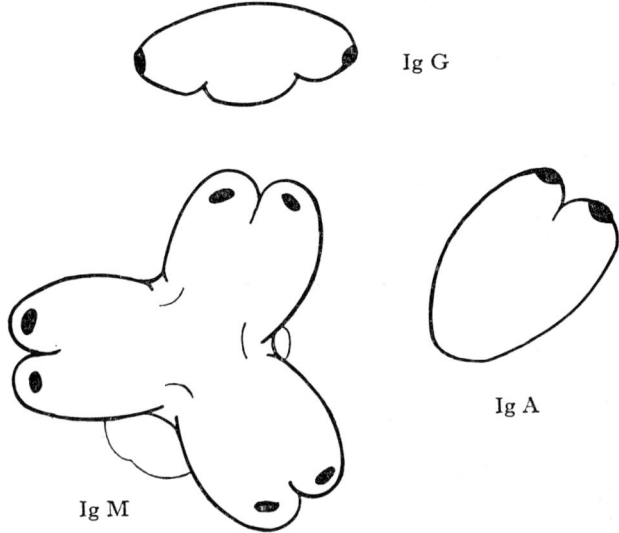

Fig. 19. Schematic illustration of the probable form of the three chief immunoglobulins.

ANTIGENIC DETERMINANTS

The picture that has been built up of antibody as a large molecule with relatively small combining sites of precise molecular structure has important implications which have led to the concept of antigenic determinant. Like so much in immunology, the gradual development of concepts of the nature of antigens and antibodies has been a matter of reciprocal or even circular interactions. Anything new learnt about antibodies allows a greater precision in understanding the essential structure of antigens, and vice versa.

With the development of Landsteiner's methods of making artificial antigens by linking a relatively large number of small organic haptens to a single protein molecule, it became evident that a small molecular configuration could be wholly responsible for immunological specificity. Further, an antibody of this sort could be wholly inhibited from precipitating the complete antigen by an adequate concentration of the soluble hapten. This technique has subsequently been extensively used for studies of cross-reactivity and serological relationships. The interaction of antibodies with haptens of small molecular weight can also be studied by immunodialysis, particularly if the hapten is coloured, contains radioisotopes, or possesses some other character which allows convenient assay of its concentration. If, on one side of a semipermeable membrane, we have a solution of antibody reactive with hapten H and, on the other, a similar solution of normal globulin, then if a solution of H is added to both sides and time for equilibration allowed, there will be a higher concentration of hapten in the compartment containing the corresponding antibody.

By the use of such techniques it has been shown that a molecule as small as a monosaccharide can significantly block a combining site but that, in some instances, the combining site can 'differentiate between' two larger molecules, e.g. an anti-dextran human antibody is more effectively blocked by an oligosaccharide of six glucose units than by one of four. In a variety of bacterial antigens, di- or trisaccharides appear to be the most important antigenic determinants. The nature of the antigenic determinants in natural proteins is unknown. In some it is necessary for disulphide links to be intact. Many synthetic polypeptides are antigenic though some, such as poly-L-lysine, are not. In some synthetic polypeptides containing three or four component L amino acids (in random mutual sequences) gel-precipitation reactions show multiple lines indicating that several different antigenic determinants occur in the molecular population that makes up a preparation of such a polypeptide. We can reasonably conclude that relatively short sequences of a peptide chain can act as antigenic determinants, but that in some or all cases secondary configurations related to folding or intramolecular bonds may be important.

It is a postulate of clonal selection theory that in the healthy

Antigenic determinants

organism significantly active antibodies are not produced against any components (potential antigenic determinants) present in accessible form in the thymus or in any other site where stem cells are differentiated to immunocytes. This should ensure that the great majority of common amino acid configurations should be unable to function as antigenic determinants under any reasonably normal conditions. The same would hold for nucleic acid components and it is probably significant that the only type of DNA readily antigenic in rabbits is phage DNA containing the base hydroxymethylcytosine, and fucosyl in place of some of the ribosyl residues.

THE FUNCTION OF A, G AND M ANTIBODIES

The functional relationships of A-, G- and M-type antibodies are still not fully understood, but it seems appropriate to conclude this chapter with a brief review of what is known in regard to function of the three types in relation to their structural differences. A certain regularity is beginning to emerge and it is worth making an attempt to define these functions.

The first antibodies to be detected when foetal or very young mammals are immunized are M immunoglobulins; so are all the common natural antibodies. When a grown animal is immunized with any standard antigen the first antibodies produced are M. With some antigens no other type develops. It is reasonable, therefore, to regard the M-type antibody (19 S) as the primary functional form. If we accept a modified Porter–Edelman structure for G antibody, in the form of an elongate flexible molecule with combining sites at each end, then the M antibody can be built up as a complex of five or six G molecules. To account for the various functional and physical characteristics of M antibody, we can picture first the folding of five G molecules into the configuration favoured by Karush's group for an equine A immunoglobulin, i.e. with the two ends carrying combining sites brought close together. This configuration may need the formation of additional intramolecular bonding and the incorporation of further oligo- or polysaccharide.

If these five primary molecules are bound into a three-dimensional configuration in which the binding forces are essentially disulphide links between the Fc regions, the product could well be identical with M antibody as we know it. Such a model is concordant with (a) the molecular weight of M antibody, (b) its susceptibility to mercaptoethanol with loss of precipitating ability, (c) the appearance of M antibody in electron micrographs, (d) the much greater effectiveness of M antibody against red cells in allowing fixation of complement and haemolysis, (e) the uniformity of the light chains from A, G and M antibodies and (f) the production of G and M antibody from the same cell. The only serious difficulty to be overcome is the clear antigenic individuality of M and G immunoglobulins and the lack of any evidence that, by dissociation of M immunoglobulin, fractions with the antigenic qualities of A and/or G can be obtained. I am not aware, however, that specific studies to test the latter point have ever been made.

Our picture of the function of M antibody is primarily to make a firm contact with antigenic molecule or particle. Most natural antigens are likely to have a surface carrying large numbers of uniform or nearly uniform antigenic determinants which will ensure that the six combining sites (of the total ten) on any side of the complex will make at least a proportion of effective contacts with antigenic determinants. Such union appears to be specially effective in initiating the very complex process we know as fixation of complement and the subsequent ingestion of the antigen–antibody–complement complex by phagocytic cells. For both the basic functions of the immune system, the recognition of foreign material in the body and its removal by phagocytosis, M antibody seems admirably adapted.

On any theory by which specific clones of immunocytes are stimulated to proliferate by antigen there must be an important danger associated with infection. In an infection there is a massive accumulation of one type of foreign antigen in the body. If such antigen could indefinitely continue to stimulate the corresponding clone of immunocytes to proliferation there would soon, in principle, be only insignificant numbers of other clones in the body and an enormous excess of specific antibody. Clearly there must be some effective and specific form of negative feedback to keep such a process within bounds. Two processes seem to be concerned.

With any intense antigenic stimulation, a large number of the competent cells are pressed into plasma cell formation. This is generally taken as prohibiting any capacity for de-differentiation—once a mature plasma cell is produced it is an end-cell, actively producing immunoglobulin (A, G or M) but incapable of further proliferation under antigenic stimulus. In this way we can have exhaustion of all clones subject to stimulation by the antigenic determinants concerned. Although most M antibody is produced by plasma cells, there is direct evidence that some cells at a certain stage after immunization are producing both G and M, while at a later stage the great majority are producing only G. The obvious implication is that a substantial proportion of cells or clones initially producing M antibody subsequently switch to the production of G. Several workers have raised doubts about the reality of the M → G switch in an individual cell, but the overall evidence is in favour of the process. Experimentally, one of the most effective ways of reducing the proportion of M-antibody-producing cells is by exposing the animal to pre-formed G antibody of the same specificity.

The significance of this effect is unclear. One way of looking at the position is to assume that all cells on primary commitment are M producers and that a proportion change spontaneously to G producers. The introduction of pre-formed G antibody will impede any antigen in the circulation from effectively stimulating any progenitor cells. There will be no further recruitment of M producers and hence no new clones of G producers. Other interpretations are possible but this seems to be the most satisfactory way of covering the salient experimental findings. The essential result is a sharp diminution in the initiation of Ig M clones with an additional but less striking effect on Ig G production.

The primary biological function of G antibody production may therefore be to prevent too great a predominance of one type of immune pattern in the immunocyte populations of the body. Other incidental virtues of G antibodies may also have emerged. Only G antibody passes readily through the placenta and (in a completely different context) any virus or toxin molecule can be rendered inactive without need for the action of complement or phagocytosis.

There may be special importance in the conditions under which the normal transition from M to G antibody fails to occur. These include (a) with polysaccharide antigens, (b) in irradiated animals under some conditions, (c) in animals given mercaptopurine, (d) in allogeneic radiation chimeras and (e) in M-type myelomas. There is little that can be said in regard to these conditions. The fact that there is presumptive damage to the immunocytes in all instances except the first suggests that the change from M to G is intrinsic to the immunocyte and that any type of damage is likely to delay or prevent the switch. The reported failure of G antibody production toward polysaccharide antigens is apparently incorrect and based on the fact that M antibody is much more readily detected, molecule for molecule, than G. In all probability there is a considerable production of Ig G, according to the usual rules.

Antibodies of Ig A type have recently become of special interest. It has long been known that in mammals generally, but particularly in ungulates, large amounts of antibody are present in colostrum and that the antibody shows certain physical differences from that in the corresponding serum. It is only since 1965, however, that it has been generally recognized that the great mass of antibody in colostrum, saliva and some other secretions is of Ig A type. It has, however, an additional antigenic quality not found in serum Ig A, which is referred to as 'transport piece' by Good's group. There is some doubt as to whether circulating Ig A is taken up by secretory cells from the blood linked with transport piece and secreted as such. Intravenous infusion of normal serum into agammaglobulinaemic children results in the appearance of Ig A in saliva. On the other hand it is reported that the protein of Ig A myelomas is not found in the globulin of parotid saliva and that Ig A labelled with ^{131}I does not reach the saliva as such, all the label being present on small molecules. All are agreed that there is a close qualitative resemblance of antibodies (that is, corresponding immune patterns) in colostrum or saliva with those in the individual's serum. In the case of *Escherichia coli* agglutinins in man there is also a close quantitative relationship even though the serum antibody was almost wholly in the Ig M fraction. It was shown many years ago that plasma cells were numerous in the interstitial tissues of the bovine udder in the early stage of lactation. The possibility that much of the antibody in colostrum is of local origin must therefore be considered, particularly in view of a recent report that 80 per cent of the numerous plasma cells found in the rat duodenum are producing Ig A. I am not aware of similar studies on mammary or salivary glands but they are obviously called for.

As things stand, it seems likely that Ig A antibodies are secreted by the secretory epithelium of the gland or mucous surface concerned but reach the epithelial cells from two sources, the circulating blood and the antibody liberated into tissue fluids by adjacent plasma cells. The relative importance of the two sources may vary greatly with the glandular tissue concerned and its physiological activity. What happens within the epithelial cell is problematical. It seems most likely that the addition of 'transport piece' to the standard Ig A is all that is needed, but the possibility of a partial breakdown and reconstruction of antibody cannot be excluded.

An intriguing finding, in view of the special relation of Ig A to lactation, is that in one investigation women showed a much higher proportion of polio-antibody in that fraction than was ever observed in men.

For a number of years it has been regarded as likely that the reagins of patients with hay fever were of Ig A type. This was based largely on the separation of the immunoglobulins by physical means and there seems to be no doubt that the immunoglobulin concerned in man has the physical qualities of Ig A. The final diagnosis is, however, an immunological one and Ishizaka and his collaborators have provided convincing evidence that at least a large portion of the reagin demonstrated in ragweed-sensitive patients by the Prausnitz–Küstner test is not antigenically Ig A. It is now referred to as Ig E, and in normal human serum is present in only minute amount. As yet there is no indication of any physiological function of Ig E, just as none is known for the other rare type, Ig D.

SUMMARY

In this picture of the nature of antibody some of the essential features of clonal selection theory can be clearly seen. Basically all that is postulated is that by some process of randomization a great variety of genetic determinants of immune pattern can be generated. This is most simply thought of as arising by a high mutability (somatic mutation) of one or more cistrons concerned with defining the immune pattern of the combining region by the amino acid sequence of the 'variable' segments of light and heavy chains. There is still a preference amongst active workers in the field to seek the origin of diversity by a process which could legitimately be called 'random differentiation'. This would lead to the same operational result by making use of some as yet unparticularized process to establish one out of many thousand other possible configurations provided in the inherited genome. In whatever fashion the genetic mechanism emerges, its effect on the hypothesis we have favoured is to determine the production of a combining site where portions of the two chains are in a determinate duplex arrangement. Such regions are incorporated into each immunoglobulin molecule and the equivalent receptors in the immunocytes. The double loop of the 'variable' segments at each end of the Ig G antibody is specialized, perhaps simply by its duplex character, to serve as a highly specific adsorptive site, but the pattern is random. It may adsorb a common constituent of the body; it may be fitted to adsorb the characteristic antigenic determinant of a virus or it may be a meaningless combination which can adsorb nothing within the capacity of living organisms to produce. It is at this point that the biological quality of selection for survival enters the picture. Pure chance determines the pattern on the combining site, but what it reacts with will determine what happens to the cells carrying the pattern as an inheritable quality. If it reacts at once with accessible body components, the cell is destroyed; if it reacts later under appropriate circumstances with determinants of a foreign protein or micro-organism, the clone concerned will flourish; if the pattern finds no determinant to react with, the cell line can respond only to nonspecific stimuli if they exist or, by taking on myeloma character, provide its own intrinsic urge to proliferation and secretion.

6 The origin of immune pattern

The central problem that has worried theorists on immunology concerns the process by which from an animal stimulated naturally or experimentally by a certain antigen, there appears an antibody (or population of antibody molecules) with a specific complementary relation to the antigen used. Until the process of protein synthesis was understood it was possible to imagine a wide variety of processes with some analogy to various craftsmen's manipulations. The protein was moulded to fit the pattern of a molecular die or the antigenic determinant was intruded into the synthetic RNA, and there were many variants of these basic hypotheses.

With the clarification of the process of specific protein synthesis in bacterial viruses and bacteria during the last decade and the mounting evidence that, in all essentials, synthesis of protein by mammalian cells uses the same mechanisms, the scope for hypothesis has been greatly restricted.

PROTEIN SYNTHESIS

Protein, including antibody globulin, is synthesized on the basis of information held in the DNA of the genome of the cell concerned. Subject only to minor disagreement on detail, the process is as follows: a protein is composed of one or more polypeptide chains, often associated with other material such as oligo- or polysaccharide, and with inter- and intra-chain linkages by disulphide and hydrogen bonds. The synthesis of each component polypeptide chain is governed by a coded length of DNA in the genome. This transfers an equivalent pattern (transcription of information) to a similar length of single-stranded RNA (m-RNA) which, in association with one or a group of ribosomes and in the presence of transfer RNA and appropriate supplies of amino acids, induces the orderly synthesis of a peptide chain, each codon of three nucleotides defining the amino acid to be incorporated. The process by which the component chains of a complex molecule, like any of the immunoglobulins, are put together is unknown. That it is genetically programmed is proven by the uniformity of the immunoglobulins produced by single clones of human myelomatosis or murine plasmacytomata. It has not, however, been proven directly that an identifiable antibody can be produced as a uniform molecular population, but at least one example has been reported where a sharp peak in the electrophoretic diagram of serum from a rabbit immunized with a streptococcal antigen corresponded to what was apparently a uniform population of antibody molecules. An accompanying statement that this result was obtained in several other rabbits of a particular breed suggests that a full analysis of these 'monoclonal antibodies' should soon be forthcoming. Indirect evidence that individual antibodies differ among themselves in the same way that myeloma proteins do is becoming stronger. When two antibodies of different specificity but the same general type are prepared in a single rabbit, there are definite differences in amino acid composition of the specifically purified antibodies. Antibody eluted from Coombs-reactive red cells from patients with acquired haemolytic anaemia nearly always shows only one antigenic type of light chain—presumptive evidence of molecular homogeneity.

Any standard antiserum contains a heterogeneous population of antibody molecules, but by appropriate manipulations it is relatively easy to obtain purified preparations of specific antibody molecules of type G immunoglobulin. The evidence that this antibody comprises only a very small number of distinguishable types suggests that these types are produced by about the same number of clones of immunocytes. This picture may be wrong but it seems to be the most satisfactory basis on which to consider currently tenable hypotheses of the origin of immune pattern.

THE POSSIBILITY OF INSTRUCTIVE PROCESSES

Perhaps the most cogent approach to the problem (following Karush) is to consider the fact that the complementary steric relationship of antigen determinant to antibody combining site is three-dimensional. The information contained in the configuration of the combining site is not explicit in any one-dimensional arrangement of amino acid residues. It is inconceivable that any instructive transfer of information in regard to the three-dimensional structure of an antigenic determinant could modify the genetic process to allow the synthesis of an appropriately modified sequence of residues to allow the polypeptide eventually to form the corresponding combining site. There are, in fact, only two possibilities.

(a) The form of the final folding of the complex immunoglobulin molecule is determined by direct three-dimensional contact with an antigenic determinant followed by 'fixation' of the impressed pattern.

(b) There is no instructive relation between antigenic determinant and combining site, and the combining site configuration is of wholly genetic origin. If it 'happens to correspond' with an antigenic determinant in the body, their three-dimensional union sets in train the various processes that are postulated by selective theories of immunity.

The first requirement, then, is to consider the probability or even the possibility of an instructive tertiary folding of immunoglobulin against a physical template of antigenic determinant. There are some very difficult problems at the physico-chemical level here. The only serious suggestion as to how the modified tertiary configuration could be fixed is that of Karush, who assumes that in the lengths of polypeptide chain concerned there are enough cysteine residues to provide a sufficiently large number of ways of producing intramolecular disulphide bonds to hold any configuration stable. Then there are the problems as to how the antigenic determinant-combining site union is dissolved once fixation is complete and how the Ig G antibody comes to be symmetrically supplied with two identical combining sites.

Evidence against the importance of S–S linkages comes from two sources. General protein chemistry indicates strongly that the position of S–S linkages is strictly determined genetically and that the sequence of sulphur-containing and other amino acid residues in the polypeptide chain in itself determines the most frequent or the only way in which disulphide unions can form. Direct study of purified antibody has shown that by careful treatment all S–S links can be broken, allowing a wholly random configuration. When such reduced antibody is allowed to re-form the disulphide linkages, a high proportion of its specific reactivity returns. This represents perhaps the strongest argument against any direct template hypothesis of the Pauling–Karush type. The fact that there are differences in amino acid content of different Ig G antibodies in the same rabbit is incompatible with any simple instructive theory, but is not decisive for the selection approach.

The general indication from all the available information is wholly against the Landsteiner–Pauling–Karush theory and, unless some unexpected new experimental approach causes a re-evaluation, instructive hypotheses can be left out of further consideration. The problem remaining is to establish the way in which a multitude of patterns can arise in a single individual. At the cellular level it is well established that standard Ig G antibody is produced by cells of the plasma cell series, that except in very rare circumstances only one antibody is produced by a single cell and that an essential part of antibody production, as stimulated by the injection of a defined antigen, involves the formation by proliferation of a clone of plasma cells. The essence of the problem is to interpret the origin of the single pattern of antibody synthesis manifested by an active plasma cell clone.

THE GENETIC BASIS OF ANTIBODY PATTERN

We have now reached the point where instructive theories of antibody production can be left out of consideration. With the evidence of the 'variable' half of the light chain in myeloma proteins and the virtual certainty that there is also a 'variable' segment which probably makes up a portion of the Fd segment of the heavy chain in both myeloma proteins (Ig G type) and antibodies, we have an important clue as to the type of genetic process that must be sought. It is perhaps still not quite fully established that the combining site is made up of portions of the variable segments of both light and heavy chains or that the physical basis of antibody diversity is, in fact, the variability of the sequence of amino acid residues in these chains. Both, however, seem to be so much more likely than any alternative that they will be accepted as a basis for all our subsequent discussion. As all who have followed the current literature on the stable and variable halves of the light chains will have realized, a genetic process of quite unusual quality must be concerned with coding for the variable segment of the chain.

There are two basically distinct possibilities in regard to the nature of this process. The first is that each pattern has arisen during the course of vertebrate evolution in analogous fashion to the way whereby the various patterns of the haemoglobin and myoglobin chains have come to vary in different species. An obvious corollary to this is that there must be a very complex set of cistrons in every cell and a mechanism for choice between them. This can be termed 'the hypothesis of polycistronic control' and will call for some introductory discussion of evolutionary changes in protein structure.

The second basic approach is to assume that the diversity of pattern arises by genetic processes taking place in somatic cells subsequent to fertilization, that is, by somatic mutation or some operationally equivalent process. At the present time there is much interest in the suggestion of Smithies that somatic recombination within an 'antibody–gene pair' offers the most economical model that would produce the required diversity. Both these 'somatic' approaches present the difficulty of (a) providing the very high mutation or diversification rates that are needed and yet (b) allowing the persistence of a standard immune pattern through an indefinite number of generations in a myeloma clone and, by implication, in an antibody-producing clone of cells. Whatever alternative or combination of these processes is responsible for the emergence of diversity of immune pattern, the actual expression of that pattern in the immunocyte will be subject to the principle of phenotypic restriction. This has been mentioned already on several occasions but it may be elaborated a little at this point, particularly in relation to the part that myeloma proteins have played in the development of immunological theory.

In any human individual there are at least twenty different immunoglobulins that can be produced, even when we confine ourselves to physical and antigenic qualities only. Every myeloma protein produces one class only. At the level of immune pattern, the individual has almost infinite potentiality to produce antibodies against foreign organic material. Any semi-purified antibody active against a single antigen is in fact a heterogeneous population of molecules of varying avidity for the antigen and of different antigenic types. On the other hand, when a myeloma protein is found with a recognizable antibody specificity, it is homogeneous in this respect. The myeloma protein described by Eisen which reacted with the artificial hapten, DNP, differed from every other 'DNP antibody' in having an extremely narrow range of affinity in combining with the hapten.

Subject only to rare and anomalous exceptions it appears to be a general rule that each immunocyte produces only one immune pattern—perhaps more correctly only one pattern of amino acid sequences in the variable chains making up the combining site—and only immunoglobulin of a single antigenic class. The nature of this process of phenotypic restriction is still uncertain. Although the three possible sources of diversity listed above are spoken of as alternatives they are not mutually exclusive and, in fact, probably the best provisional conclusion is that all three processes play a part. Before attempting to apportion their roles in producing a diversity of variable chains it is desirable to say something about the general quality of these processes.

The evolution of change in protein structure

Information on the theme of the changes in protein structure arising in the course of evolution will be drawn mainly from the report of a Symposium in 1965, 'Evolving Genes and Proteins'. With the development of satisfactory methods of obtaining the full amino acid sequence of small and medium-sized polypeptide chains, much attention has been turned on the species differences in small proteins and peptides such as insulin, the fibrinopeptides, pituitary hormones, cytochrome C and haemoglobin. Cytochrome C (104 residues) and the α and β chains of globin (141 and 146 residues) are only slightly smaller than the light chain of immunoglobulin (214 residues). Both are functionally very important proteins with a long evolutionary history. Cytochrome C, which is functionally and to a large extent chemically similar in yeast and man, has presumably existed for 2×10^9 years, and haemoglobin for perhaps 400 million years. In the process both have undergone great changes in their amino acid composition.

Over the whole series of organisms from yeast to man, cytochrome C has 51 of its 104 residues present in the same positions. The others are variable and the number of differences is roughly proportional to the evolutionary distance between the forms concerned. In the haemoglobin chains, all of which, including the single myoglobin chain, are presumed to have had a single evolutionary origin, only 8 per cent of the residues are in equivalent positions in all chains. The changes must have arisen by mutation plus the processes of recombination, selective survival and genetic drift which allowed the replacement of one form by another. The evidence suggests that in the vast majority of instances the mutation in question was a transition in which a single base pair in the DNA was altered.

Evolutionarily effective mutations in globin chains seem to have occurred about once in seven million years but, as Ernst Mayr pointed out, many millions of mutations must have taken place in the relevant region of the genome of individuals over the same period but for one reason or another failed to replace the existent pattern. It is reasonable to assume that the retention of nearly half the residues in cytochrome C, virtually since the origin of aerobic organisms, means that these are functionally necessary, or at least that there is no biologically possible way by which they can be replaced with an equally effective amino acid. In the globin chains an examination of the number of alternative amino acids which are known to be able to occupy the various positions gives something very close to a Poisson distribution with a mean of 2·1. Random processes clearly play an extremely important part.

In addition to these changes in the detailed sequence of amino acid residues, there is a second evolutionary process of great importance for understanding the history of the haemoglobins and potentially of the immunoglobulins. This is the duplication of genes in the course of evolution with subsequent independent mutation. In normal human beings, haemoglobin contains α and β chains and, in the foetus, α and γ chains. All three chains are obviously of common origin but differ sharply in amino acid sequence. Each must be represented separately in the genome and in the case of the γ–β relationship there must exist a mechanism by which, in the course of differentiation, one cistron must be closed down and another activated. The three cistrons clearly result from duplication of a primitive gene at least twice and in all probability at very different geological periods. Most geneticists believe that this process of gene duplication with subsequent independent mutational changes has played a major part in the development of functional proteins. In discussing the evolution of the immunoglobulins we can take it as almost axiomatic that similar processes have been involved. This does not, however, necessarily mean that the diversity of immune pattern has been so produced.

Somatic mutation in vertebrates

In any discussion of somatic mutation as a source of variation in protein pattern, it is important to seek evidence on two points: (*a*) the legitimacy of comparing somatic and germinal mutations and (*b*) the frequency of somatic mutation of the type in which we are interested. Once again it is necessary to emphasize that only by refined genetic methods is it possible even in principle to differentiate between the various processes that can give rise to inheritable changes in somatic cell lines. Irrespective of whether they arise by point mutation, by deletions or inversions, or by any form of somatic recombination, provided they are qualitatively random in character the result can be accepted as 'somatic mutation' in the broad sense.

There is no doubt about the occurrence of somatic mutations in a wide variety of organisms and there is at least some evidence to suggest that they are of the same quality as germinal mutations. I have frequently quoted Fraser and Short's paper on fleece mosaics in sheep, which implies that in a mammalian species a single easily recognizable mutation occurs with approximately the same frequency ($10^{-7}\pm$) per cell in any stage of development of the fertilized ovum from the 2-cell stage onward. Mutant forms of fleece of basically similar character can also arise as a result of mutation in germ cells.

When somatic mutation occurs in a cell of a fully differentiated organism, it is always difficult to recognize its occurrence. If we accept a reasonable figure, say 10^{-6}–10^{-8} for the likelihood of mutation involving any particular locus per cell per generation, the most that can happen initially is that one cell amongst a million or more unchanged cells either dies or changes one of its functions. If it normally secretes a protein recognizable by its enzymic activity and, as a result of mutation, now secretes a protein antigenically similar but without enzymic activity, the modified enzyme molecules will represent 0·0001 per cent of the amount of active enzyme and will be quite undetectable. Only in quite exceptional circumstances can somatic mutational change in a single cell be detected. For a mutant to become demonstrable it must for one reason or another proliferate more extensively than its unchanged congeners so that a large number of descendants can manifest the change. The possibilities are:

(a) that the mutation directly involves some function controlling proliferation of the cell and allows rapid proliferation of neoplastic character;

(b) that, as a result of mutation, a stimulus present in the internal environment can stimulate the mutant cell to proliferate. This is the basic process postulated by clonal selection theory.

There is, however, a third situation in which a mutation (c) produces a functional change in a cell without influencing its proliferative potential. If subsequently an unrelated mutation of type (a) or (b) occurs allowing preferential proliferation of the cell, the function related to mutation (c) will become demonstrable. There are now many instances in which malignant tumours, notably hepatoma and bronchial carcinoma, have shown striking metabolic abnormalities, presumably as a result of this process.

Somatic genetic processes in relation to the diversity of the 'variable' segments

There are some obvious resemblances between the diversity of amino acid structure in proteins like cytochrome C or haemoglobin from a wide range of species, and the diversity found in the Lv (variable) segments of Bence Jones proteins and, by reasonable extension, in antibodies. In any attempt to equate the two processes, however, there are obvious difficulties particularly in regard to the time scale concerned. If a diversity of structure about as great as would be seen in the whole range of past and existent cytochrome C is needed to produce the required number of patterns, it must be produced in a few months instead of in one or two billion years.

The origin of immune pattern

It has become conventional to say that perhaps 10^4 immune patterns would be needed to account for the range and flexibility of the immune response. On the line of thought we are following, mutations would be required in a particular cistron controlling a peptide chain of 107 residues, that is, of 321 nucleotide pairs. By the time of birth, stem cells, thymocytes and lymphocytes might make up about 1 per cent of the cells of the body and, in a newborn child, would number about 3×10^{10} cells which would have required approximately twice that number of replications to produce them. If we adopt Orgel's figure of 10^{-8} 'errors' per nucleotide pair per replication, there would have been an average of 600 changes at each point in the cistron. For any given cell, however,

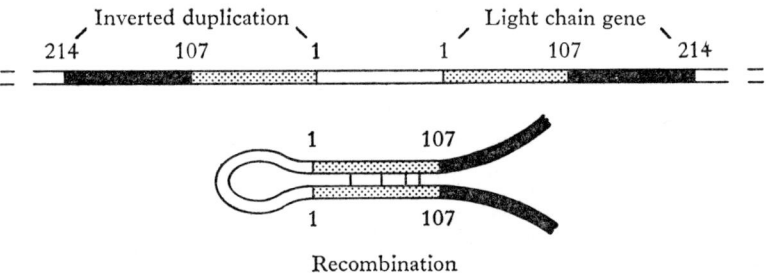

Fig. 20. Smithies's 'scrambler hypothesis' for production of diversity by intra-chromosomal recombination of duplicated 'variable' genes.

with about thirty-two generations from the fertilized ovum there would be only a 10^{-4} chance of its differing by one single nucleotide pair replacement, 10^{-8} of two being present. All the rest should have the inherited quality—or more probably one of the two inherited qualities since the individual is sure to be heterozygous. If the calculation is even remotely correct, a much higher rate of mutation or some other type of change is called for. Mutation at the rate of 10^{-4} per nucleotide pair would be needed if virtually every differentiating cell were to show some change from the ancestral patterns. This does not seem to be impossible and if something of this degree of heightened mutability has been evolved for this particular cistron—and one can think of some local anomaly in the supply of DNA polymerases and repair enzymes at the site—none of the other difficulties is insurmountable.

If, in addition to accelerated point mutation, there is also avail-

The genetic basis of antibody pattern

able opportunity for somatic recombination—of the type suggested by Smithies in 1967, or in some other guise—a much wider range of patterns could be developed in the short period between fertilization and birth. Smithies makes no mention of somatic point mutation and considers that given a series of *ad hoc* but reasonable assumptions his 'scrambler' hypothesis of somatic recombination could allow the emergence in a single individual of a whole range of differences in Lv chains, equivalent to those seen in a comprehensive collection of Bence Jones proteins from many different patients.

Two comments may be relevant. (1) The recombination postulated must presumably take place at some period of embryonic development before the differentiation of immunocytes and with a relatively high frequency. After differentiation it must cease or occur at a very low rate. (2) As with the alternative of hyperactive point mutation concentrated on 'hot spots' within the variable segment, the changes produced by recombination will be wholly random in character from the point of view of the antigenic determinants with which the derivative immune pattern will react.

The feature in which any postulated process of randomization of pattern differs from every other type of mutational change is that there are no positive metabolic or other requirements for pattern in the 'variable' peptide chain. The pattern is required only in relation to factors external to the cell. The special type of selection for survival that it will undergo, according to our hypothesis, in the thymus or in any other organ of equivalent function is of quite a different quality from anything that involves a functioning component of the cell. Changes that in any other protein would necessarily lead to breakdown of cell or organism are in this context quite acceptable. Their action is nil unless they are brought into effective contact with something specifically adsorbable.

It is an interesting point that if mutational changes occur as frequently in multiplying somatic cells as in germ cells, there must be a constant wastage of cells through one or other functional lack. But, even if as many as 1 per cent of cells quietly died in every tissue, the effect would probably be recognizable only with very elaborate technique.

Whatever hypothesis is adopted to account for the generation of diversity in immune pattern and in the amino acid sequence of the variable chains, there seem to be two necessary conditions to provide the observed phenomena. The first is some form of phenotypic restriction by which only one of the alleles in a heterozygote is active. If the 'variable' cistron is on the X chromosome, the Lyon phenomenon would fit the circumstances admirably. At some stage in early embryonic life each cell in a female mammal elects at random to inactivate one X chromosome subsequently visible in interphase as a Barr body. Once the decision is made by the cell, its descendants are permanently controlled as to X characters by whichever X chromosome remains active. About half the cells have a paternal X, half the maternal one. Such restriction is not known for any autosomal chromosome pair but there seems no reason why specific types of phenotypic restriction should not occur.

The second condition is more questionable. At first sight it seems obvious that there must be a hypermutability (in the broad sense) of the relevant genes during embryonic development followed by stabilization once differentiation to immunocyte has occurred. If, however, one remembers that the effect of any inheritable somatic change is negligible unless it results in preferential proliferation of the phenotype, the necessity for postulating stabilization of the gene after differentiation becomes minimal. Even at the high rate of 10^{-4} mutations per necleotide pair per generation, in ten cell generations of a proliferating immunocyte only 3 per cent of the thousand descendants would have mutated. This assumes that all 320 nucleotide pairs were equally susceptible, while in actuality the percentage would probably be much smaller. There is no suggestion as to how frequently per cell generation Smithies's scrambler process occurs. It could hardly be more frequent than 10^{-4} per cell generation. Amongst the population of an established clone, mutants arising since its establishment would represent only a minute proportion unless they had some proliferative advantage. It would be impossible to detect in practice the fraction of 1 per cent which had undergone a significant change.

The relative importance of the processes of diversification in the origin of immune pattern

It has already been emphasized that the three processes that may be involved in producing the diversity of antibodies and immunoglobulins are not mutually exclusive. We have only to look at the multiplicity of genetic markers on human Ig G from a single individual to be certain that there must be polycistronic determinants for immunoglobulins. Most modern writers, too, are impressed with the evidence that each light chain is composed of *two* units of 107 amino acid residues and that in all probability the heavy chain of Ig G can be thought of as composed of four similar units plus the polysaccharide unit. Multiple cistrons arising by duplication is the most appealing implication.

The problem of accounting for the known diversity of structure in the Lv segments of human Bence Jones proteins is usually accepted as being equivalent to interpreting the diversity of immune pattern amongst antibodies. Provided there is a realization that other aspects of the immunoglobulin molecule may have some modulating influence on immune specificity, this is probably correct. Whatever the genetic mechanisms responsible, it is certain that their overall result is unique. No remotely similar phenomenon is known, and rather strained analogies therefore become permissible. Various types of intragenomic recombination can be imagined which would facilitate diversity. In microbial genetics, mutational processes of very high frequency have been observed and even within a limited region of a single cistron there are some loci vastly more mutable than others. Clearly, somatic recombination could involve a gene or portion of a gene which was also subject to abnormally high levels of point mutation at some regions.

From our present point of view the requirement is not to attempt any decision between alternatives but to assess the part different processes may play and to suggest the lines of work that can be expected progressively to clarify the position.

Most of those who have attempted a single interpretation have postulated processes which would allow a single cell to produce any one of a wide variety of immune patterns. One such hypothesis calls for a relatively small number of genetic loci being concerned

The origin of immune pattern

in determining pattern, the diversity springing from the various combinations that can be produced. If, for instance, the number n of loci involved in determining antibody specificity was 15, some 33,000 (2^{15}) patterns might be possible, provided a process of randomized phenotypic restriction were operative. The results of such a process would be operationally identical with a set-up in which n is much smaller and mutational changes are freely operative. Most who favour such a view would think of the antigenic determinant as entering the cell and in some fashion instructing the cell as to the correct combination to be allowed phenotypic expression. To do so would need 33,000 ready-made molecules of each possible type to act as sensors of the antigenic determinant's three-dimensional configuration, and for each to have an individual 'circuit' to ensure de-repression of the proper allele of fifteen different loci. This is biologically inconceivable.

A slightly different approach would be to postulate a direct genetic specification of the combining site and to assume that a battery of 10^4–10^5 small cistrons carried the information needed in the genome, one for each pattern. If the repressor for each cistron had the quality of the three-dimensional combining site, one might postulate that union of antigenic determinant with the repressor would activate the cistron. This hypothesis is operationally indistinguishable from a simple instructive one and equally unattractive.

These two hypotheses derive essentially from Lederberg's suggestion that subcellular selection was a legitimate alternative to clonal selection. Both require two extremely cumbersome postulates that sterically correct sensors must be present in each cell for all the antigenic patterns with which the animal can react and, to account for tolerance, that a very large number, perhaps half, of these sensors must be blocked by each one of the 'self' determinants to which the animal is tolerant.

It is highly improbable that these or any similar views have any relevance to the real problem. The relative importance of polycistronic information developed in the course of evolution and the processes of point mutation and recombination or other intragenomic processes in somatic cell lines, however, will remain subject to debate for a long time. The most significant evidence bearing

The genetic basis of antibody pattern

on the part played by gene duplication is probably to be drawn from the antigenic character of heavy chains in human Ig G, while from the point of view of somatic cell processes the retention of a standard length and many stable sequences in the Lv chains is probably the most critical aspect. Both will be discussed, but it is perhaps of no great importance from the strictly immunological angle to try to reach any definite conclusion. It is inevitable that future developments will bring modifications of opinion at the genetic level but these may have little bearing on aspects of immunology susceptible to experimental study.

It is the essential theme of this book that immunology as a science has advanced far enough for us to be certain that any general approach will contain the central features of clonal selection theory:

(*a*) a genetic origin of pattern information;

(*b*) a randomized process determining phenotypic expression (somatic mutation or random differentiation);

(*c*) population dynamics of immunocytes determined by the results of specific antigenic contact.

Within that framework there is plenty of scope for modification to keep in line with new developments in cytogenetics and protein chemistry.

The significance of the stable components of the variable chains

In ascribing immune pattern to diversity in the variable segments, no mention has yet been made of the probable significance of the fact that most of the 'variable' segment of the light chain is constant in character and has many sequences in common between species as far apart as mice and men.

In the first place this immediately rules out any suggestion that completely random base-changes in DNA are involved. If single changes in nucleotide pairs are mainly responsible they must be highly concentrated in certain positions in the cistron. The main point in favour of Smithies's 1967 hypothesis is the possibility of obtaining changes of this sort of somatic recombination between two 'half-genes' of similar general character.

The conservative elements of the variable segments could also have a bearing on a quite distinct set of phenomena. The disproportionately large size of the whole Lv segment, compared with the small extent of a typical combining site, suggests the possibility that more than one potential combining site might be present on a single immunoglobulin molecule. It would, for instance, not be too disconcerting to find a monoclonal myeloma protein or antibody showing two quite unrelated specificities. Quite small fragments of a haptenic complex, such as that of dextran, can block a combining site.

If our hypothesis is correct that the combining site is a small $10 \pm$ sector of duplex where equivalent portions of the variable sequences on light and heavy chains come together, one might well find that several quite distinct antigenic determinants could find appropriate regions with which to make effective contact. What is of special interest is the situation that would arise if a substantial sequence of constant character were associated with adjacent labile residues and the stable sequence had a significant adsorptive power for a certain range of related antigenic determinants. It could emerge that for some particular range of chemically related antigenic determinants of high evolutionary significance, a set of complementary combining sites might be developed by relatively few point mutations involving the adjacent labile positions of the variable chains. One has in mind the special problems of histocompatibility that are raised in chapter 13. On such a formulation, one could well believe that if a mouse histocompatibility determinant A reacted with a combining site sequence a of the type described, then if a point mutation produced a modification of the antigenic determinant to A^1, although it would fail to react actively with combining site a, yet a single change in one of the adjacent variable residues could allow it to do so. Some such interplay of stable and labile positions will almost certainly have a major role in determining the initial proportions of progenitor immunocytes that will react with this or that general type of antigen.

This is merely another implication of the contention that the sequence of amino acids in the combining site is wholly genetic in origin and has no instructive relationship whatsoever to the antigenic determinant with which it reacts. The only mandatory condition in regard to the range of reactivity of a given clone is that it shall *not* react significantly with any accessible determinant natural to the animal producing it. Within those limitations it may

The genetic basis of antibody pattern

react significantly with any antigenic determinant that can find a sequence of appropriate complementarity on the combining site. Any argument against clonal selection theory based on the fact that 'too many' cells or molecules from a normal animal react with a single antigen must not ignore this situation.

THE HEAVY CHAIN ANTIGENS OF IMMUNOGLOBULIN G

From the genetic point of view, the work largely centred on Kunkel's group at the Rockefeller University on the multiplicity of antigenic types in the Ig G of all normal human beings is of special importance. Omitting any reference to A, M or D immunoglobulins and confining ourselves to Ig G, we find four serologically different types of heavy chain, We, Vi, Ne, Ge. These are present in all normal Caucasians. In addition there are within each group 'Gm' factors. A man We and Gm(a f) will produce globulins which are (a), (f) or (−) in respect to these factors. There are other factors associated with Vi (b g) and Ne (n^+ n^-). There is evidence that antibody specificity may be associated with any of these but there are some restrictions which may but do not necessarily mean that capacity to produce a given antibody is always associated with one antigenic type. There is no evidence that involves the combining site of an antibody or the very poorly defined variable region of the heavy chain in these antigen-defined genetic qualities. So far as I am aware, no one has yet produced an authoritative interpretation of this antigenic diversity in the heavy chains of the same individual. The findings could be interpreted as depending on the existence of a series of, say, twenty complete cistrons each coding for one type of Ig G heavy chain.

In view of the close correspondence in physical and chemical features of the Fc segment of all G heavy chains, the postulated twenty cistrons must have arisen by duplication. This seems unduly cumbersome when one has the rather clear evidence that the halves of the light chain are so similar in general structure that they must represent a far distant duplication of the cistron concerned, with subsequent independent point mutation in each. It seems much more likely that, as several workers have already suggested, all parts of the immunoglobulin molecule are derived from a single

The origin of immune pattern

primitive unit of 100–110 residues, equivalent to a primitive myoglobin molecule in the haemoglobin series. Two of these are concerned in the light chain, four in the heavy chain, with the possibility not yet finally excluded that in some immunoglobulin molecules one unit may be common to both chains. It would be completely premature to suggest what sort of a genetic and synthetic mechanism would be needed to account for chromosomal relationships, for the 'choice' of units for expression under rigid

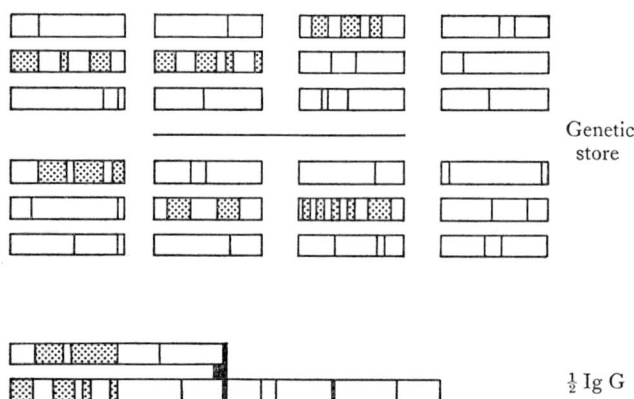

Fig. 21. A way of visualizing the store of genetic information in an immunocyte and the way by which the information is expressed in light and heavy chain of Ig G under a process of phenotypic restriction. 'Variable' segments are shown with broad dotted bands.

phenotypic restriction and for the synthesis of light and heavy chains and their fabrication into immunoglobulin molecules. It is, however, a reasonable guess that perhaps ten to sixteen such cistrons present in each cell of the individual could provide the information needed for the construction of all the *antigenic* variants of heavy chain pattern.

Until it is replaced as a result of adequate experimental data, the hypothesis that the combining sites are solely composed of determinate portions of the variable segments in heavy and light chains still seems the most satisfying available. If it is accepted, the diversity of *antigenic* pattern of Ig G will have only a minor secondary influence on *antibody* pattern which is wholly a responsibility of the 'variable' chains.

THE GENETICS OF CAPACITY FOR ANTIBODY PRODUCTION

In summary, I have regarded antibody pattern as being derived (*a*) by random choice from the small number of cistrons (perhaps two to eight) that will define the variable segments of the light and heavy chains of the differentiating immunocyte, and (*b*) as a result of a high level of somatic mutation in the chosen cistron(s).

This still allows genetic factors in the conventional sense to play a significant part in defining the range of antigenic determinants for which the individual can produce effective immune patterns. Despite the random character of their emergence, immune patterns have an important determinate element in the presence of a number of stable sequences in the 'variable' segments responsible for the combining site. The existence of such stable groups is based not only on studies of the light chain sequences but also by analogy with the species differences that have evolved in standard proteins like haemoglobins and cytochromes, and with the results of Benzer's fine-structure work on phage mutation.

All immune patterns must be derived from the small number of relevant cistrons present in the fertilized ovum. It is obvious that some changes are more likely to occur than others and that some will be very unlikely to be derived from one starting pattern although readily obtainable from another. It would be expected, therefore, that one might find inbred strains of animals showing well-marked individuality in the type of their responses to a range of antigens and that even with outbred animals there should be many occasions on which failure of antibody response to one antigen should occur without any weakness being apparent against some others.

There are many such examples in the literature and anyone with experiences of experimental immunization will know that one will always obtain a wide range of titres, often with some below significant level, when a considerable group of animals is uniformly injected with a standard antigen. There has been less extensive work on pure line animals.

Recent work with pure line guinea-pigs and synthetic polypeptide antigens has added a new facet to the problem of genetic differences in capacity to produce antibody. A certain hapten–polylysine complex may be effectively antigenic in one strain of guinea-pig but completely inactive in a second (non-responder) strain. This can be shown not to be due to any inability to produce the necessary immune pattern, since complexing the hapten-polylysine to a protein carrier produces antibody against both carrier and the hapten. The genetic difference here is concerned with some phase of the preliminary process by which the antigen acts as a stimulus to the synthesis and liberation of significant amounts of antibody.

SECONDARY MUTATION IN ESTABLISHED CLONES OF IMMUNOCYTES

By any acceptable hypothesis the cistron(s) coding for immune pattern must be abnormally labile at some stage of embryonic development. It would represent economy of hypothesis if that lability persisted through the proliferative phases of the immunocyte. In this section the pros and cons will be discussed.

Every classical antiserum against a conventional antigen is highly heterogeneous. The proportion of Ig M, Ig G and Ig A antibodies will vary characteristically from one stage of immunization to another but at almost every stage all three are present. In human beings, both K and L types of light chain are found and several electrophoresis bands for light chains from any subpopulation. Amongst all this heterogeneity it is hard to obtain evidence of secondary somatic mutation and it is best to look first at the myelomas.

When we are interested in mutant forms of protein there are two inbuilt difficulties: (a) we can only deal effectively with highly purified preparations and (b) the mutants we might expect to find will be in very small yield compared with the standard protein. Proteins are not easy to purify from associated proteins, and myeloma protein, for instance, needs strenuous treatment to eliminate more than traces of normal immunoglobulins or any other proteins not identical with the main mass of the myeloma proteins. The latter would include secondary mutants if they occurred. It may be significant that all the myeloma light chains tested by Cohen and Porter in starch electrophoresis showed in addition to a single very heavy band a single, much weaker, additional band one place on the negative side of the main band with some trailing between them. Subject to the exclusion of purely technical artefacts this would be consistent with the occurrence of a reasonably high incidence of single amino acid replacements by point mutations since the clone was initially established.

It is now well known that there are fairly numerous cases in elderly people of what has been called 'monoclonal gammopathy' without symptoms or radiological signs of myelomatosis bone lesions. These may persist for years but a proportion eventually develop malignant characteristics. Such patients might supply valuable material to determine whether the change to malignant character was associated with change in the amino acid sequence pattern.

Until homogeneous antibody populations can be obtained in reasonable quantity, direct examination of specific chain patterns is not likely to be productive. If our general point of view is correct, when an antigen is introduced into the body it has opportunity to contact a wide randomly established range of immune patterns carried by the immunocyte population. Depending on accidents of local concentrations and availability of patterned cells, it is likely that a wide range of separate clones will be stimulated with variable effectiveness. This will hold particularly for 'good' antigens which are 'good' presumably because they can react with a relatively wide range of patterns. These *a priori* deductions are in fact entirely in line with what has been observed in regard to the heterogeneity of specific antibodies.

Under the circumstances it becomes impossible to find functional evidence for the occurrence of secondary mutation in established clones of immunocytes. There are many instances in which secondary stimulation of a previously immunized animal with a related but not identical antigen gives rise to antibody different in quality from what would be produced by primary and secondary stimulation by either antigen alone. This may mean that secondary mutation has occurred, but it is much more likely that complex conditions for selective survival amongst the many clones of cells responding to the primary stimulus, and available for further selective response to the secondary one, could be responsible.

A superficially related problem arises from two types of experiment concerned with the repopulation of heavily irradiated animals or sequences of irradiated animals used in successive transfer experiments. The Harwell group showed by karyotype studies of heavily irradiated animals that, on occasion, decisive evidence could be obtained that almost the whole haematopoietic and lymphopoietic system had developed from a single surviving cell. The second line of approach was to pass stem cells through heavily irradiated hosts with the production of Till–McCulloch clonal nodules in the spleen, and to show that by repeated such passage commenced with a single nodule, reconstituted animals of relatively normal immune competence could be obtained. In both instances we have a situation in which one stem cell is provided with almost the same capacity to proliferate as the zygote or one of its early descendants. It is merely establishing in an unusual fashion the axiom that any relatively primitive cell possesses the whole repertoire of genetic information contained in the genome of the zygote.

7 The role of macrophages, eosinophils and other auxiliary agents in relation to adaptive immunity

There cannot be the slightest doubt that defence of the integrity of the body against parasitic invasion from the environment or anomaly from within requires much more than the functioning of the system of adaptive immunity with which this book is concerned. In all probability the polymorphonuclear leucocytes and the monocyte–macrophage system are in the direct line of the relatively nonspecific defence processes that have been an evolutionary necessity since the advent of the Metazoa. Their part in defence against bacterial infection and in the removal of damaged and effete cellular material is fundamental and in a sense the facilitation of some of these processes by opsonization is merely an evolutionary afterthought.

It is equally evident that throughout the vertebrates one finds eosinophil cells of characteristic morphology which in some only vaguely understood fashion are associated with immune reactions. So, too, are the basophil leucocytes and mast cells, but the significance of these 'pharmacologic time bombs' is even more obscure. Finally, we have the extraordinary system of laboratory phenomena which has been developed from Ehrlich's 'complement' or Bordet's 'alexine'. Just as has been observed in the study of blood coagulation, a dozen or more factors are concerned in complex adsorptive and enzymatic interactions. The development of these studies is something to chasten every laboratory biologist. It is more than probable that every biological phenomenon we study at some accessible level is at least as complex as either. From our present angle, however, all that we are concerned with is the relationship of complement to phenomena within the conventional field of immunology.

The aim of this chapter will be mainly to summarize the evidence *against* ascribing any major role to these components in the process by which immunocytes and antibody come into being and exert their specific immune functions. Their ancillary roles in the various processes that have a major immunological component have, however, provided fascinating subjects for investigation and must be covered even if only in summary fashion.

THE MONOCYTE–MACROPHAGE SYSTEM

When Aschoff's formulation of the reticulo-endothelial system in 1922 became well known, it was regarded as almost self-evident that the cells of the system were responsible for antibody production. It was evident that all particulate antigens as well as a wide variety of non-antigenic foreign materials were taken up by macrophages and, if antigen was responsible for the production of antibody, the macrophage was the obvious site for its synthesis. With the recognition of the plasma cell series as the major and probably the only producer of antibody in more than trace amounts, the role of the macrophage has been reduced to that of an auxiliary whose exact function is problematical. Interpretations may still range from those which regard the macrophage as the cell in which the most important initial stages of antibody formation take place to those by which the macrophage's only function in immunity is to lower antigen concentration to a biologically tolerable level.

Perhaps the basic facts are: (*a*) Antibody production is a function of organs in which macrophages, lymphocytes and plasma cells are conspicuous and well-intermixed components.

(*b*) After appropriate injections of antigen, significant amounts are found to be present in all types of macrophage, but not in lymphocytes or plasma cells.

(*c*) Conversely, in a recently immunized animal, antibody (that is immunoglobulin) is present in large amount in plasma cells and is detectable in the germinal centres. None is found in typical macrophages although with immunofluorescent technique some littoral cells show evidence of immunoglobulin.

(*d*) Under carefully defined conditions, evidence has been obtained that exposure of cell suspensions containing macrophages to antigen can give rise to material with higher specific immunogenetic power than the original antigen. This modified antigen may contain low molecular weight RNA as an essential component.

(e) Within lymphoid tissue there is a system of dendritic phagocytic cells capable of concentrating both antigen and antibody on their cell surface. For a variety of reasons that will be discussed, I believe that these cells are of primary importance in the process of antibody production. Their origin is uncertain, and from the functional angle they are so distinct from the classical monocyte–macrophage series that they are being considered here under a separate major heading.

The relevant types of phagocytic cell

Current usage is to refer to the mononuclear phagocytic cells of the blood as monocytes and to those of the tissues as macrophages. There are, however, very well marked differences amongst the phagocytic mononuclear cells in different tissues and it must remain an open question as to how legitimate it is to lump them into a single group. The following tabulation is concerned merely with the immunological significance of the different groups.

Blood monocytes. These have typically an indented reniform nucleus, numerous mitochondria and usually show lysosomes in the cytoplasm. The evidence is conclusive that the monocytes circulating in the blood are nearly all cells recently generated from stem cells in the bone-marrow. It is not excluded that the stem cells concerned have the morphology of small lymphocytes and are the same stem cells which, entering the thymic environment, would differentiate to immunocytes. Monocytes are mobile and leave the blood through intercellular junctions in the capillary endothelium. They accumulate in any area of subacute inflammatory change, whether produced by immunological activity or otherwise. In the tissue they take on the tissue macrophage form and may actively proliferate. There is still controversy as to whether the mononuclear cells infiltrating regions where a delayed hypersensitivity reaction is taking place are solely monocytes or include both lymphocytes and monocytes.

Large macrophages of the spleen and lymph nodes. The classical macrophages in lymphoid and other tissues are usually considerably larger than blood monocytes and much less uniform morphologically. In electron micrographs the most characteristic feature is the wide variety of cytoplasmic granules, some physiological (phagosomes, mitochondria, etc.), and some representing ingested material or its debris. In many, some rough-surfaced endoplasmic reticulum can be seen.

When an isotopically labelled antigen is injected locally and the draining lymph node is examined at appropriate times by autoradiography, early uptake of antigen is predominantly in the littoral cells of the peripheral sinus and of the lymph channels in the medulla and in macrophages present in the diffuse areas of the cortex. There is relatively little in the lymphoid follicles. In the next day or two some of the label in these cells disappears, presumably by digestion of the antigen. In the spleen such cells are numerous throughout the red pulp and are concentrated at the immediate periphery of the Malpighian areas of white pulp.

Peritoneal macrophages. When a suitable mild irritant such as liquid paraffin is introduced into the peritoneal cavity of any of the laboratory rodents the exudate produced contains large numbers of actively phagocytic mononuclear cells. Small and medium lymphocytes are also present and a number of authors have commented on the difficulty of clearly differentiating the two types morphologically. A fairly good functional separation can be obtained on the basis that cells that do not attach to glass are lymphocytes. Macrophages and polymorphonuclears rapidly develop a firm attachment to glass. Morphologically the peritoneal macrophages are mostly larger than blood monocytes.

There is evidence that a population of peritoneal cells from an immunized animal can transfer antibody-producing ability to a suitable test recipient but, where a differential study of cell types was possible, this facility was absent from the macrophage fraction.

A great deal of work has been done on various aspects of the functional activity of macrophages from the peritoneal cavity. The general conclusion has been that such cells have no intrinsic capacity of specific immune reactivity but that their behaviour is greatly influenced by the presence of 'natural' or 'immune' opsonins in the experimental system. For example, washed peritoneal phagocytes from the rabbit will take up foreign red cells only if these are opsonized by treatment with normal rabbit serum. The opsonins are relatively highly specific and are removed by appropriate absorption with the antibody concerned. It is sometimes possible to confer specific capacity to phagocytose a particulate antigen, e.g., foreign erythrocytes, by treating the peritoneal macrophages with serum containing cytophilic antibody. Under certain conditions, macrophages can be stimulated to destroy ingested living bacteria but the same enhanced activity is also shown against quite unrelated bacterial species.

Even if the peritoneal macrophage is neither a producer of antibody nor has any specific capacity for antigen recognition, its reactions may well have important implications in regard to a more primitive type of recognition of foreignness and of defence against micro-organismal invasion.

At the technical level there has been much interest in work, largely due to Fishman, in which attempts have been made to establish the nature of the apparent association of macrophages and lymphoid cells in antibody-producing tissues. The basic experiment has been to expose a population of peritoneal exudate cells to an antigen (phage T2), extract RNA from the treated cells and apply this to a culture of lymph node cells. In about 20 per cent of such experiments, minute amounts of specific antibody were demonstrated and all controls were negative.

There seems to be little doubt that from mononuclear phagocytic cells that have taken up antigen, material can be extracted which is more immunogenic than the equivalent amount of original antigen and, in the techniques used, the modified antigen is associated with RNA. It must still remain doubtful whether it is justifiable to regard this as a model for all antibody production in the body. Discussion of its significance will be deferred until the next chapter.

Kupffer's cells of the liver. These are very numerous in the sinusoids of the liver and appear to possess cytoplasmic projections actually spanning the lumen of the sinusoid. They are highly active in removing particulate foreign matter and effete red cells from the circulating blood. There appears to be no direct evidence that Kupffer's cells have any immunological function.

Alveolar phagocytes of the lung. Since such cells can be readily obtained by washing out the bronchial tree of guinea-pigs and rabbits, they have been used in a variety of studies and show a number of differences from macrophages of the peritoneal cavity; for example, they contain higher concentrations of acid phosphatases and other hydrolytic enzymes found in lysosomes than any of the other types.

Such cells play an important part in dealing with micro-organisms and other foreign particulate matter entering the lung but, again, no special immunological function in our sense has been ascribed to them.

The origin, movements and transformation of the mononuclear phagocytic cells

There is a current disinclination to make definite statements about the origin of a cell population specified by such a functional criterion as capacity to ingest foreign particles. By implication the population, here the mononuclear phagocytic cells, is a homogeneous system with a common developmental history. This is something that can never be established by the techniques that are nowadays obligatory. The most powerful is to find some way of labelling nuclei of a definable cell group with tritiated thymidine or some other DNA label and to examine the organism at successively later stages by autoradiography. There are always many difficulties in interpreting the results of such experiments but, with the macrophages, there is the special difficulty that these ingest nuclear fragments of damaged cells, particularly lymphocytes. The presence of label in a macrophage will therefore be almost as likely to have been derived from ingested material as to have been passed on from an ancestral cell.

Some limited evidence can be obtained in experiments in which distinctively labelled cells from one animal are transferred to another in which for one reason or another they are acceptable. The label may be a radioisotope, karyotypic marker or a histocompatibility antigen. By experiments of this general type, what appears to be good evidence has been obtained that (*a*) Kupffer's cells may be derived from thoracic duct lymphocytes, (*b*) when a lethally irradiated mouse is saved by the administration of bone-marrow cells, the phagocytic cells subsequently obtained from the peritoneal cavity are of donor origin and (*c*) the cells which migrate from capillaries to give macrophages in a lightly traumatized area are not derived from circulating small lymphocytes but come perhaps wholly from bone-marrow.

All these statements are applicable only to the special circumstances of the experiment concerned but, taken together, they suggest that the bone-marrow contains cells that have potentiality to produce any type of macrophage and that, while the great majority of small lymphocytes have no such potentiality, the possibility is not excluded that, under special circumstances, thoracic duct lymphocytes may give rise to descendant macrophages. Although the evidence is far from conclusive, there is a mounting opinion that the small lymphocyte-like cells in the bone-marrow may, for the most part, represent stem cells in the strict sense of being able to give rise to lymphocytes, macrophages and granulocytes. In addition there are hints from human pathology that in the absence of a functional thymus no 'lymphocytes' are seen in the bone-marrow.

It is at least conceivable that one of the reasons for the almost complete failure to obtain a clear picture of the interrelationships of wandering mesenchymal cells is that, in fact, morphological type is simply a reflection of functional activity and that, within the series, the normal sequence of specific differentiation along one or other of the paths from stem cells to specialized end-cell may, under appropriate circumstances, be interrupted by de-differentiation. Depending on the completeness of that de-differentiation and the local *re*-differentiating stimulus, a new line of differentiation may take place. This interpolation in a discussion of macrophage origins is admittedly based simply on the absence of definitive experimental evidence and can be refuted (or confirmed) if new experimental approaches are developed.

From the general immunological point of view, probably the most important outstanding problem in the cellular field is the origin of the mononuclear cells found in the tissues in the areas of delayed hypersensitivity and other subacute inflammatory reactions. The current disinclination to call such cells anything other than mononuclear cells is an indication of how difficult it has been to decide what type of blood cell, lymphocyte or monocyte has given rise to them. The pros and cons will be considered on p. 245.

In more chronic conditions the development of mononuclear phagocytic cells to epithelioid and giant cells is well known.

Opsonization

An opsonin is a serum component which facilitates the ingestion of foreign particulate material by phagocytes; either polymorphonuclear leucocytes, or the various types of mononuclear phagocytic cells. In general, opsonin is synonymous with antibody or perhaps, more accurately, with adsorbed and partially denatured immunoglobulin. It is characteristic that when autologous proteins are administered to an animal the only one actively taken up by the phagocytic cells is immunoglobulin, necessarily partially denatured during the process of purification. The presence of homologous (or other) serum may be necessary even for the phagocytosis of synthetic particles such as polystyrene, and it is of much interest that the component of normal serum responsible for the opsonization of polystyrene particles is a specific one that can be removed by appropriate absorption.

This may be an appropriate place to attempt to assess the significance of opsonization in relation to macrophage function and antibody production. There is good evidence that antitoxin production in young animals is facilitated if very small amounts of antibody are administered artificially or received physiologically from the mother, before active immunization with toxoid is begun. This is reminiscent of Jerne's first theory of antibody production but most immunologists, probably now including Jerne himself, would interpret the findings differently.

In all mammalian and avian species, newborn animals receive antibody from the mother. The method of transfer and the type of antibody transferred will differ with the species. In many mammals, including man, transplacental passage is limited to Ig G-type antibody while, for those mammals in which transfer by colostrum is important, Ig A-type antibodies will predominate. In either case, a representative sample of the circulating antibodies of the mother will be received. The range of patterns will probably cover antigenic determinants of all the common micro-organisms the mother has encountered. This will ensure that when such micro-organisms begin to enter the tissues of the newborn animal they will be opsonized and readily taken up by phagocytes, both polymorphonuclear and mononuclear. The primary function of the macrophage is to get rid of potentially dangerous foreign material by ingestion and enzymic breakdown to molecules which can either be contributed to the metabolic pool or prepared for excretion by one of the natural routes. As indicated earlier, another important function may be to reduce the concentration of all circulating antigens to a level that will prevent its undue activity at the immunological level. There is no evidence to convince me that the large macrophages of liver, spleen, lymph node and lung have any other significant immunological function than these. The results of Fishman and others can be best regarded as an indication that unspecialized phagocytic cells can carry out rather inexpertly a process characteristic of the specialized antigen-retaining reticular cells of primary lymphoid follicles.

THE DENDRITIC PHAGOCYTIC CELLS OF LYMPHOID TISSUE

The primary lymph follicle of lymph node or other peripheral lymphoid tissue can be thought of as a spongy reticulum of supporting cells whose dendritic processes are in part directed along a light mesh of reticulin fibres. Within this framework lie the relatively closely packed small lymphocytes, in life probably a mobile mass of amoeboid individuals. These reticulum cells are actively phagocytic.

If a lymph node is examined three to seven days after the administration of a labelled antigen such as flagellin, label is conspicuously concentrated in the lymph follicles. It is held in the dendritic reticular cells fairly regularly dispersed throughout the follicle, and electron microscopic study points to most of the antigen being concentrated on the surface of the dendritic processes. When a germinal centre develops in the lymph follicle the usual effect is for the region showing label to be compressed into a cap on the outer side of the germinal centre. Basically similar appearances are to be seen in the lymph follicles of spleens in animals given antigen intravenously.

Studies of the presence of immunoglobulins in lymphoid tissue, using appropriate fluorescent antibodies for their detection, have consistently shown a reticular distribution of immunoglobulin within germinal centres. Unlike the situation in any isolated plasma cell, which shows only a single type of immunoglobulin, that present in the germinal centre is characteristically heterogeneous. Everything combines to suggest that antibody, both locally produced and circulating, is accumulated on the surface of these dendritic phagocytic cells and may in fact play a major part in retaining antigen in a situation where it is specially accessible to contact with committed immunocytes. It is in line with current opinion to believe that the retention of antigen in the surface layer of such dendritic cells may provide a particularly suitable means of stimulating any appropriately patterned cell receptors carried by small lymphocytes. The rapidity with which small lymphocytes move from one lymphoid cell collection to another throughout the body has been described earlier.

Basing our interpretation largely on the results of the group led by Nossal and Ada at the Hall Institute, special importance is attached to these reticulum cells of lymphoid follicles. They are actively phagocytic, are subject to the normal benefits of opsonization and are protected from too great an uptake of any individual antigen by a protective screen, in both spleen and lymph node, of standard macrophages. The special attributes of these cells, which are of significance for their role in antibody production, are:

(*a*) their capacity to retain antigenic label much longer than do standard phagocytes, most probably because of a less active lysosome mechanism for breakdown of ingested material;

(*b*) concentration of antigen at the cell surface and particularly at the surface of the dendritic processes. If the pictures published of the distribution of one labelled antigen, flagellin, can be given a general application, one can assume that each such cell in a lymph node carries on its surface a sample of most or all of the antigens that have been derived from the lymph node's area of drainage during the lifetime of the cell;

(*c*) if the accumulation of small lymphocytes in primary follicles is a mobile 'bag of worms', as seems likely from the *in vitro* behaviour of lymphocytes, large numbers of contacts between any given deposit of antigen on a dendritic process and a great many individual lymphocytes become inevitable;

(d) the frequently described picture of a rim of small lymphocytes forming a rosette around a macrophage could well represent an example or analogue of the process by which antigen carried on a reticulum cell surface can stimulate a lymphocyte with appropriate receptors.

Although we regard this as the standard intervention of the macrophage series in the process of antibody formation, the possibilities cannot be excluded, first, that antigen not held on a macrophage surface may be effectively immunogenic, and second, that other types of macrophage in special circumstances may play a similar role.

One final remark may be made in relation to the phenomena of tolerance to be discussed in a later chapter. If, by any means, cells capable of producing normal antibody reactive against antigen A are eliminated from the lymphoid cell population of the body and there is no opsonin for A in the circulation, this absence would in itself greatly reduce the chance that the antigen could establish itself on the reticular phagocytic cell surfaces.

EOSINOPHIL LEUCOCYTES

Eosinophil leucocytes are well-defined cells present in all mammals and characterized by large cytoplasmic granules staining strongly with acid dyes. The granules are specialized lysosomes containing a variety of enzymes of which the most unusual is a very stable peroxidase of unknown function. In electron micrographs the most conspicuous feature is a large crystalloid of high electron density in each granule. Apart from the fact that it is protein in character, nothing is known of the chemical nature or functional activity of the crystalline material. Eosinophils develop in the bone-marrow and spend on the average only a few hours in the circulation. The cells are moderately mobile, leave the circulation through endothelial cell junctions, and are attracted to and phagocytic for antigen–antibody complexes. In the tissues, eosinophils are present in considerable numbers in the submucosa of the intestinal tract and other situations exposed to foreign antigens and, by implication, the site of frequent antigen–antibody interaction.

Specific experimental work on the movement of eosinophils from the blood into tissue has been principally concerned with their entry into lymph nodes activated by antigen. It has been shown that eosinophils appear usually about the cortico-medullary junction of the node within a few hours of antigen being administered. In order to account for this accumulation, it is necessary to postulate some product of cellular activity associated with antigen–antibody union which presumably modifies local capillary endothelium so that circulating eosinophils are more or less specifically held and can pass by diapedesis into the tissues. The very rapid accumulation observed by Litt must, on current interpretations of the process of antibody production, result when antigen in the phagocytic reticulum cells makes contact with any reactive lymphocytes, well before there is proliferation and development of plasma cell clones.

The only positive suggestion as to the substance mediating the attraction of eosinophils to the site of an antigen–antibody reaction is derived from R. K. Archer's experiments in horses. Infiltration of skin areas with histamine caused a local accumulation of eosinophils within 30 hours, the intensity of the response being linearly related to the dosage of histamine used. Experiments with species other than the horse have not confirmed this, and general opinion is that some other product of antigen–immunocyte reaction must be involved.

Blood eosinophilia is characteristic of a variety of allergic states and of acute worm or protozoal infestations, all of which in human beings are associated with immediate skin reactivity of histamine type. There is also a fairly regular accumulation of eosinophils in the tissues containing metazoan parasites.

There is no accepted interpretation of eosinophil physiology but it must obviously be concerned in one way or another with the immune process. The fact that granules disintegrate when phagocytosis of antigen–antibody aggregates occurs with liberation of many enzymes suggests that the basic function of the eosinophil is as a mobile scavenger to assist in clearing up areas of subacute damage associated with immune responses. As in all such systems, one must postulate a system of controls and feedback to ensure an adequate production of eosinophils in the bone-marrow, to regulate the level in the circulation and to channel circulating cells to the tissues where they are required. There is no substantial information in regard to any aspect of these controls.

The striking association of eosinophilia with extensive metazoan infections may speculatively be ascribed (*a*) to the long persistence of antigenic material difficult for the body to dispose of, (*b*) a relatively high content of A-type antibody with its characteristic tendency to fix to tissues and react to circulating antigen with histamine liberation and (*c*) the common absence of G-type antibody with its blocking activity against sensitivity reactions.

MAST CELLS AND BASOPHILS

It is rather depressing to find that the vast early literature on anaphylactic shock contained no reference to mast cells. Current opinion seems now to be firm that anaphylaxis is the symptom complex resulting from the discharge of the battery of pharmacologically active substances stored in the mast cell. These include heparin and histamine in all mammals, serotonin in mice and rats, and the slow-reacting substance of Kellaway and Trethewie in the guinea-pig.

Mast cells are common in all types of loose connective tissue and the standard experimental material is the omentum and peritoneal lining of the rat. They show only minimal evidence of mitosis as such and are usually assumed to arise by heteroplastic transformation of fibroblasts. In the course of a large number of histological examinations of mouse thymuses I found, not infrequently, massive areas of heteroplastic transformation of cortical thymocytes to mast cells. There is no indication as to the nature of the process causing the extraordinary transformation from fibroblast or thymocyte to mast cell nor is there any established function for the mast cell in the body's economy. It is the only known source of heparin in the body but there is no evidence that the anticoagulant action of heparin has any physiological function.

Since it is well accepted that histamine liberation is probably responsible for the first phase of inflammatory reactions, it will probably emerge that mast cells in some way facilitate local processes of defence and repair. Their capacity to discharge their granules and liberate histamine when stimulated by antigen–antibody reactions in various situations may be no more than a general response to a mildly damaging stimulus. There are a number of pathological conditions in which mast cells are conspicuous and some, such as urticaria pigmentosa, in which histamine liberation is responsible for symptoms, but none provides any significant clue as to physiological function. Anaphylaxis in its various forms seems always to be an experimental artefact—'a creation of the hypodermic needle'—or a rare accident in genetically abnormal individuals.

The only conclusion one can reach is that the mast cell and the basophil leucocyte are so widely present in vertebrates that they must have some function that is significant at the evolutionary level. Whatever that function may be it does not appear to have any aspects which can be meaningfully related to the general theme of adaptive immunity.

COMPLEMENT

Since the classic studies of Bordet, Ehrlich and Wassermann, the concept of complement as an essential part of the mechanism of immunity has progressively been replaced by rather uncertain decision that the classic phenomenon of complement lysis of red cells is a laboratory artefact of no real significance for immunity.

The circulating blood plasma is an immensely complex mixture which, as R. G. Macfarlane has noted, achieves a miracle of 'peaceful co-existence with a vast surface area of the normal vascular endothelium'. When, however, trauma introduces the biological necessity of rapidly enforcing haemostasis in preparation for repair, a process involving at least twelve components leads to localized fibrin deposition; while at appropriate points platelet aggregation, kinin activation with modified endothelial stickiness and vascular contraction are co-ordinated with the fibrin formation to ensure haemostasis. When infectious processes with or without trauma are initiated, there are doubtless equally complex processes set in action and there can be little doubt that the variably large number of components, co-factors and inhibitors that have been described as being concerned with immune haemolysis by 'complement' represent a similar range of plasma factors, perhaps including some of those in the haemostatic group, whose co-ordinated function has as yet escaped recognition.

Research on complement seems to have failed to attract anyone with a capacity to look beyond finding a new 'component' but one can feel optimistic that an acceptable biological approach equivalent to R. G. Macfarlane's cascade view of the clotting mechanism will eventually emerge. As they stand, the C^1 factors $1p$, $1q$, $1r$, $1s$, 2, $3a$, $3b$, $3c$, $3d$, $3e$, $3f$, 4 and the co-factors Ca^{++} and Mg^{++} are biologically meaningless.

Certain strains of mice lack complement in the sense that, because of the absence of part of the $C^1 3$ complex, their fresh serum has no lytic activity. No one has demonstrated any inefficiency in meaningful immunological reactions in such strains.

Possibly all that can usefully be said is that when a complex of antigen and antibody is formed in the body it is liable to adsorb a variety of enzymically active components to produce an even more reactive aggregate. There are considerable differences in the ease with which antigen–antibody complexes adsorb complement in the diagnostic immunologist's conventional sense. A certain compact bulk of denatured globulin appears to be necessary. A single M-type antibody molecule attached to a red cell provides a nidus for the initiation of the sequence of enzymic actions that culminate in the production of a tiny hole in the surface membrane of the red cell through which haemoglobin can leak out. For lysis to be initiated with G (7S) antibody there must be sufficient antibody molecules for at least one pair to be attached adjacently to each other. In other systems involving the production of antigen–antibody aggregates there is equally an optimal size of the individual aggregates for complement fixation.

There is direct evidence that adsorption of complement components *in vivo* increases the activity of phagocytosis and the speed of killing of bacteria after ingestion. Under appropriate conditions, antigen–antibody–complement complexes can be shown to adsorb to certain red cells (the immune-adherence phenomenon). For the most part this is a laboratory artefact but it is closely related to the mechanism by which drug reactions producing haemolytic anaemia or purpura are mediated (see p. 284).

In the course of several types of autoimmune disease or other types of immunopathology there is a sharp reduction in the measurable complement activity of the patient's serum. This has been observed particularly in systemic lupus erythematosus (SLE) and in kidney disease. Evidence that this results from fixation of complement in regions where auto-antibody has become attached to tissues can be obtained by the use of specific anti-human complement used in immunofluorescence tests. In practice, a serum against globulin β1c which is a component of $C^1$3 is used. With such methods, fixed complement can be detected in the kidneys in SLE nephritis and in the skin in SLE. A related finding is that synovial fluid from joints showing lesions of rheumatoid arthritis shows lower complement levels than normal synovial fluids. It is usual to ascribe a significant role to complement in the production of damage by antigen–antibody combination in both experimental and autoimmune situations. So little is known about the pharmacological activity of complement components that such statements are essentially meaningless.

Even if 'complement' appears to have little relevance as such to the interpretation of adaptive immunity, its importance remains unimpaired at the laboratory level as a reagent in complement-fixation tests for the measurement of antigen–antibody reaction.

8 The immunocyte and its response to specific stimulation

THE NATURE OF THE IMMUNOCYTE

It is logical to adopt Dameshek's term 'immunocyte' for the cells directly concerned in immune responses but it must be recognized that a fully satisfactory definition of the term is not yet possible. It is a useful but perhaps oversimplified procedure to define an immunocyte as any cell that can be specifically stimulated by an antigenic determinant and that either itself produces antibody or is a potential ancestor or collateral of cells that can produce antibody. If a cell is to be specifically stimulated by an antigenic determinant it must carry a sensor, a receptor capable of recognizing and responding to the antigenic determinant in question. It would be unreasonable to look for such a specific receptor in any other terms than equivalence to the combining site of antibody globulins. This does not necessarily mean that the receptor is identical with A, G or M antibody as found in the circulating plasma, but since the light chain is common to all the immunoglobulins and appears to play an essential if minor part in the specificity of the combining site we should expect it to be present as part of any specific receptor. If only a limited portion of the Fd fragment of the heavy chain is needed to produce the combining site of a receptor there would be the further possibility that an immunocyte could conceivably be reactive to antigen without presenting evidence of the presence of any of the standard antigenic markers of the immunoglobulins.

At the operational level, a cell can be identified as an immunocyte (*a*) if it can be shown to be synthesizing antibody, (*b*) if it responds demonstrably and specifically to contact with antigen—and any effect due to adventitiously adsorbed antibody is appropriately excluded—and (*c*) if immunoglobulin can be shown to be present in the cell and, again, the possibility of its adsorption from the environment excluded. As in all immunological reasoning, only positive identification of an immunocyte is possible. As a rule,

Response to specific stimulation

reactivity to one or, at most, a very small number of antigens is all that can be tested. Morphologically similar cells that do not react might, if they could be tested, react with one of the many thousand other possible antigenic determinants. Another characteristic difficulty arises from the fact that in a wide range of experimental manipulations a large population of cells, usually in the range 10^6–10^8, is tested for immune activity of one sort or another. A positive finding means only that the population contains some of the immunocytes in question. It does not necessarily follow that because the population contains a large majority of one morphological type that particular cell is the immunologically effective one.

There are, however, methods by which the immunological reactivity of single cells can be recognized. Chapter 3 discussed the methods by which active production of antibody by isolated plasma cells can be demonstrated. Here we are concerned with the more interesting problem of detecting immunocytes at stages where no active production of antibody is taking place. In any form of clonal selection theory it must be postulated that as soon as a cell has been differentiated to an immunocyte it must have developed at least one of the immunoglobulin receptors that are within its genetic capacity to produce. There may well be a genetically predetermined predominance of certain immune patterns in the newly differentiated immunocytes but this has not been demonstrated as yet by any experimental technique. Where we are concerned with any standard foreign antigen we can expect only very small numbers of reactive cells in a population of millions. Highly sensitive methods are necessary for their detection. In practice the experimental approach is to look for cells reactive with a given antigen in animals which, as far as is known, have never been in contact with that antigen. An alternative is to devise methods of detecting very small amounts of immunoglobulin in lymphocytes without regard for its precise immunological reactivity. The presence of immunoglobulin, more correctly the presence of antigenic determinants specific for immunoglobulin, is prima facie evidence, but no more, that the cell has a specific immune function.

THE PRESENCE OF IMMUNOCYTES IN UNIMMUNIZED ANIMALS

Reactions of immunological quality can be observed in unimmunized animals by three main types of technique:

(a) Graft-versus-host reactions; for example, that shown by chicken lymphocytes deposited on the chorioallantois of an unrelated strain.

(b) The Jerne–Nordin technique of detecting cells capable of producing haemolytic antibody against heterologous red cells by plating in agar containing the appropriate red cells. Discrete 'plaques' of haemolysis are produced around each antibody-producing cell.

(c) Stimulation of cells, typically small lymphocytes, to dedifferentiate to blasts preparatory to proliferation, either by specific antigen or by antibody against immunoglobulins characteristic of the animal from which the cells are obtained.

The graft-versus-host reactions introduce many factors outside the scope of this book, and consideration of those that are relevant will be deferred until surveillance is discussed in chapter 13.

The significance of Jerne's antibody-plaque technique

If a mouse is immunized with sheep red cells and four days later the spleen is removed, it can be shown that many cells in the spleen are actively producing haemolytic antibody. Jerne's technique is, in outline, to prepare a suspension of single cells from the spleen, mix them in warm liquid agar with an excess of washed red cells and pour the mixture on the surface of a plain agar plate. After 1 hour incubation the plate is 'developed' by exposure to guinea-pig complement for another 30 minutes. Small circular areas of haemolysis are each centred on a single cell often recognizable as a plasma cell. The reaction is specific for the type of red cell used for immunization.

Normal mice spleens contain small numbers of cells capable of producing such plaques. The number varies widely from one individual to another and the average value from strain to strain. It is very much lower in neonatally thymectomized animals. At least rabbit, sheep and pig cells have been used for test and appropriate experiments have shown that the number of normally reactive cells and the increase by antigenic stimulation are specific for the individual cell type. Suitable experiments have failed to show single cells haemolytic for two distinct red cell types.

The following interpretation follows that suggested by Jerne, but is equally compatible with the results from several other laboratories. Progenitor cells reach or arise in the spleen in very small numbers. These cells are probably subject to low-level nonspecific proliferation possibly, as suggested on p. 177, by a side-effect of the specific stimulation by antigen of other immunocytes. With the entry of the corresponding antigen perhaps after preliminary uptake and processing by splenic macrophages, a proliferation of plaque-forming cells occurs. Where the number of progenitor cells can be assayed by inoculation of normal isologous spleen cells into a heavily irradiated mouse, it can be shown that localized areas of 100-1,000 plaque-forming cells develop, each area from a single progenitor. If two different antigens are used the separate areas each contain only one type of antibody-producing cell. It appears still to be an open question whether the progenitors of these clones of proliferating antibody-producing cells are identical with the 'normal' plaque-forming cells or are non-antibody-producing but reactive to antigen. The fact that, in certain situations, lymphocytes can be stimulated by antigen to divide and to synthesize cytoplasmic protein but not immunoglobulin points to the second alternative. There is, however, nothing to negate the possibility that a plasmablast proliferating slowly for nonspecific reasons may be *specifically* stimulated by antigen to accelerate its proliferation.

The antibody detected by Jerne's technique is wholly M in type and, as such, much more haemolytic than G-type antibody of the same specificity. As far as information is available it appears that all 'normal' antibodies are of M (19S) type. The Jerne technique has already been modified in various ways to detect other types of antibody. Anti-red cell Ig G antibody can be detected by treating with anti-mouse-globulin serum before the addition of complement. Other antigens can be used if, like many bacterial antigens, they can be firmly adsorbed to the red cell surface. In such experiments the red cells used in the test plates have been appropriately treated with the antigen.

In vitro *stimulation of lymphocytes to mitosis and blast formation*

As a by-product of attempts to produce rapid separation of red cells from leucocytes by agglutinating red cells in citrated or defibrinated human blood with kidney bean extract (phytohaemagglutinin) it was found by Nowell that leucocyte cultures from cells isolated in this fashion showed enlargement and mitosis. Subsequently it became evident, to the surprise of most haematologists, that the cells involved were largely or wholly small lymphocytes. The use of phytohaemagglutinin for this purpose has greatly increased the ease with which blood cells can be karyotyped, but the immunological significance of the phenomenon is far from clear. There is adequate evidence that human small lymphocytes can be stimulated to undergo blast transformation to take up tritiated thymidine and to undergo mitosis *in vitro* by phytohaemagglutinin and anti-human lymphocytic serum made in the rabbit; when two populations of lymphocytes from different individuals are mixed, a significant amount of blast transformation occurs, and when persons with a positive tuberculin test or with anti-streptolysin O in their serum are donors, their lymphocytes react respectively with tuberculin and streptolysin O *in vitro*. Claims that the reaction can be obtained with any antigen against which an individual has produced antibody, or that, on stimulation, specific antibody is produced have not been adequately confirmed.

It is probable that effective analysis of what is obviously a very important phenomenon will have to be carried out in experimental animals. So far it has proved much more difficult to obtain reproducible results in animals, and the present discussion is almost wholly based on work by Sell and Gell reported in 1965. In discussing the nature of antibody, mention was made of the antigenic qualities of human immunoglobulins and their constituent chains. In experimental animals there are similar 'allotypic' differences between the immunoglobulins of different individuals. In rabbits, Ig G is made up of heavy chains which can carry any one of three antigenic determinants A_1, A_2, A_3, while the light chains also have three possible determinants A_4, A_5, A_6. Genetic studies indicate that qualities A_1, A_2, A_3 are co-dominant alleles of locus a, while A_4, A_5, A_6, are similar alleles at the locus b unlinked to a. In a heterozygous rabbit we may have the combination A_1, A_3, A_4,

A5, and in such an animal the Ig G will show the four types A1 A4, A1 A5, A3 A4, A3 A5. Everything suggests that when an anti-A4 serum is made by immunizing a rabbit with a genotype lacking A4, the antibody reacts only with the light chain of an immunoglobulin of the appropriate allotype.

TABLE 3. *Stimulation of lymphocytes by anti-allotype sera*

Anti-allotype sera	Lymphocytes from		
	A2, 3/5, 6	A1, 1/5, 5	A2, 3/4, 4
Anti-A5	+(x)	+(x)	—
Anti-A6	+(y)	—	—
Anti-A5 + anti-A6	+(x+y)	+(x)	—

A schematic table based on Sell and Gell's results. x and y are the proportion of lymphocytes undergoing blast transformation.

When lymphocytes from a rabbit are exposed *in vitro* to an antiserum in a goat against rabbit γ-G globulin, the lymphocytes show blast transformation and thymidine uptake just as in the analogous human experiment. It is of much more interest that similar effects, but involving a smaller proportion of lymphocytes, can be produced by anti-allotypic sera produced in rabbits on lymphocytes from an animal of appropriate genotype. The effect is specific; an anti-A1 serum will only stimulate lymphocytes from rabbits with 1 in their genotype, and can be additive in heterozygotes (see table 3). Unlike the position with human cells, mixing of allotypically different lymphocyte populations does not induce mutual blast transformation. Further, none of the new protein synthesized during the blast transformation can be identified as immunoglobulin and, finally, lymphocytes from neonatal rabbits possessing only maternal allotypes in their immunoglobulins and making none of their own react with antisera corresponding to their genotype and the antigenic types of immunoglobulin that they will *subsequently* produce.

The implications of these facts are of first-rate importance for immunological theory and provide the first direct evidence for the presence of *genetically determined receptors of immunoglobulin character on lymphocytes* (including cells from very young animals) showing no other evidence of immunoglobulin production. They point, too, to the existence of phenotypic restriction allowing the production of only one type of light or heavy chain by any given cell in a heterozygous animal. The 'choice' as to which of two alternatives will be produced appears to be a random one. The next implication is that both heavy (Ig G type) and light chains are or may be present in the receptors. It does not, however, establish whether light and heavy chains are combined in the receptors in the same fashion as in immunoglobulins.

One might summarize by saying that experiments of this type confirm the lymphocyte as an immunocyte of which the immunoglobulin production is determined by genetic information, with phenotypic restriction to single chromosomes and that the first phase of specific stimulation is mitosis and proliferation, not immunoglobulin production. This is all precisely in line with clonal selection theory as formulated in 1958. There are, however, several areas still to be cleared up. It is not established that the antibody specificity of the receptor is present before the capacity to produce immunoglobulin develops, and there is no evidence for or against the contention that the combining site of antibody may have a genetic determination distinct from that of the antigenic determinants of light and heavy chains.

In the rabbit, mixtures of lymphocytes theoretically capable of reacting one with the other show no increase in blast transformation and when lymphocytes from a rabbit hyperimmunized against a foreign allotype are exposed to the corresponding allotypic serum only a few cells show a response.

There is thus only a limited amount of direct experimental evidence to support the contention that cells can carry specific immune patterns without having had any contact with the antigens used to detect them. Nevertheless the evidence in its limited fields is unequivocal and there is no valid evidence that is equally unequivocal in locating any source of immune pattern other than the genetic mechanism of the cell.

THE PHARMACOLOGY OF ANTIGENIC STIMULATION

General principles

Before considering the influence of antigen on cell receptors it is of interest to look at the modern approach to the nature of drug action. In general, there is recognition that a cellular receptor must be postulated for any response being investigated and that the action of drugs will depend on the effective concentration of drug in relation to receptor and the affinity as judged by k_1/k_2—respectively the association and dissociation constants for drug–receptor substance interaction. In terms of Paton's 'rate' theory, stimulant action is proportional to the rate of association between drug molecule and receptor; receptors become free for further stimulation by dissociation. If a drug is rapidly and almost irreversibly adsorbed, for example, in the action of nicotine on ganglion cells, there is a primary stimulation followed by a state experimentally indistinguishable from competitive inhibition.

Paton's point of view was used by A. Shulman to discuss the nature of pharmacological differences between drugs of the same general structure but differing in the nature of the substituents at appropriate positions in the molecule. The series he used were substituted glutarimides acting on the CNS (probably on cells of the ascending reticular formation) and giving a range of activity which, having regard both for drug structure and dosage, covered convulsant, analeptic, anti-convulsant, and hypnotic actions. Analysis of competitive actions between, for example, hypnotic and analeptic drugs indicated that common receptors were involved with results that could be quantitatively covered by appropriate elaboration of Paton's point of view. The dissociation constant k_2 is of primary importance in determining whether a drug functions as agonist, partial agonist or antagonist. On Shulman's view, a hypnotic is such by virtue of its power to block an endogenous stimulant.

This introduces a point of much importance both for pharmacology and immunology—the necessity of recognizing that any postulated cell receptor must in one way or another be associated with some normal cellular function. The clonal selection theory adopts the reasonable view that the immuno-receptors are in fact a specially evolved type of organelle integrated into the cell structure for the specific purpose of immune reaction. This does not, however, eliminate the possibility that such receptors may be stimulated in some nonspecific fashion or that there may be a 'final common path' for both immuno-receptor and some other type of receptor adapted, for example, to react to a thymic or other hormone.

Another feature which at present seems to be unique to the immunological field is the possibility of effectively replacing a genetically determined receptor with antibody present in the circulation. Such cytophilic antibody must always present a major difficulty in interpreting cellular reactions to antigen.

In interpreting immunological reactions, pharmacological principles are probably specially relevant in relation to the action of antigen on the genetically determined receptors of immunocytes. Basically similar considerations, however, will be equally relevant to the action of antigen on antibody more or less adventitiously attached to cells as exemplified, in all probability, by the liberation of histamine in passive anaphylactic experiments and from basophil leucocytes from allergic subjects following contact with the specific antigen. From this it is a simple further step to become involved in the cytotoxic action of antibody on cells carrying the corresponding antigen, and the reactivity and toxicity of antigen–antibody complexes.

Application to immunocyte stimulation

In interpreting the nature of cellular immuno-receptors, we must necessarily use soluble antibody as a conceptual model but be prepared to find the same sorts of relatively minor types of specificity difference that have been demonstrated between antibody reactions *in vitro* and the response to delayed hypersensitivity tests.

In regard to specific adsorptive capacity it is now well known that in an antiserum produced in response to immunization with an appropriate hapten–carrier combination there are antibody molecules for which, when tested with the hapten, association constants vary over a 100–1,000-fold range. In other words, for any given hapten there are many more or less similar configurations of combining sites with which reaction is physically detectable, but the chance of specific pharmacological response will presumably become increasingly rare as the association constant becomes smaller.

Other factors to be considered at the pharmacological level will be (*a*) the physical properties of the carrier of the antigenic determinant in so far as it influences the kinetics of association and dissociation and (*b*) the number and accessibility of the cell receptors. By hypothesis there are no immuno-receptors at all until the cell line has been differentiated in the thymus or elsewhere and it is reasonably certain that the number of receptors will be low until antigenic stimulation has occurred. (*c*) At the receptor–drug (antigen) reaction level we are only concerned with the initiation or blocking of stimulation. Once stimulation has been achieved, the result in terms of cell behaviour will depend on the physiological state of the cell, particularly as determined by the state of the internal micro-environment in the immediate neighbourhood of the cell.

At the present time it is not practicable to apply conventional pharmacological approaches to all the situations of interest. Attention may, however, be drawn to the following points elaborated either in the immediately following sections or in later chapters, all of which have pharmacological relevance.

(*a*) The influence of antigen dose (and age of the animal) in determining tolerance or positive immune response.

(*b*) The ability of specific antibody to prevent the initiation of a primary response to antigen in much smaller dose than is necessary to block a secondary response.

(*c*) The fact that in the presence of an adequate concentration of an immunosuppressive drug, a dose of antigen that would otherwise act as an active stimulus to antibody production can produce tolerance, presumably by destruction of the reactive immunocytes.

THE RESPONSE TO SPECIFIC ANTIGENIC STIMULATION

When we are concerned with the general problem of the responses of immunocytes to their specific antigen we have to work mainly on indirect evidence derived from the behaviour of large cell populations from immune animals. It is legitimate, however, to develop the implication of these experiments in the light of what has been drawn from the work we have just been considering on cells from unimmunized normal animals.

It is our contention that the result of contact of an immunocyte with the corresponding antigenic determinant will depend on a variety of factors involving the antigen, the physiological state of the cell and the internal environment in which contact takes place. The effect may be (*a*) mitosis and proliferation, (*b*) accelerated differentiation to the plasma cell series, (*c*) development to a 'memory' clone of lymphocytes, (*d*) surface damage with liberation of pharmacologically active cell products or (*e*) death with autolysis and/or pyknosis of nuclei.

As in so much of immunology, supporting evidence for each aspect of this statement is limited to a small number of well-worked out experimental situations plus fragmentary pieces of confirmatory evidence from a wide variety of sources.

Mitosis and proliferation

The primary postulate of any selective theory of immunity must be that, under some circumstances at least, contact of antigen with lymphoid cell of appropriate immune pattern must stimulate its selective proliferation. The evidence that this occurs *in vivo* will be considered later. Here we limit ourselves to *in vitro* studies, notably those of Dutton and his collaborators. Their work indicates that spleen cells from a rabbit immunized some months previously and 'primed' *in vitro* by a brief exposure to antigen show within 24 hours a rapid uptake of labelled thymidine. The technique is a versatile and convenient one and has allowed the recognition of some important additional points. The first is that stimulation of such cell suspensions is not necessarily specific. Phytohaemagglutinin, zymosan and staphylococcal extracts were all effective. If the cell suspension was irradiated, priming with antigen gave rise to only a minor uptake of label. Evidence of a specific effect could, however, be established by mixing such primed but inactive cells with normal unprimed cells themselves incapable of taking up more than trivial amounts of label. The mixture showed a greatly increased uptake. The irradiated cells had clearly been specifically stimulated to produce a transmissible agent, presumably as a first stage to the initiation of DNA synthesis which, though inactive in the irradiated cell, was available to initiate the process in adjacent unstimulated cells. The simplest, though not of course the only interpretation, is that the primary effect is to liberate one or a number of pharmacologically active agents which provide the more immediate stimulus to mitosis. This would ascribe the nonspecific stimulation by phytohaemagglutinin, etc., to a similar type of activation and is in line with its known effects on human lymphocytes. This effect by which adjacent cells are stimulated as a result of specific antigen–cell interaction is likely to become important for understanding the interaction between thymus-dependent cells and immunocytes of other primary origin.

In several instances it has been shown that the initial protein synthetic activity induced by contact with antigen is not associated with increased immunoglobulin production but is mainly or wholly production of structural cellular protein. Most of the detailed work on blast transformation has made use of phytohaemagglutinin stimulation, and it remains to be proved whether this process has any close relationship to the proliferative activity induced in primed cells appropriately stimulated by antigen. As far as it is relevant it is clear that in the first stages by which a lymphocyte develops into a pyroninophil blast cell there is no more than trivial development of the endoplasmic reticulum which characterizes the plasmacytic series. If it is true that the progenitor immunocytes associated with delayed hypersensitivity should be differentiated quite sharply from those from which antibody-producing cells arise, some of these difficulties disappear. If the blast transformation involves only cells of the delayed hypersensitivity series no plasma cell formation would be expected.

Accelerated differentiation in the plasma cell line
The data from experiments by Jerne's antibody-plaque technique and from Nossal's studies on the rat popliteal node seem to be best interpreted on the basis of slowly multiplying blast cells being stimulated to combined proliferation and progressive differentiation to mature plasma cells. There is still scope for eventual interpretation of the phenomenon of plasma-cell clone production in terms involving transfer of information from genetically deter-

mined cells to neutral 'nurse cells'. The pros and cons of this point of view are discussed in another section. From the present approach the alternatives are (*a*) the stimulation of a blast cell to give by proliferation a clone of plasma cells, or (*b*) the stimulation of an immunocyte to produce alone or, in addition to (*a*), transferable units of information (equivalent either to transforming principle (DNA) or to virus RNA) which can induce cells not in the same genetic line to give rise to a plasma cell clone.

Development of a memory clone of lymphocytes
The appearance of germinal centres is a characteristic sign of immunological activity, and there is evidence from immunofluorescence studies that germinal centres may be associated with antibody or immunoglobulin production at a low level. So far as one can deduce from indirect evidence, a germinal centre represents a centre of replication arising from a stimulated immunocyte. Germinal centres arise only in lymphoid tissue, and a large proportion of the newly formed cells pass to the blood and are widely distributed throughout the other lymphoid tissue of the body with the exception of the thymus. The simplest way to account for persisting immunological memory is to accept the production by each germinal centre, as it arises, of a large clone of lymphoid cells, a large proportion of which lodge as small or medium lymphocytes in various peripheral lymphoid tissues. In the absence of new entry of the corresponding antigen the survival of the clone (and of 'memory') will depend on (*a*) the numbers of lymphocytes produced during the immunizing episode and (*b*) the existence and extent of nonspecific stimuli to random immunocyte proliferation.

The relative absence of 'memory' in circumstances where antibody production is almost or wholly confined to Ig M has not been adequately explained, and interpretation has been complicated by the report of at least one example of a wholly Ig M secondary response. There is some basis for the suggestion that any immunocytes in which a significant proportion of receptors are blocked by union with antigenic determinant are incapable of giving rise to small lymphocyte descendants. They may become plasma cells, but these are end-cells and, once the stage of the mature plasma cell is reached, there is no evidence that this can by de-differentiation or otherwise ever become capable of mitosis and proliferation. In chapter 10 the effectiveness of specific antibody, particularly in the form of Ig G, in inhibiting further recruitment of Ig M antibody producers and perhaps accelerating the switch from Ig M to Ig G producers, is described. This may allow a proportion of the immunocytes to proliferate as memory cells which would otherwise have gone on to mature (end-cell) plasmacytes producing Ig M.

Stimulation of lymphocytes to produce pharmacologically active products of cell damage

Much of the recent discussion on cell damage associated with immune reaction has centred on the function of lysosomes. These are organelles visible in electron microscopic sections of a variety of cells. They are characterized primarily as containing acid phosphatase and a variety of other hydrolytic enzymes and seem to represent a heterogeneous group of structures. They are specially characteristic of polymorphonuclear leucocytes and macrophages but may also be found in lymphocytes and most other cell types. It has been suggested that they arise from pinocytosis vesicles and represent essentially organs for intracellular digestion.

A variety of cytotoxic influences can induce discharge of the lysosomes which may be either the immediate cause of cell death or one of the manifestations of the process. None of the defined components of lysosomes have specific pharmacological effects but it is probable that, associated with their disruption, proteolytic enzymes capable of producing peptide kinins, etc., will be activated.

Other aspects of cell damage possibly concerned in immune reactions are all somewhat uncertain. The part played by histamine is undoubted but general opinion is that the liberation of histamine is wholly a function of mast cells and basophils. The nature of the relationship, if any, of mast cells to immunocytes is problematical but there is no doubt that they can, in an immunized animal, be stimulated to liberate histamine and degranulate. The existence of the change from thymocytes to mast cells in some strains of mice may suggest that all immunocytes have some capacity to liberate histamine on stimulation but this has not been demonstrated.

Most of the information that bears directly upon the reaction of lymphocytes with antigens to which some of the cells in a population are sensitized is clouded by the heterogeneity of all natural cell populations and the impossibility of obtaining more than a partial purification of any particular cell type such as small lymphocytes. Peritoneal exudates on which much of the work has been done are particularly difficult to interpret.

Further difficulties have arisen recently from the finding that nonspecific stimulation of lymphocytes by phytohaemagglutinin can result in a cytotoxic reaction against foreign cells, a reaction in which there is no overt evidence of antibody or immune patterns playing any part whatever.

Without being able to provide complete documentation for each component of the interpretation, the following account seems to be in accord with the experimental facts.

Any lymphocyte is a relatively vulnerable cell and when combination of antigen with antibody or immune receptor takes place on the cell surface, stimulation or damage results. In the presence of complement, destruction probably mainly by autolysis is common, provided the antigen–antibody reaction is a vigorous one. It is immaterial, in broad terms, whether the lymphocyte carries antigen on its surface or antibody (which may be either immune receptor or attached cytophilic antibody) or even whether a preformed antigen–antibody complex of the right physical character becomes attached to the cell surface. In every one of these situations there is evidence that damage may occur—often not readily demonstrable unless complement is present.

There are at least two types of experiment which indicate that antigenic stimulation of some of the cells in a lymphocytic population can produce similar results in normal cells. One is the uptake of tritiated thymidine; the other, adhesion of lymphocytes in culture when cells from a sensitized animal are exposed to the sensitizing antigen. In both cases it appears that specific stimulation by antigen produces, concomitantly with the effect being studied, liberation of active substances which confer presumably by simple pharmacological action the same effect on any normal lymphoid cells in the system. Probably closely related is the capacity of distinct populations of mouse lymphoid cells to react with mutual damage if they differ by major histocompatibility antigens even without any type of cross-immunization.

Death of immunocytes following reaction with antigen
It is obvious that in the body there is a high mortality of lymphocytes, particularly evident in the thymus but probably also occurring in all other regions. Death and autolysis is the normal fate of probably 99 per cent of lymphocytes: antigen–antibody contact on the surface will, under many circumstances, be the extra stimulus which determines the actual time of cell death. Indirect evidence suggests that once a clone of cells is developing to mature plasma cells it has entered an irreversible path but, equally, there is no evidence that an excess of antigen has any damaging effect on plasmablasts or plasma cells actively synthesizing antibody. In the discussion of tolerance in the next chapter it will be assumed that tolerance represents either the elimination of all reactive immunocytes or their direction into the irreversible plasma cell development.

GENERALIZATION OF THE RESULTS OF IMMUNOCYTE–ANTIGEN INTERACTION

At this stage it seems appropriate to try to provide a formulation of the results of effective contact between immunocyte and the corresponding antigenic determinant which can be used in the interpretation of such phenomena as delayed hypersensitivity and desensitization or antibody production, tolerance and auto-immune disease. In all of these, antigen–cell contact is obviously a critical step in the phenomena. In essence it is based on the central theme of the clonal selection approach that the combining site of antibody or cell receptor is a pattern produced by a random genetic process.

As in many other aspects of biology it is extremely difficult to present the general characteristics of immune reactions in any sort of a logical sequence. In this attempt to generalize the results of immunocyte–antigen interaction it will be necessary to anticipate some of the discussion in later chapters but it is felt that in its turn the attitude schematized in figs 6 and 22 will be helpful in later discussions.

The importance of avidity
If the pattern of the combining site as it emerges on differentiation is wholly random, then, for any given antigenic determinant,

whether it is carried by a self-component or only on foreign macromolecules, there will be a range of newly differentiated immunocytes with avidity ranging from nil or negligible to a maximum determined by the still unknown potentialities of amino acid residue disposition in the combining site. One can be certain, however, that the distribution of immunocytes graded by avidity for a given antigen determinant will show a peak for those with minimal avidity and a progressive diminution of numbers as avidity increases (fig. 6). The highly avid combining site must always be very rare for the same reason that the chance of being dealt a complete suit in a hand of bridge is vanishingly small.

The process by which antibody against any antigenic determinant is developed will depend on the circumstances that allow cells with avidity in the higher ranges to be stimulated to multiply on contact with the antigenic determinant. Since the patterns by hypothesis are wholly random, capacity to combine with the antigenic determinant is the only quality which is relevant.

Our problem is to devise a means of predicting the result of combination between cell receptor and antigenic determinant under various defined conditions. From first principles, one could feel confident that both the concentration of antigenic determinant, and the avidity of interaction between combining site and antigenic determinant, would play a part. From our general knowledge of immune reactions we can also be certain that the response of an immunocyte is not simply proportional to the product of concentration and avidity. Both the way in which the antigenic determinant is presented to the cell and the physiological state of the immunocyte obviously play a part.

In an attempt to find a useful way to express the situation fig. 22 has been devised in which the ordinates and abscissae are the avidity of antigenic determinant–combining site union and the effective concentration of antigenic determinant respectively. Avidity between antigenic determinant and combining site has been extensively studied by Karush, Eisen and others using soluble haptens as antigenic determinant. It can be expressed as an adsorption coefficient, K_a, but as there is only limited quantitative experimental work it will often be necessary to use some qualitative index of higher or lower avidity. The term 'effective concentration of antigen' (or antigenic determinant) represents a complex function of concentration and time of exposure as qualified by the physical presentation of the antigen determinant to the cell. No single value can be attached to it in any physiological situation and information from *in vitro* studies can only be used cautiously and at the qualitative level in interpreting natural situations.

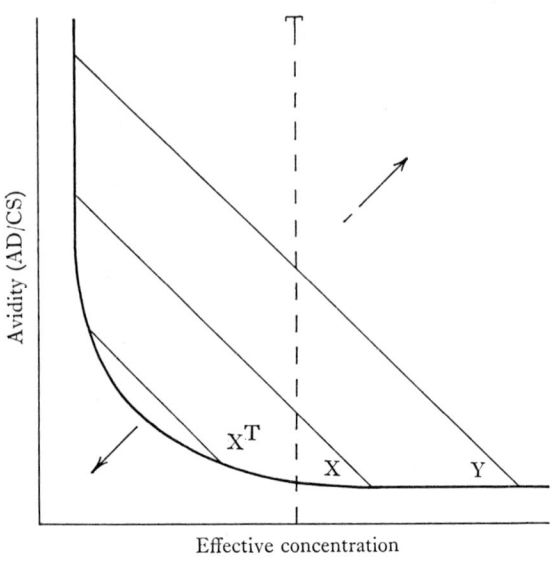

Fig. 22. To illustrate the concept that the result of specific contact of antigenic determinant and immunocyte may be either destructive or stimulating to specific activity, depending (*a*) on the affinity of receptor–A D union, (*b*) on the 'effective concentration' of the antigenic determinant and (*c*) on the physiological state of the immunocyte.

Destruction is more likely above and to the right of the diagonal line; proliferation and antibody production, below and to the left.

A wide variety of experimental approaches shows that small doses of antigen tend to promote proliferation and antibody production, while larger ones lead to tolerance and paralysis. On this basis, fig. 22 has been constructed.

It is obvious that if there is no antigenic determinant in the system or if the combining site has no avidity for it then there can be no response. There will therefore be a threshold for any response indicated by the rectangular hyperbola. On this can be drawn diagonal lines which can be taken as marking the zone on one side of which proliferative and antibody-producing responses to contact with antigen determinant will predominate while, on the other, destruction will be characteristic. The arrow indicates, upwards and to the right, increasing likelihood of destruction (producing tolerance and paralysis) or lesser degrees of damage associated with liberation of pharmacologically active agents (perhaps concerned with delayed hypersensitivity reactions). Downwards and to the left the arrow indicates that above the null thresholds the smallest concentration of antibody is likely to be the most effective in provoking antibody production and the production of memory cells.

Changed cell reactivity

Irrespective of whether immunocytes undergo their primary differentiation in the thymus or elsewhere, there is general agreement that their first stage is one in which it can react with antigen but not by production of antibody. This has been called by various names: 'progenitor immunocyte', 'uncommitted cell', 'antigen reactive cell', or 'X cell'. For simplicity we shall use 'X cell', following Sercarz and Coons.

The effect of contact with antigen determinant is to convert an X cell into a Y cell (for which 'committed cell', 'plaque-forming cell' and 'memory cell' are approximately equivalent terms). Further antigenic stimulation will provoke Y cells to give rise to a clone of plasma cells (Z) or further generations of Y cells (memory cells).

There is evidence that X cells can be prevented from effective stimulation to Y cells either by the presence of preformed antibody of the same specificity or of an excess of the antigen concerned. Cells in the Y state are significantly less susceptible to either. In the diagram, therefore, line Y lies considerably to the upper right of line X.

It is an essential postulate of this approach that the general rules expressed by fig. 22 will hold under any circumstances where immunocytes and antigenic determinants react, with the necessary qualification 'other things being equal'. To a first simplifying assumption 'other things' will act by changing the position of the diagonal that lies at right angles to the double-headed arrow.

Response to specific stimulation

There are two sets of controlling factors which need special consideration, the local tissue environment and the effect of somatic mutation on an immunocyte line. The influence of drugs and hormones may also be important but is not immediately relevant.

In addition to factors which can modify the process that controls the response, there are implications of fig. 22 for the temporal course of antibody production and the relative avidity of antibody at different stages that are of great interest.

The local environment

The special features of the thymic environment have already been discussed. On general grounds, one would expect that somewhat similar situations can occur in germinal centres of lymph nodes and spleen, i.e. the standard position of the diagonal is displaced downward and to the left.

The other environment of special interest is the complex anatomical situation of the granuloma produced by antigen injected with Freund's complete adjuvant, and the draining lymph nodes. As will be discussed at a later stage, there are several pointers that favour the hypothesis that immunization with Freund's complete adjuvant results in a higher proportion of high-avidity immunocytes and antibody than is the case without adjuvant. This would mean that in the environment of the Freund granuloma and its draining lymph nodes the diagonal of our diagram is moved to the upper right. Despite what must be a relatively high antigen concentration, immunocytes of high avidity can proliferate to give memory cells and antibody-producing cells.

Any such statement has as a corollary that immunocytes of high avidity can arise and that they do not normally proliferate as a result of simple contact with antigen. On the random origin of pattern hypothesis we are using, in the uncommitted lymphocytes of the body there will be a range of immunocytes including some very rare ones with extreme avidity. One must assume that when a union of high avidity takes place in the germinal centre there is a strong probability that the cell will be destroyed and become visible as a necrotic pyknotic nucleus. We can reasonably assume that a small concentration of thymic hormone will be associated with primary nodules and germinal centres and that it will be absent in the Freund granuloma. Following this, our hypothesis becomes that in the complex antigen-containing environment of the Freund granuloma the most avid cells are allowed or even stimulated preferentially to multiply instead of being lethally influenced, as would be the case under more physiological conditions.

Somatic mutation

Quite apart from the origin of immune pattern there are other possibilities of results arising from somatic mutation. If the local environmental changes or drugs can shift the diagonal line of our diagram, it is reasonably certain that there are also somatic mutations that could result in equivalent positive or negative cellular changes. If the mutation favours destruction of the cell concerned, nothing more will be heard of it but, as is the case in every evolutionary situation, if the mutation favours proliferation under the existent conditions, the mutant form will become evident. In the present circumstances only a mutation shifting the diagonal towards the upper right will have any significance. If, for example, such a mutation involved a cell capable of reacting with an autologous red cell antigen freely present in the thymic environment, movement of the line XT in the upper right direction would result in the escape from the thymus of *low avidity* cells capable of producing the equivalent incomplete antibody recognizable by a positive indirect Coombs test but not producing haemagglutination or haemolysis *in vitro* (see fig. 26).

It is immaterial how rare may be the concurrence of such a mutation with an immune pattern of the appropriate quality. Only one cell may be needed to initiate a pathogenic clone and there is evidence already that in a majority of cases of warm-type haemolytic anaemia the antibody that can be eluted from the patient's red cells is of monoclonal origin.

Combination of a similar mutation with immune pattern directed against a foreign antigenic determinant would rarely become evident but could be suspected whenever an individual being immunized gave an exceptionally active antibody response. There is a recent report which could be interpreted as a particularly striking example in which a burst of what appeared to be monoclonal antibody was seen in one of several rabbits immunized by a streptococcal antigen. No information as to the avidity of the antibody–antigen union in this case was provided.

Another possible field in which examples may be found is in the drug-induced purpuras and haemolytic anaemias in which binding of drug by antibody is demonstrable. Most of these diseases involve only a small proportion of those taking the drug and the likelihood is that only those persons who in one way or another can produce a highly avid type of combining site will be candidates for this type of drug reaction.

The significance of avidity changes in the course of immunization
Eisen has pointed out that, strictly speaking, 'affinity' is the correct term to use when one is discussing the intrinsic association constant for the reversible binding of simple antigenic determinants by antibodies. 'Avidity' is a looser term used by conventional immunologists to cover the overall binding activity of an antigen with perhaps many different types of determinant and a heterogeneous antibody population. It is convenient, however, when one must deal with a variety of situations to use 'avidity' at times with the strict meaning of affinity and at other times in the looser sense.

From the studies of dinitrophenyl (DNP) haptens and antibodies made in various laboratories and summarized in Eisen's 1964 Harvey Lectures, two points arise of special significance for our general approach. These are (*a*) that when a rabbit is injected with a single small dose of a DNP-immunogen in Freund's complete adjuvant, the avidity of the antibody present in the circulation rises about a hundred-fold in a six-week period and (*b*) that when 20–50 times that dose is given the rise in avidity does not occur.

This combined situation is of special interest in relation to the standard diagram of immunocyte response (fig. 22). With a very small circulating concentration of antigen, progenitor immunocytes of very high avidity for DNP-lysine will occasionally be stimulated by antigen to commitment and, at once, become more resistant against destruction by antigen contact unless a high concentration of antigen is encountered. If the concentration of antigen is very low the likelihood of effective stimulation of committed cells will be higher for cells with more avid immune receptors than for cells of low avidity. The figure shows that there will therefore be a build-up of high avidity antibody as long as the effective level of circulating antigen is maintained very low, as is the case where it is being slowly liberated from a Freund granuloma.

We have already (p. 121) adopted the point of view that as long as antibody is circulating the likelihood of a progenitor immunocyte being committed is very small. The subsequent history of a primed animal is therefore dependent almost wholly on the behaviour of committed cells and their descendants. New progenitor immunocytes that could react are prevented from doing so by the presence of antibody. As far as this particular reaction is concerned the thymus has no function. One might have predicted in fact the recent finding from Miller's laboratory that when a neonatally thymectomized mouse is supplied with adequate numbers of thoracic duct lymphocytes from normal syngeneic mice it produces antibody in normal fashion. Cells once committed are independent of any thymic control and do not require fresh recruitment of primary immunocytes.

AVIDITY AND DELAYED HYPERSENSITIVITY

Much of the interest in the functional significance of avidity for immune reactions stems from the hypothesis of Karush and Eisen that delayed hypersensitivity represents the result of reaction between antigen and very low concentrations of highly avid circulating antibody. This was presented as an alternative to the dominant theory that delayed hypersensitivity and the closely related homograft immunity were cellular reactions. On the whole, the evidence points away from the importance of antibody, avid or otherwise, in delayed hypersensitivity but an extension of the concept of heterogeneity in avidity to the immunocytes could be highly relevant.

A quantitative study of desensitization of guinea-pigs using crystalline human serum albumin points strongly against the suggestion that delayed hypersensitivity is essentially a reaction between high affinity antibody and antigen. The central feature of the results is that when sensitized guinea-pigs are desensitized with human serum albumin intravenously they will remain reactive to large enough challenge doses even while significant amounts of antigen can be shown to be present in the circulating plasma.

All investigators are agreed that when the challenge dose of antigen is deposited intradermally the immunological reactant, be it antibody or cells, reaches the site from the circulation. The presence of small amounts of antigen in the circulating plasma would undoubtedly remove the postulated minute amounts of high affinity antibody. On the alternative theory which we favour, there are in the circulation lymphocytes derived from the lymph nodes draining the antigen deposit, which are immunocytes *vis à vis* human serum albumin. These cells will have variable avidity for antigen but, when effective contact is made, changes in the cell surface of a circulating cell will result in a very high probability that it is removed from the circulation, presumably in lymphoid tissue. This variable avidity or affinity may well involve both differences in the pattern of the combining site and of its relative accessibility to antigen in cells with the same combining site.

As Silverstein and Borek point out, their results point to a heterogeneity of affinity in the lymphocytes responsible for delayed hypersensitivity. If one accepts Spector and Willoughby's general interpretation of the tuberculin and similar reactions, movement through the local vascular endothelium is primarily nonspecific. When, however, specific immunocytes of high enough reactivity (avidity) enter the region where the antigen is present in relatively high concentration, they suffer a damaging reaction. This results in the release of a variety of pharmacologically active reagents. Among the effects of these on record are modification of the cell surface of other lymphocytes and monocytes leading to their diminished mobility and retention in the area of the reaction, and increased permeability of the local capillary endothelium allowing the entry of further specific immunocytes and other mobile blood cells.

On this view, the administration of a desensitizing dose of antigen intravenously will greatly reduce the proportion of circulating high avidity immunocytes and, to a progressively lesser extent, those of lower avidity for the antigen in question. A glance at fig. 20

will make it evident that in such partially depleted animals a higher local concentration of antigen will be necessary to produce a demonstrable damaging reaction.

THE ORIGIN OF THE PLASMA CELL

Plasma cells are the major producers of antibody and the most striking histological feature of a secondary immune response is the rapid production of clones of plasma cells. The evidence is clear that plasma cells arise as clones derived from blast cells. They are characteristically found in close relation to small blood vessels and a number of histologists have claimed that they arise from perivascular cells. There is no doubt that when primed lymphoid cells from spleen or lymph node are placed in Millipore chambers in an isologous host, or injected into a heavily X-irradiated host, they respond to specific antigen by the production of numerous plasma cells. The precise origin of such cells is still unknown.

There is no shadow of doubt (*a*) that thoracic duct lymphocytes in which plasma cells and blasts are rare carry the information needed to allow antibody production, (*b*) that such cells can be converted into pyroninophil blasts which can undergo mitosis and (*c*) that most antibody is produced by cells of the plasmacyte series. There is no adequate evidence against the view that a small lymphocyte stimulated by antigen and in the right physiological environment will become a pyroninophilic blast from which proliferation and differentiation in the plasma cell series can develop. Equally it must be emphasized that there is no unequivocal positive evidence that this actually occurs.

A second possibility arises if there is any process by which genetic information capable of directing antibody pattern can be transferred to another somatic cell line genetically lacking that information. If antigen passes to a lymph node and there stimulates an appropriately patterned immunocyte to produce large numbers of information transfer units, we can conceive of these passing to any available blast cells and directing them to develop along the plasma cell line. There is no direct evidence in favour of this interpretation but a good deal of puzzling indirect evidence and nothing to veto it unequivocally.

Response to specific stimulation

At the present time it seems desirable to keep any ideas of inter-cell transfer of information in the background and to put the main emphasis on the experiments by Jerne's technique, which point rather directly to a direct proliferation to plasma cells of genetically determined lines. The process already mentioned on several occasions by which immunocyte–antigen reactions can modify adjacent cells may be relevant here. There are indications that a quiescent immunocyte of non-thymic origin needs to be activated in some way before it reacts with its corresponding antigenic determinant. The simplest way this could occur in a lymph node situation where a variety of antigens are likely to be available is for reaction by a thymus-dependent cell with *its* antigen to provide the nonspecific stimulus needed.

9 Antibody production

In this chapter we are concerned with the actual process of antibody production and only incidentally with the special character of antibody and the qualities that differentiate one antibody from another. It will be impossible to avoid some overlap with earlier and later chapters. What is being attempted is to bring together what has been discussed earlier in regard to the patterns of immune specificity and the cells concerned in immunity and to describe them in action. As everywhere in immunology it is impossible to provide a general interpretation that can be tested against each of the major areas available for study. Variability and heterogeneity are of the essence of the problem, there are 'good' antigens and 'poor' antigens in the sense of the amount required to provoke a measurable response and, for most antibodies to 'good' antigens, methods of assay are almost all still at the level of functional titration rather than truly quantitative estimation.

It follows that data obtained by the use of a good antigen like phage $T2$ or $\phi X 174$ are very hard to compare with those obtained with a pure soluble antigen of relatively low antigenicity such as bovine serum albumin. The choice of what is to be taken as most significant in the observations must therefore be rather intuitive than logical—a choice in fact among possible formulations of those which require least distortion to cover phenomena distant from those on which they were primarily developed.

ANTIBODY PRODUCTION FROM THE SELECTIVIST APPROACH

'The production of antibody' is a rather equivocal phrase particularly when one adopts a thoroughgoing selectivist approach. On this view, any immunocyte that can react with an antigen is a producer of antibody in the sense that the cell receptors have all the essential immune pattern of an antibody. Further, there is increasing evidence that all lymphocytes of the immunocyte series release

Antibody production

small amounts of immunoglobulins into their environment. The synthesis is of quite a different order of magnitude from the massive production of immunoglobulin by developing or mature plasma cells.

In general this chapter deals with the production of effective amounts of antibody by cells of the plasma cell series. This is a matter that can be looked at from several points of view, depending essentially on the type of experimental observation being considered.

1. For many types of experiment, what is convenient to follow is the amount or concentration of immunoglobulin or some physical fraction such as the conventional 'γ-globulin' of simple electrophoresis. At this level we have two important questions to put: (a) What are the homeostatic mechanisms that keep the dynamic equilibrium concentration of γ-globulin in the blood approximately constant in health? (b) Is all γ-globulin antibody in the sense of carrying specific combining sites or are there wholly nonspecific globulins as well?

2. We have already described the physical differences among the three types of immunoglobulin having antibody function and indicated broadly the functional significance of the differences between A, G and M immunoglobulins in antibody function. There is a great deal to suggest that their specificity, their combining sites, are essentially identical or, more correctly, that they will show the same range of heterogeneity in each type. At this level we have three major questions: (a) What determines in a given immune response whether A, G or M is produced? (b) What changes in addition to M to G are possible within the same cell line? (c) Are there individual homeostatic mechanisms for each type?

3. It is axiomatic that, for the production of substantial amounts of antibody, an antigenic stimulus is necessary. This holds as much for a selection theory of antibody production as for an 'instructive' one. It is also evident that some antigens are much more effective stimulants to antibody production than others, and that the physical state of an antigen and its administration with or without adjuvant substance may also have great effect upon the antibody response. At this level we have the questions: (a) What is the process by which antigen initiates the sequence which leads to antibody forma-

tion? (b) What part do the cells which *par excellence* take up foreign material, macrophages and polymorphonuclear leucocytes play in the process? (c) What are the actual antigenic determinants concerned?

4. Finally, we have the striking difference between the primary and the secondary immune response, particularly when certain types of antigen are used. Since an active secondary response is the most characteristic form of antibody production and has been the most extensively studied, it will be convenient to begin the discussion of antibody production with this theme.

THE SECONDARY-TYPE RESPONSE

If a rabbit or a rat has been immunized some months previously with an antigen, bovine serum albumin or *Salmonella* flagella for example, and now has a minimal or no detectable antibody titre, it will respond predictably and strongly to a second injection of the same antigen. If the injection is made locally, e.g. into a hind footpad, the regional lymph node will rapidly enlarge and, by three to four days, there will be a greatly increased proportion of plasma cells in the node. Antibody, almost wholly of Ig G type, will appear and show a rapidly rising titre in the blood.

A situation closely resembling this, though ostensibly a primary response, has already been described for the rapid increase in cells producing Ig M antibody in the spleen of a mouse immunized by sheep red cells. Analysis of the situation in the lymph node following a secondary stimulus leads to the same conclusion. The entry of antigen results in the rapid proliferation of cells to form clones, the members of which become progressively closer to the mature plasma cell type.

The plasma cell is unequivocally the major producer of antibody and its intracellular structure with complex endoplasmic reticulum is specialized for this function. The indications are that proliferation and antibody production take place concurrently until the descendant cells have reached the morphological character of mature plasma cells. Once that stage has been reached, proliferation ceases but antibody synthesis may continue for some time. The fate of the large numbers of plasma cells present at the height of a secondary immune response has never been quantitatively followed. There is a progressive diminution in numbers, presumably by death and autolysis, but individual plasma cells labelled as the product of a defined immune response may persist for as long as three to six months. Direct and circumstantial evidence both make it almost certain that the plasma cell is a differentiated end-cell incapable of giving rise to any type of descendant cell.

The origin of plasmablasts

What is still controversial is the nature and origin of the cells from which the plasmablast proliferation arises. There seem to be two formulations that cover a wide range of facts and represent two broad currents of opinion.

(a) In the previously immunized ('primed') animal, the antigen is rapidly taken up by a variety of phagocytic cells of which the most significant are the dendritic reticulum cells intimately associated with lymph follicles in lymph nodes, spleen and elsewhere. Here, a proportion of the antigen is converted to a more effective form of antigenic stimulant. A popular interpretation is that in the phagocytic cell partial proteolysis occurs and the antigenic determinant, with a few adjacent amino acids, becomes linked to a low-molecular-weight strand of RNA. This material is probably concentrated on the surface of the macrophage including its dendritic processes. A lymph follicle can be visualized as a moving three-dimensional crowd of lymphocytes from which large numbers are moving away mainly by efferent lymphatics to be replaced by approximately equal numbers arriving by the bloodstream and entering the follicle by passage through the thickened endothelium of postcapillary venules. With changing populations and as a result of their incessant active mixing movement, sooner or later lymphocytes capable of responding to a given antigen will make contact with that antigen presenting on the reticulum cell surface. Contact initiates proliferation and presumably influences both the mobility and reactivity of the cell. Either within the lymph follicle or in the course of its movement elsewhere the stimulated cell becomes a pyroninophil blast and the progenitor in the right environment of a clone of plasma cells.

This formulation can be summarized as the stimulation of a

small or medium pre-adapted lymphocyte, i.e. a committed immunocyte, by processed antigen to become a blast and initiate a plasma cell clone. Such a sequence has not been directly established but the importance of lymphocytes in allowing antibody production is undoubted.

(b) There is a need for a constant replacement of immunoglobulins in the circulation, irrespective of specific antigenic stimulation, and the second set of opinions would postulate that in some essentially random fashion some immunocytes are stimulated to take on the blast form, divide for one or two generations and produce small amounts of whatever antibody they are genetically capable of producing. The suggestion has already been made that when an immunocyte is specifically stimulated by the corresponding antigenic determinant the stimulus is mediated by the release of pharmacologically active material which could have a similar nonspecific stimulatory effect on adjacent lymphocytes. This would ensure that in any individual exposed to a natural environment there would be a random population of nonspecifically stimulated immunocytes, ripe as it were for specific stimulation. Just as in the spleen of the mice in Jerne's experiments, contact with antigen greatly accelerates the proliferation and differentiation of these cells. From this point of view it is immaterial whether the antigen is presented directly to the cells or after processing in macrophages. The most important evidence in favour of this approach is due to Nossal and Mäkelä, who found that when tritiated thymidine was given an hour before antigen most of the new plasma cells present four days later were labelled. This provides a prima facie case for the claim that the antigen was only effective in stimulating cells already in the stage of DNA synthesis for proliferation. The main weakness in this argument is that it does not wholly exclude early transfer of DNA or its molecular components from a disintegrating primarily labelled cell to others.

(c) A third possibility, that regularly or occasionally there may be a transfer of information from a cell that received it genetically to other cells capable of subserving a 'nurse' function, is better deferred.

THE PRIMARY IMMUNE RESPONSES

There is a strong current tendency to minimize differences between primary and secondary responses and to look solely for quantitative reasons for the differences actually observed. On the simplest form of selection theory one might divide the type of primary response to be expected into three categories:

(a) in which, for some genetic reason, a relatively large range of combining sites can react with the antigenic determinant in question;

(b) in which previous experience with natural (bacterial or other) antigens has increased by a specific process the number of cells which can react with the chosen antigenic determinant;

(c) in which only rare configurations of the combining site will react significantly with the chosen antigenic determinant.

Only in the third circumstance is there likely to be a clear-cut differentiation between primary and secondary responses. In practice it will always be difficult to differentiate between (a) and (b) when we are looking for a reason why a given antigen provokes an active primary response only slightly less active than a secondary one. On the other hand there are instances where the primary response seems to have a different quality from the secondary. In my own early work I was greatly impressed by the contrast between a first intravenous injection of staphylococcal α-toxoid in a rabbit and the second, two to three weeks later. The first response is minimal and delayed, the second, after a lag of about 40 hours, rises exponentially for 3 or 4 days.

There are few examples in which the difference is so evident but there are many indications that cells are functionally changed after first contact with antigen. Strictly speaking, to obtain a true primary response, an antigen should be given in a single brief 'pulse' and in one way or another be immediately eliminated or removed. An intravenous injection of toxoid may come much closer to this ideal than, for example, any immunizing situation that involves a persisting deposit of antigen or in which the antigenic determinant is not susceptible to rapid breakdown by tissue enzymes. If, at a guess, to 'commit' an immunocyte requires rapid de-differentiation and perhaps two successive divisions within two

The primary immune responses

or three days, then what is technically a secondary response could regularly be produced as a result of the primary infection or inoculation of antigen.

In line with our earlier discussion, the qualitative differences between primary and secondary response can be ascribed to an increase in the number and accessibility of immune receptors and a more 'robust' response to antigenic stimulation. Simple quantitative factors may well be even more important: there are simply more immunocytes available for stimulation by the antigenic determinants. This is probably the main or only reason for the

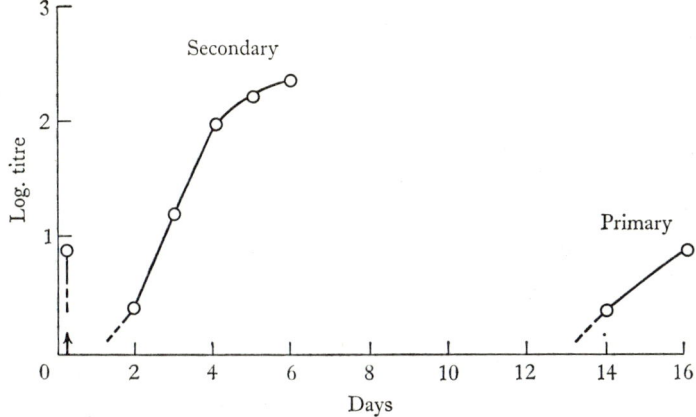

Fig. 23. Primary and secondary antitoxic response to α-staphylococcal toxoid. From F. M. Burnet (1941), *The Production of Antibodies*. Melbourne: Macmillan. Both injections given intravenously at day 0.

difference when the stimulus for the primary response is of such a character that significant amounts of antigen persist in the body for more than two or three days.

There is no reason to believe that the ways in which antigen can reach the receptor of the primarily reactive cell differ from those at work in the secondary response. The essential difference is that immunocytes of the right type are fewer in number and the requirements for stimulatory contact more strict. It is probable that the avidity of the cell receptor must be above a certain level for any stimulation to occur but also that any contact with more than minimal concentrations of antigen will have an inhibitory or destructive effect.

Foetal and neonatal production

The former generalization, that no antibody could be produced in the embryo, is no longer valid. Recent work on sheep, pigs and cattle in which there is no transfer of immunoglobulins from maternal to foetal circulation has established this quite clearly. The period of gestation at which the embryo becomes competent to produce antibody varies very markedly from one antigen to another but with a phage antigen an antibody response was obtained in foetal sheep by injection at the earliest stage, 60 days, that was experimentally feasible.

In unimmunized foetal ungulates, very small but definite amounts of Ig M develop and foetal or neonatal antibody is also at first wholly Ig M. The rather patchy evidence is all consistent in indicating that the process of tooling up for antibody production goes on at least from the period when lymphoid cells appear in the thymus. Depending on the species, there is a transfer of maternal antibody to the offspring either *in utero* or after birth by way of colostrum and milk. On current information, the antibody that passes into the later human foetus is Ig G, while that concentrated in the ungulate colostrum is Ig A. This passively transferred antibody appears to act as a temporary shield against infection and under its cover the further development of the mechanism for active immunity proceeds.

There have been suggestions that nonspecific γ-globulin was produced during the foetal and neonatal period but there is no valid evidence that the situation is any different in principle from that obtaining in postnatal life.

The change from Ig M to Ig G antibodies

Current interest in the primary response is concentrated largely on the characteristic switch seen, at least with predominantly protein antigens, from initial production of Ig M (19 S) antibody to Ig G (7 S). There is no evidence as to whether a similar switch from M to A may also occur.

In virtually every type of experimental immunization that has been reported the antibody first produced is of M type. This holds also for all 'natural' antibodies and for the antibody liberated by the splenic cells that produce Jerne plaques against sheep red cells. The characteristic methods of demonstrating the difference between M and G antibodies, susceptibility or resistance to the inactivating effect of 2-mercaptoethanol, are only applicable to antibodies which are conveniently demonstrable in tests made *in vitro*. This excludes Ig A antibodies and any Ig A or Ig M antibodies not demonstrated by the test being used.

There are some types of antibody which predominantly remain of M type; notably those produced in response to bacterial polysaccharides. It is probably an important correlate that these are also antigens which do not give any evidence of immunological memory. An animal that has responded to pneumococcal polysaccharide antigen and subsequently lost or almost lost its titre will respond to a second injection of the same type in what is apparently exactly the same fashion as a previously uninoculated animal of the same age. Recent work, however, indicates that this finding is, in part, a technical artefact. Following a first immunization, some Ig G antibody is produced appearing as usual a few days after the first appearance of Ig M antibody. Previous failure to recognize the Ig G production is due to the physical differences between the two types of antibody in relation to the distribution of somatic antigen on the bacterial surface. When compared on a molar basis, Ig M antibody may be up to a thousand times more effective than Ig G antibody in bactericidal action or as agglutinin. This depends apparently on the larger number (probably ten or twelve) of combining sites on the Ig M antibody compared with two on the Ig G molecule. On the bacterial surface, an Ig M antibody is therefore able to establish two to four points of attachment to antigenic determinants and, following appropriate collisions, to a similar number on another bacterium. By contrast, Ig G antibody can make only a single contact at each combining site, so providing a very much weaker bridge between two bacteria.

Following secondary immunization there is increased production of Ig G antibody, but the observed result is still dominated by Ig M. There is 'memory', even if it is not easily recognized, for Ig G production but the Ig M response retains the primary character.

Antibody production

The evidence suggests that the same cell line and probably the same individual cell can produce first M and later G antibody and this will be accepted as a provisional conclusion in our discussion. Direct evidence for this is limited to one set of experiments and many workers would still prefer to hold that Ig M and Ig G producers are more distinct than is accepted here.

The most important recent finding is that by administration of specific Ig G antibody to an animal producing M antibody there is induced a sharp change to G production and an almost complete inhibition of further M production. This phenomenon has some important implications. Since the effect is not given by any unrelated antibody the action must in some way involve the antigenic determinant. There is no doubt that most of the effect is a simple inhibition of the ability of antigen to act as a primary stimulus to what we have called 'progenitor immunocytes'. In addition there is presumptive evidence that the circulating Ig G antibody is able to switch some of the Ig M-antibody-producers to Ig G antibody production. This is doubted by some authors and it is not easy to provide a satisfactory explanation of the switch if it occurs. Whatever the details, there soon develops a situation in which the majority of active immunocytes are producing Ig G antibody and are committed as end-cells while an increasing concentration of G antibody will automatically prevent antigen from making initial contact with newly differentiated cells of appropriate pattern. These points follow fairly directly from the experimental data but to account for the existence of memory cells within the same framework requires some ingenuity.

'Memory cells' is a commonly used term for the cells in a previously immunized animal which, while not producing demonstrable antibody, are available for stimulation with the active antibody production characteristic of the secondary response. Always with the reservation that the actual situation is bound to be more complex than any hypothetical model, it is convenient to think of these as arising from uncommitted or committed immunocytes which, after stimulation by antigen, do not go on to form a clone of plasma cells. Either because they are cleared of antigen at an early stage or for other reasons, these cells in an appropriate internal environment can proliferate, perhaps in the form of a

The primary immune responses

germinal centre, to give rise to large numbers of descendant lymphocytes with the ancestral immune pattern—reserving the possibility that a proportion may have undergone somatic mutation.

THE POSSIBILITY OF TRANSFER OF IMMUNOLOGICAL
INFORMATION BETWEEN SOMATIC CELLS

For many years there have been insistent suggestions that somatic cells might transfer immunological information from one to another. In bacteria and viruses there are several processes by which such transfer can occur, the first to be discovered and the one most potentially relevant to immunological discussion being type transformation in pneumococci. In this, segments of DNA pass to and can be re-incorporated into the genome of suitable recipient individuals. A second phenomenon, which has often been accepted as a possible prototype of information transfer between somatic cells, is the infectivity of nucleic acid from some RNA viruses. This has a legitimate claim for consideration since the phenomena are shown with many of the small RNA viruses which infect mammalian cells. The third approach is to accept the accumulating evidence that under some conditions hybridization and segregation can occur in somatic cells.

The reasons for postulating the existence of one or other of these processes are not very substantially based on experiment. The experimental observations that are reported have almost all been obtained in an attempt to establish a preconceived idea rather than to elucidate an unforeseen observation. Most have arisen in attempts to implant immune capacity on nonimmune cells by treating them with extracts of immune cells prepared in the way by which 'infectious RNA' was obtained from some of the smaller animal viruses.

Another reason for considering the possibility arose from efforts to explain within the limits of a rigid clonal selection theory the occurrence of a proportion of cells producing more than one type of antibody, the so-called 'double producers'. If a given clone of immunocytes can produce only one pattern of antibody or immunoglobulin, the existence of a small proportion of double producers in doubly immunized animals would call for some explanation

Antibody production

in terms of transfer of immunological information between two independent lines of somatic cells. With the recognition that any acceptable present-day version of immunological theory is of necessity complex and flexible, the difficulties tend to disappear or at least become less urgent. One important possibility of understanding how nominally unrelated viruses used as antigens could on occasion react with a single type of combining region has already been raised. There are various other possibilities implicit in the interpretation of immune specificity developed in chapter 6.

In many ways it might be wise to postpone any consideration of transfer of immunological information until the experimental evidence for its existence becomes unequivocal and fully accepted. To discuss the three possibilities listed above can only be justified on the grounds of wide interest in the problem and the fact that there are recorded observations which appear to require explanation in terms of one or other process.

The most acceptable approach is probably to use the existence of somatic cell hybridization under certain conditions in tissue culture as a justification for assuming that immune pattern can be subject to recombination and segregation by fusion of somatic cells. The actual circumstances could only be guessed at and the overriding quality of phenotypic restriction makes any simplification highly artificial. We are forced to assume that of any alleles only one will be functional and if, for simplicity, we assume that only one gene in each cell is relevant to immune pattern, the cells taking part in recombination could be represented as *ao* and *bo* where *o* is a nonfunctional allele.

Suppose we have an antigen in the form of a single molecule containing two antigenic determinants *A* and *B*. This will stimulate cells of *ao* and *bo* clones respectively and in the appropriate lymphoid tissue we shall have proliferating cells of both clones in close proximity. If recombination and segregation can occur, these conditions could well be optimal. We assume segregation would be at random and would result in a ratio of $1\,aa\quad 1\,bb\quad 2\,ao\quad 2\,bo\quad 3\,ab$ plus nonviable or inert *oo*. The phenotypic ratio at equilibrium would be $1\,a\quad 1\,b$ and $1\,ab$ but, as there will never be complete recombination there should always be something less than 33 per cent of *ab*. If, however, *ab* is more actively stimulated than *ao* or *aa* by *AB* antigen, which is not unreasonable, then a higher proportion of the double producers could be found.

There may be special limitations on the types of somatic cell that can undergo recombination and segregation and if the restriction of extensive double producers to antigenic determinants carried on the same molecule is valid, the restriction may well be to cells producing the same type of antibody G, M or A and perhaps to cells in equivalent physiological states. Since with a single molecule as antigen, antigenic determinants *A* and *B* must be handled in precisely the same fashion, these requirements would be fulfilled much more readily than when two unrelated antigens were inoculated simultaneously.

The two subcellular possibilities that have been canvassed can be expressed in more or less similarly simplified terms:

(*a*) Until much more is known about the genetic determination of the combining site, the form that any equivalent of pneumococcal transforming principle could take must remain completely unknown. Probably all that can be said is that unless the combining site or region is controlled by a single small genetic unit, a process of this sort is virtually inconceivable. The only qualification is that if there was a clear survival gain from the existence of cell-to-cell transfer of immune pattern, a process might conceivably have evolved for the immunocyte series alone. The lack of any biological analogy would then have less weight.

(*b*) If immune pattern could be transferred to another cell in the form of informational RNA this would imply that, like virus RNA, it fulfilled the dual function (i) of messenger-RNA in directing specific protein synthesis and (ii) of replicating to produce more RNA of the same pattern. It is also implicit that it should, in one form or another, provide information to enforce the development by the 'infected' cell and its descendants of the elaborate endoplasmic reticulum with its membranes and ribosomes characteristic of the mature plasma cell. By analogy with bacterial situations this would presumably demand a variety of information needed for the synthesis of necessary enzymes. It could, however, require no more than a signal to some 'operator' that could set the cell on the same road to differentiation as plasma cell, in a fashion analogous to what must occur in active antigenic stimulation.

Antibody production

None of the direct evidence for transfer of immunological information is both unequivocal (in excluding alternate explanations) and adequately confirmed. Most of what has been published as evidence of transfer by RNA is now regarded as representing the action of antigen modified in macrophages to units comprising antigenic determinant, peptide of perhaps minimal size, and low molecular weight RNA possibly of the type used for amino acid transport. An important recent experiment by Friedman has shown that a cold phenol extract of immunized mouse spleen has a minor effect in stimulating corresponding antibody production in normal mice but none in mice rendered specifically tolerant to the antigen.

It is probably best to maintain a sceptical approach to all suggestions of informational transfer between immunocytes and to seek other interpretations of awkward facts. The whole situation will probably remain obscure until a satisfactory means of growing pure clones of functional antibody-producing cells *in vitro* is developed and methods become available for full sequence-analysis of the immunoglobulins they produce.

THE ORIGIN AND HOMEOSTASIS OF IMMUNOGLOBULINS

There is no accepted doctrine in regard to the existence of immunoglobulins (as defined solely on physical and antigenic qualities) which lack combining sites. At the present time what evidence there is points very much against the possibility but it cannot be regarded as absolute. Until it was shown that at least three Ig G myeloma proteins were carriers of immune reactivity, it was possible to hold that these proteins lacked any combining site. It is still, of course, possible that this holds for some but not for others. The evidence to date, however, is that the light chains of myeloma proteins are structurally similar to each other and to the light chains of antibody. In addition, the finding that both light and heavy chains in mixed antibody populations can carry tyrosine molecules capable of specific reaction with hapten by the affinity-label method and that this corresponds to the variable portion of the light chain in Bence Jones proteins, gives solid reason for assuming that what is found in myeloma light chain can be transferred with only minimal reservations to the situation in antibody of normal physiological origin.

Our discussion will therefore adopt the viewpoint that all immunoglobulins conforming to the standard antibody structure are, in fact, antibodies in the sense that they carry two regions homologous with combining sites whether or not there is any antigenic determinant known or conceivable which would unite significantly with them. It seems, in fact, that if the structure of immunoglobulins that we have adopted is correct, 'nonspecific γ-globulin' could arise only as a result of gross error in the synthesis of the polypeptide chains. The failure of a given preparation of immunoglobulin to react with any available antigen is meaningless and a definite decision could only follow a demonstration (*a*) that the combining site had a specific genetic determination distinct from that of light and heavy chains and (*b*) that a physical difference could be shown between immunoglobulins which corresponded to one set having combining sites and the other lacking them.

On the interpretation we are adopting, non-antibody γ-globulin represents those immunoglobulin molecules which carry specific patterns nonreactive against the limited number of antigens that the experimenter has available for test. They can be regarded as a more or less random mixture of all the types of antibody a given individual can produce. The problem that arises is whether this random mixture results from a large number of small specific stimuli or is synthesized under the influence of some nonspecific process.

Our preference is for the second alternative although the evidence is probably inadequate to justify the choice. There is evidence, for instance, that when a specific response occurs there is a variable but often large increase in immunoglobulin which does not react with the antigen used. Freund's complete adjuvant given without additional antigen causes a rise in globulin not related to the antigens of the incorporated acid-fast bacteria. It has been claimed that 'immunization' of an animal heavily irradiated on the preceding day gives rise to an increase in γ-globulin but not of precipitable antibody. Some have also claimed that lymphocytes can be stimulated by phytohaemagglutinin to produce some additional γ-globulin.

Antibody production

A thoroughgoing genetic approach to antibody production would almost require that a proportion of the random patterns generated would not react with anything present in the body fluids and tissues nor with anything reasonably likely to be introduced into the tissues from outside. These, however, would be just the patterns required to help deal with any 'new' antigen which might appear and there is an easily recognizable biological requirement that a proportion of cells with such potentialities and a low concentration of the antibodies they produce should be retained in the body.

We are virtually forced, therefore, to assume that there is some way in which a nonspecific stimulus to proliferation can affect all clones of immunocyte without discrimination. There is a constant loss of lymphocytes across mucous membranes which is almost certainly nonspecific as well as the well-known losses in thymus and in lymphoid tissue which may have a specific element, and in one way or another these losses must be made good. One can hardly avoid postulating a series of homeostatic controls governing the total content of immunocytes in the body. On the positive side this would mean a continuing production of Ig M antibodies to maintain the natural antibodies of the blood. On the negative side the natural corticosteroids could well play the major role.

At several points the capacity of agents liberated by antigenic stimulation of a cell to activate adjacent cells has been described or suggested. If this activation is able to stimulate low-grade DNA synthesis and proliferation and to leave these cells temporarily more highly reactive to contact with their 'proper' antigenic stimulus, a number of experimental findings would be clarified, notably recent findings that an interaction between thymus-dependent and non-thymus-dependent immunocytes is necessary for the production by the latter of certain types of antibody.

It is an interesting point that, if the concentration of immunoglobulins acting on an appropriate sensor provided the necessary feedbacks to stimulate either lymphopoietic and antibody-producing activity or an increased corticosteroid output to diminish the immunocyte population, we should have the basis for a homeostatic control. There appears to be no evidence for or against such a concept which would provide a natural corollary to the specific feedback provided by Ig G antibody. Clearly there must be a complex process by which the A, G and M ratio is held constant or modified according to need, but no effective experimental approach has been described.

It is quite certain that mechanisms controlling the level of immunoglobulins in the body will be uncovered in the future. The existence of both congenital and acquired agammaglobulinaemia as pathological states in man points strongly to the presence of some unitary mechanism or substance necessary for the development of plasma cells and the production of immunoglobulins in more than minimal amounts. Elsewhere it has been suggested that this may be a hormone related to whatever tissue in the mammal corresponds to the bursa of Fabricius in birds. If such a hormone exists it presumably plays a major part in maintaining a standard level of immunoglobulins in the circulation.

THE ROLE OF ANTIGEN

In any formulation of a selective theory of antibody production the function of antigen becomes wholly that of a specific stimulus which, acting through an appropriate receptor, initiates cellular response. This may be positive—for example, proliferation of the immunocyte to produce either plasma cells actively synthesizing antibody or memory cells—or it may yet be shown that direct conversion of lymphocyte to an antibody-synthesizing form can occur. Negative responses exemplified by destruction and perhaps non-destructive inhibition of immunocyte function are more relevant to the subject of tolerance (chapter 10), but must always be kept in mind.

The presentation of antigen as stimulus

There are innumerable substances or organic structures which can serve as antigens and their effectiveness as stimulants to antibody production must depend on many factors. Bovine γ-globulin is a very 'poor' antigen in mice when it is completely soluble and undenatured and provokes unresponsiveness to the 'good' antigen that results when the bovine γ-globulin is partially aggregated. The physical condition of the antigen and the way in which it is presented are both obviously important. The intravenous route is standard when one wishes to induce tolerance. The production of a localized deposit of antigen by adding Freund's adjuvant to the inoculum can, in general, be relied upon to produce antibody in quantity.

Included in the 'presentation' of the antigen, and probably the main feature determining the outcome, are the relations of concentration and time of exposure to the antigen. Details are still to be worked out but the general picture that emerges, for example, from Mitchison's experiments, is that effective contact of an antigenic determinant with a cell receptor on a previously unstimulated cell will have a certain probability (P) of initiating a positive response and the reciprocal ($1 - P$) probability of initiating inhibition or destruction. In the fraction P where positive action has been initiated, subsequent contact presumably with other receptors may have partial or complete inhibitory effects. In fig. 22 in the discussion of avidity in the previous chapter (p. 180) P will increase at right angles to the diagonal in the lower-left direction and conversely the ($1 - P$) probability of destruction in the opposite direction. The size of P will almost certainly increase with the age of animal at least from mid-embryonic life till adolescence and with the relative maturity of the cell concerned. It will also differ greatly with the nature of the antigen concerned. A bacteriophage such as $\phi X 174$ seems to have a high value of P in nearly all circumstances including embryonic life. Purified soluble plasma proteins on the other hand have a relatively low value of P in mice and in young rabbits. The difference between the physical form of a complex virus and a soluble protein will, of course, be highly relevant.

In this discussion it is implicit that the characteristic negative response is functional and, probably, physical elimination of the cells concerned. These are therefore not subject to secondary effects. Positively stimulated cells are, however, activated to proliferation and differentiation. They remain susceptible to further stimulation by the corresponding antigenic determinant and the one thing we know about such cells is that with adequate exposure to high concentrations of antigen they can be functionally eliminated. It follows that in every situation where antigen is by one means or another maintained for a significant period of days or weeks in the body we have a highly complex dynamic situation in action. At all stages, a proportion of competent cells committed or uncommitted will be eliminated by reaction with antigen. Some uncommitted cells are stimulated to direct production of Ig M antibody, others in perhaps two or more sequential steps to proliferate either to antibody-producing plasma cells with eventual elimination of the line, or to 'memory cells' with continuing potentialities of reaction with the antigenic determinant.

If this analysis is correct we have an adequate theoretical basis to account for the dependence of the curve of antibody response on a host of factors: species, strain, sex and age of the animal immunized, physical and chemical characteristics of the antigen and the route concentration and time sequence in which it is presented. We may add to this two aspects discussed elsewhere: (a) genetic factors determining the readiness with which certain antigenic patterns can be produced by the individual and (b) the capacity of circulating antibody (7S, G) to block the action of antigen as stimulus and to 'turn off' 19S, M antibody production. Taken together, these factors provide an explanation of the need for quite extraordinary standardization of all experimental particulars if quantitatively uniform antibody responses are to be obtained.

When we look more closely at the function of antigen it soon becomes evident that the impact of antigen on the immunocyte is often, and as far as classic antibody production is concerned, possibly always, mediated by macrophages.

It has already been discussed in another context that macrophages, especially the dendritic macrophages of lymph follicles, serve to prepare antigen to function as an effective stimulus to proliferation and antibody production. With the usual reservations about the possibility of alternative formulations, current opinion can probably be represented as follows. In order to be capable of stimulating antibody response the antigenic determinant with a pattern complementary to the receptor of the immunocyte must be in an appropriate physical form. The most effective conformation appears to be the antigenic determinant attached to part of a peptide chain, perhaps no more than one amino acid, to which in its turn a low-molecular-weight RNA, possibly s-RNA, is attached.

The major function of a dendritic macrophage is to maintain this complex in functional antigenic form on the surface of its projections for several days. The evidence suggests that less specialized macrophages quite rapidly destroy the antigenicity of any antigen which is basically protein in constitution.

At the evolutionary level the significant immunological needs are probably (*a*) the elimination of mutant somatic cells as they arise, (*b*) defence against micro-organismal invasion including both 'mopping up' of the first attack and prevention of re-infection thereafter and, possibly, (*c*) control of situations that arise in connection with pregnancy where two antigenically different organisms are in a close organic relationship. None of these is particularly close to the standard experimental situation in which a highly purified antigen is injected in relatively large amount by a single route. All results from such artificial situations must be carefully considered in the light of the realities that are relevant to the evolutionary process. So long as this is kept in mind the simplifications and abstractions of experimental work are fully justifiable.

Hapten-carrier antigens

The first type of study to be mentioned involves the use of simple haptens of known chemical structure such as dinitrophenyl (DNP) which are not themselves antigenic but become so when they are attached either to a suitable natural protein such as ovalbumin or to synthetic polypeptide. There are two important findings. If the hapten is attached to a synthetic polypeptide of L-GLU, L-ALA and L-TYR, the compound is antigenic and produces a corresponding antibody primarily directed against the hapten. If, however, the same hapten is attached to a synthetic polypeptide made up of D-amino acids it is not antigenic but when used as a test antigen it can be precipitated by antiserum made against the L-polypeptide complex. The second point is that when wholly synthetic antigens of this type are tested in guinea-pigs it is very rare to find all the test animals responding. If two sets of pure line guinea-pigs are used it is usual to find a certain pattern of response in one line and quite a different one in the other. Using non-responder guinea-pigs which produced no antibody to DNP-polylysine, Green and Benacerraf showed that complexing this to a carrier protein gave immunogenic material. Specific anti-DNP-producing cells could be demonstrated so that there was no genetic inability to produce the immune pattern.

Taken along with other evidence it seems that some preparatory process is needed to bring what is injected into a form that can directly stimulate antibody production. Following Benacerraf, the most likely interpretation is that the carrier peptide or protein must be broken down by intracellular enzymes in the macrophage that takes it up, so as to leave an antigenic determinant attached to an amino acid or small peptide to which low-molecular-weight RNA can be attached to give the 'directly antigenic' complex. The differences between individual guinea-pigs may well be due to differences in their capacity to break down the carrier, but genetically determined differences resulting in the presence or absence of appropriate patterns on the immunocytes may also be relevant in some instances.

The effect of adjuvants

It has become almost a habit amongst immunologists to use Freund's complete adjuvant (F.C.A.), (a mixture of liquid paraffin, an emulsifying agent, 'Arlacel', and killed acid-fast bacilli) to enhance the action of any type of antigen used for experimental immunization. In general a longer lasting, higher titre, antibody response is given than when the antigen is injected alone. It is equally effective in increasing the ease with which delayed hypersensitivity is produced and its use is essential if 'autoimmunization' by homologous organ tissue is to be achieved. The action of F.C.A. is certainly complex. The water-in-oil emulsion induces a complex granuloma containing many cell types including macrophages, plasma cells and lymphocytes. Within this, the inoculum persists almost indefinitely, allowing a continuing release of antigen which, after the first day or two, continues at a low level for a very long period. There is experimental evidence that, at least as far as the course of antibody production is concerned, the effect of a single injection of antigen in F.C.A. can be reproduced by following up an initial injection of antigen alone with a prolonged series of small daily injections.

There are, however, qualitative as well as quantitative differences when F.C.A. is used and there are probably additional factors yet to be demonstrated experimentally. Raffel, for instance, has suggested that constituents of the tubercle bacillus may deflect the process of differentiation of the immuno-competent cell to allow the appearance of these qualities. This may be part of the truth but it does not fit easily into a selective approach.

The established qualitative differences after F.C.A. immunization which call for explanation are the emergence of immunocytes and antibody of higher avidity, and the appearance of unduly large amounts of 'nonspecific' immunoglobulin. Even in that statement there is a clear suggestion that there has been disorganization of normal homeostatic processes by this unnatural presentation of antigen. Under such circumstances it seems preferable to look for a change in the selective process rather than a meaningful deflection of differentiation.

The following suggestion may have experimentally testable consequences. The environment, either within the Freund granuloma or somewhere in the sequence of draining lymph nodes, is such that there is a movement of the normal balance between proliferative and destructive responses to immune stimulation toward the former. In terms of fig. 20 a proliferative response is obtainable when the product of avidity multiplied by effective concentration of antigen is higher than would be allowable in the absence of adjuvant. If, at the same time, antigen–immunocyte contact under F.C.A. conditions resulted in a much more effective or widespread nonspecific stimulus to proliferation of adjacent randomly distributed immunocytes, the observed conditions would be fulfilled.

Another point to be borne in mind is that long-continued release of very small amounts of antigen will induce a chronic proliferation of immunocytes under specific stimulation. Within these clones the possibility of (minor) somatic mutation, including movement to higher avidity, is always present. Again, the special local conditions might allow the proliferation of immunocytes with these secondarily avid receptors.

In one way or another, clones reactive with the deposited antigen may arise which would never become available under more physiological conditions. These may include clones with undue avidity for the antigen used and, when conditions are extreme,

The behaviour of 'good' antigens

A comparatively recent development in academic immunology has been the study in relatively pure form of the antigens which for many years have been recognized by medical microbiologists as being particularly effective in producing high titre antibody. Typical examples of such 'good' antigens are bacterial flagella, influenza virus and certain bacteriophages. All these when used in the form of the natural organized material give a very rapid primary response, antibody being detectable in from one to three days. When, however, the same antigenic determinants are presented in molecular form in the two first examples there is a significantly longer period (7–10 days) before antibody is demonstrable. Similar experiments have not been recorded for bacteriophage. In both investigations the antibody produced by the molecular units was 7 S in character and, as far as currently incomplete data are available, only the molecular form, when given to neonates and continued at intervals, can provoke complete or almost complete tolerance.

In this response to a very good antigen, we may well be seeing the 'standard' form of the immune process developed to deal with pathogenic micro-organisms in the course of vertebrate evolution. The most direct interpretation may be as follows:

(*a*) Contact of the natural antigen with an uncommitted immunocyte, either directly or by way of a macrophage, will in a high proportion of instances result in stimulation of the cell to produce Ig M antibody, often of relatively low avidity.

(*b*) Contact of the monomer with immunocytes will commonly result in tolerance, especially when the animal is in the neonatal period.

(*c*) Taking up of the monomer by phagocytic reticulum in the lymphoid follicles provides a modified antigenic stimulus producing especially, but probably not exclusively, G-type antibody.

These results bring the findings into relatively close relationship to those observed with soluble antigens such as foreign γ-globulins. The behaviour of well centrifuged human γ-globulin in the mouse

Antibody production

is discussed in chapter 10. It merely underlines the frequency with which contact of antigen with immunocyte must be lethal when large amounts of antigen are present and how much more effectively immunity is produced when the antigenic determinants are carried by organized or insoluble antigens. In this connection we can probably homologize denatured and partly aggregated foreign γ-globulin with the organized form of the microbial antigens.

10 Immunological unresponsiveness

Under the term 'immunological unresponsiveness' it is convenient to include all those phenomena in which, by one manipulation or another, an animal fails to produce the immune response regularly given by an equivalent untreated animal. It was first noted in regard to the failure of an animal to reject genetically distinct cells implanted neonatally, but much recent work has made use of simpler antigens. Unresponsiveness can be recognized by the use of any of the techniques used to demonstrate immune reactions and can be manifested as follows:

(a) Absent or diminished antibody production after a standard antigenic stimulus.

(b) Failure to reject a graft of allogeneic tissue.

(c) Failure to eliminate a viral infection, sometimes associated with abnormal absence of symptoms.

(d) Absence of the usual tissue reaction to challenge after a normally sensitizing injection.

Unresponsiveness or tolerance has now been recognized under a wide variety of conditions, the most important of which are:

(a) Physiological unresponsiveness resulting either:
    (i) from the presence of circulating antibody or
    (ii) from simple depletion of lymphocytes.

(b) Neonatal tolerance resulting:
    (i) from the implantation of living sources of antigen, allogeneic cells or certain viruses in embryonic or neonatal life or
    (ii) appropriate administration of non-living antigen in adequate amount at the neonatal period.

(c) Immune paralysis induced in postnatal life by doses of antigen, the amount needed varying widely with the type of antigen, the mode of administration and the species of animal used.

(d) The unresponsiveness of irradiated animals and of animals under the influence of immunosuppressive drugs.

Each of these will be discussed separately, but as a guiding line to the discussion it is important to remember that all immune processes are very complex and where there is an unexpected failure to produce antibody it is likely that more than one factor is at work. It should be remembered, too, that whenever purified or rare antigens are being used it is almost regular to find gross discrepancies in the antibody titre resulting from uniform immunization even in homozygous animals.

The approach to be adopted has necessarily been foreshadowed in earlier chapters and it may be convenient to summarize here the main points of the interpretation to be placed on the rather heterogeneous phenomena included within the general field of immunological unresponsiveness.

(*a*) Immunocytes under stimulation by antigen may respond positively or negatively, the decision being determined both by antigenic factors—concentration, sequence and mode of presentation—and by factors involving the immunocyte: maturity, local environment, presence of immunosuppressive drugs, recoverable damage from irradiation.

(*b*) Cells proliferating as plasma cell clones rapidly become irreversibly committed as end-cells and once their antibody-producing activity is ended they have no further existence.

(*c*) The presence of significant amounts of circulating antibody greatly diminishes or annuls any capacity of the corresponding antigen to act as a primary antigenic stimulus.

(*d*) Very small amounts of circulating antibody by opsonizing antigenic molecules or particles may greatly increase the primary response to a given antigen, particularly in young animals.

PHYSIOLOGICAL UNRESPONSIVENESS

Inhibition by immunoglobulin G antibody

The inhibitory effect of antibody, especially of 7S Ig G type on primary-type stimulation, has been mentioned earlier, along with the probability that it may also have an effect in switching cells from Ig M to Ig G antibody production. One widely used experimental example of unresponsiveness is the repeated administration of sheep red cells to rats, starting immediately after birth. A detailed examination of this type of unresponsiveness by Rowley and Fitch in 1965 led them to conclude that the inhibitory effect of antibody and the end character of Ig G-producing plasma cells were the most important factors in the observed failure to produce more than small amounts of antibody.

This conclusion is based largely on the behaviour of plaque-forming cells in the spleen. These are cells capable of producing Ig M antibody against sheep red cells. If 10-week-old rats in three categories are tested (*a*) for serum antibody and (*b*) for the number of plaque-forming cells in the spleen, the results will be as shown in table 4.

TABLE 4. *Tolerance to sheep red cells in rats*

	Antibody	PFC per spleen
Normal untreated	0	40–100
SRC twice weekly since birth	±	200–500
1 injection SRC at 7 weeks	+ +	100,000 ±

SRC = Sheep red cells.   PFC = Plaque-forming cells.

The picture that emerges from such findings can be expressed as follows: There are probably several antigenic determinants in the sheep red cells but it is reasonable to assume that they behave in similar fashion and, for ease of discussion, refer to a single antigenic determinant, S. Immunocytes with the complementary s pattern are probably present in the spleen from birth and are being steadily reinforced from the thymus. For the first two weeks they are highly susceptible to specific elimination by contact with S but as the system matures a complex balanced condition develops. Antigen in various stages of processing by macrophages will be constantly present in the spleen and there will be a continuing entry of progenitor immunocytes. Some of these will be stimulated to produce Ig M antibody and become plaque-forming cells; more will be eliminated by antigenic stimulation at too high a level; others, for unknown reasons, will soon switch to Ig G production. Once a significant amount of Ig G antibody is present the number of plaque-forming cells falls rapidly and no fresh cells are recruited to this function.

Once an established production of Ig G antibody is under way the antibody will not interfere with its own production by cells already in action. Depending on its concentration, however, it will shield a large proportion of any newly arising competent immunocytes from being committed by antigen to M → G antibody production. With cessation of antigen injections the content of both antigen and G antibody will steadily fall, a proportion of memory cells will persist and the situation will return to one equivalent to that which follows a primary immunizing injection. A new injection of antigen will give a secondary-type response. This is one form of partial tolerance, and similar factors will undoubtedly play a part in other manifestations of incomplete unresponsiveness.

High-level and low-level unresponsiveness

An example of different type may be taken from Mitchison's analysis of the response of mice to a wide range of doses of bovine serum albumin. He studied both the direct production of antibody and the subsequent response to a standard challenge by antigen (bovine serum albumin) in Freund's complete adjuvant. In this system there are two zones of partial tolerance or paralysis —a large dose (10–100 mg) given three times weekly gives a brief rise followed by a fall and partial paralysis. Very small doses give only a very slow, low-level response and leave the recipients strongly paralysed from an early stage. Interpretation of this will follow analogous lines. If we first consider progenitor immunocytes making initial contact with antigenic determinant, then at any level of antigen concentration there will be the two possibilities— of positive response on the one hand, committing the cell to proliferation and antibody production, and of negative response to damage and elimination, on the other.

The essential point to be remembered is that a cell once killed cannot thereafter be stimulated positively. On the other hand there is abundant evidence that even when an immunocyte has been set on the road to antibody production it can be overwhelmed by a large enough dose of antigen. The general impression from both the rat–sheep red cell and the mouse–bovine serum albumin systems is that, for progenitor immunocytes, primary contact with antigen present in more than minimal amount is always more prone to produce paralysis by elimination than immune commitment to antibody production or memory cell formation. There are undoubtedly circumstances, too, in which self-sterilizing antibody-producing end-cells are more readily produced than memory cells.

In an earlier section, the possible role of Mowbray's factor in facilitating specific elimination by contact with antigenic determinants in the thymus was mentioned. Mowbray's experiments have not been fully confirmed nor have they been extended by the author himself. It seems likely that there may be uncontrollable factors involved but it does appear that, under some conditions, injection of an α_2-globulin fraction from bovine serum given before injection of antigen will prevent antibody production and leave at least a partial degree of unresponsiveness to the antigen used for some weeks afterwards. Search of various organ extracts for such an agent gave positive results only with the thymus.

It is biologically reasonable that there should be a hormonal factor which would raise the probability of destruction of immunocytes by specific antigenic contact and that this agent should be present in the thymus. Until the experimental results have been confirmed, however, no emphasis can be laid on this concept.

EMBRYONIC AND NEONATAL TOLERANCE

Natural twin tolerance

It is of the essence of the clonal selection approach that a Darwinian process of proliferation, mutation and selection is part of the natural history of the lymphoid cells of the body. To a large extent this concept is derived from a mass of experimental data that has been obtained by the use of antigens and of manipulations that are remote from any contingency that could be relevant to evolutionary development. The first development of ideas of self and not-self in an immunological connotation came, however, from a consideration of natural phenomena—the occurrence of twin chimeras in cattle and the persisting tolerated infection seen with lymphocytic choriomeningitis virus in an endemically infected population of mice.

When twin calf embryos arise each from a separately fertilized ovum, their blood groups will usually be genetically distinguishable. If they had developed separately calf *A*, when inoculated a few months after birth with blood from calf *B*, would produce agglutinins and haemolysins against *B* blood cells and any *B* cells from the inoculum which might have persisted would be destroyed. In practice, however, the twin placentas A and B fuse at an early stage and there is a mixing of all the circulating cells and antigens of the two calves. The calves are born each with the same mixture of two genetically distinct types of red cell and, in general, the proportion of the two remains reasonably constant through life. Occasionally, progressive changes in proportion may occur but this is probably for other than immunological reasons.

The fact that the genetically 'wrong' cells persist without provoking immune response and, in fact, behave precisely as the animal's 'own' cells, provides the main evidence for the view—central to clonal selection theory—that normal unresponsiveness to the body's own potential antigens is not a directly genetic character but is generated by processes taking place during the embryonic phase and persisting at least till early adult life.

In all examples of persisting tolerance, whether to normal or chimeric antigens, it appears to be mandatory that the antigen should persist. Detailed study of the allotypes of human globulin and their antibodies has shown that when a mother is Gm(a$^+$) and her child is Gm(a$^-$), a considerable proportion of the children produce anti-Gm(a) antibody. This indicates that tolerance induced by the presence of the maternal Gm(a$^+$) globulin in the early months of life does not persist long after the elimination of the maternal antigen. There is presumably a delicate balance of probability toward the end of the first year as to whether the remaining traces of maternal antigen will or will not find cells capable of being positively stimulated.

As a control to this result we may mention the findings in a large series of children who had had multiple transfusions necessarily resulting in the entry of γ-globulin of a variety of allotypes. A high proportion produced antibody, but never against an antigen present on their own γ-globulin. Tolerance to a persisting antigen obviously lasts indefinitely.

Intrinsic immunological tolerance

Since Owen's demonstration of the double blood groups found in certain twin calves it has been implicit that an active process of similar quality must be responsible for the tolerance of the body for its normal components. I stated this more explicitly in 1954 by saying that 'recognition of self is something that needs to be learnt and is not an inherent genetic quality of the organism'.

It is only in 1968 that final unequivocal proof of that statement has been provided as a result of the work of Beatrice Mintz on the production of 'allophenic mice'. She has shown that when fertilized ova from mice are at the stage of 10 or 12 cells—early blastomere—they can be manipulated *in vitro* so that two such blastomeres can fuse and reorganize to form a single larger blastomere. This can then be transferred to the uterus of a suitably receptive fostermother and with correct technique it will develop to a healthy mouse containing components of both the parental strains. This is just as practical with mice of different coat colour or of different major histocompatibility antigens as with syngeneic embryos.

The fact that an allophenic mouse which is a composite of two distinct H2 types can be normally viable and fertile shows at once complete mutual tolerance. Whatever is incorporated into the structure of a new mammalian embryo and can persist, whether by hybridization or by this type of laboratory manipulation, will become completely tolerated by the organism as it develops. In the allophenic mice there is no suggestion of a choice between one or other histocompatibility antigen; both are demonstrable by appropriate experiment.

It has been rightly said that this is *intrinsic* immunological tolerance precisely equivalent to natural tolerance. It must replace the various demonstrations of *acquired* immunological tolerance as the experimental basis of the concept of the natural tolerance of self-components.

Persisting tolerated infection

The existence of persisting tolerated infection by lymphocytic choriomeningitis virus in mice has been extensively studied and the phenomena observed are of great interest. In all probability, serum hepatitis virus behaves very similarly in man and there is obvious relevance to the persistence of rubella virus from early foetal infection until after birth. In the context of theoretical immunology, however, these phenomena are not specially revealing and may be passed over with this brief mention.

Homograft tolerance in mice

Since Medawar's team showed in 1953 that tolerance to homografts could be induced experimentally in mice, a very large amount of work has been published on this theme. The basic experiment is to allow a mouse of strain A to accept a skin graft from strain B, tolerance being induced by implantation of B cells of suitable type into newborn A-strain mice. In practice, for reasons to be mentioned later, the actual strains to be used for such an experiment must be properly chosen and an adequate dose of B cells, preferably from bone-marrow or neonatal spleen rather than from adult spleen, given intravenously on the first day of life. When 'runt disease', that is, graft-versus-host reaction, is avoided by attention to these points, long-lasting tolerance with complete retention of the homograft is the rule. This tolerance is specific: an A mouse tolerant to B will reject skin from a third strain as readily as a normal mouse.

From experiments of this type, two main generalizations have emerged. The first is the relation between age and the dose of cells needed to produce tolerance. A very small dose given immediately after birth will sensitize or show no effect. An adequate dose is needed to give satisfactory tolerance, and a rapid increase in the number of cells needed takes place with each day of life. For mice over a week old it is usually impossible to induce tolerance by a single injection. A sufficient degree of unresponsiveness to allow retention of homografts can be induced in older mice but only by repeated intravenous injections of bone-marrow or spleen cells.

The second generalization is that persisting tolerance is always associated with colonization of lymphoid tissue by donor cells, i.e. chimerism. This does not necessarily imply that tolerance may not persist for a variable time after elimination of donor cells or that every chimera is fully tolerant to all tissues of the donor line. Split tolerance can be very readily shown by giving small numbers of spleen cells from male strain B to neonatal females of strain A. Such mice become almost 100 per cent tolerant to grafts of male A skin but a much smaller proportion will accept B skin (either male or female) if, as will usually be the case, there is a major histocompatibility difference between A and B. Partial tolerance and split tolerance will presumably depend on the extent to which antigen is liberated both by the tolerigenic implant of spleen or other cells and by the test grafts, and on the still incompletely understood intensity of the destructive action of competent immunocytes against the graft. It is well known that a partially tolerant mouse may retain an already established homograft but reject a new transplant of skin of the same allogeneic character. The situation under such circumstances may be visualized as follows.

Relatively small numbers of B cells implanted in thymus and spleen, and the established B skin graft, are liberating small concentrations of the relevant histocompatibility antigens. Any newly differentiated A immunocytes which are highly avid, that is, closely complementary in pattern to the B histocompatibility antigens, will be destroyed on contact. Other immunocytes capable of less avid reaction will escape from the thymus and some will reach peripheral lymphoid tissues. At the time the new test homografts are made there will be, by hypothesis, no avid fully complementary immunocytes to any of the specific antigens of the graft. There are, however, some immunocytes capable of less avid reaction with the histocompatibility antigens. In the case of a major histocompatibility difference between graft and host, the proliferation of weakly reactive immunocytes will be adequate to bring enough of them into close enough contact with vulnerable graft cells to produce a mildly damaging effect. This may include the allogeneic inhibition effect described by Hellström and other workers at the Karolinska Institute. The specific tissues of an *established* graft of B skin are separated from the bloodstream by intact vascular endothelium and the graft is in a much less vulnerable position than one in the process of attachment.

Split tolerance in which an H2 difference leads to rejection, but a simple Y (male) antigen difference is tolerated, presumably depends either on the minor character of the antigenic difference in the antigen or on the small amount of it liberated from the tissue.

Immunological capacity in the foetus

During the early years of work on perinatal tolerance it was accepted almost universally that the embryonic animal, mammal or bird was incapable of producing antibody or mounting any other type of immune response. It had, however, been known for many years that plasma cells were conspicuous in foetuses infected with congenital syphilis and it was shown experimentally in Australia as early as 1953 that a foetal sheep could reject a skin homograft in typical fashion. More recently, extensive work on foetal sheep at various stages of development has shown a curious progressive development of immune capacity. When a suitable bacteriophage is used as antigen, a foetal lamb will produce antibody from the 60-day stage onward. This is in fact the earliest stage at which it was found possible to give the immunizing injections *in utero*. On the other hand, diphtheria toxoid and *Salmonella typhi* vaccine are not immunogenic until at least 6 weeks after birth.

The lamb is born, proverbially well advanced in development compared with a mouse or rat, after a gestation period of 150 days. It is of interest, therefore, that there is a period before the 75th day of pregnancy when a homograft can be accepted and retained indefinitely. From 85 days onward, however, it is regularly rejected.

Graft-versus-host reaction
The other main point of interest in neonatal tolerance is in regard to graft-versus-host reaction or its absence. In a large number of combinations, if strain A is injected neonatally with spleen cells from strain B, the host animal will develop a characteristic runt disease with failure to gain weight, roughened fur and chronic diarrhoea. At an early stage there is enlargement of the spleen followed later by general atrophy of lymphoid tissues. The syndrome is ascribed to the proliferation of implanted B immunocytes capable of reacting with histocompatibility antigens of the host strain A and, in the process, damaging host lymphocytes and other cells. There are also combinations where adult spleen cells can be used to confer tolerance on neonatal hosts without risk of subsequent runting and many more combinations in which adult bone-marrow or embryonic spleen and liver cells can produce effective neonatal tolerance without subsequent harm.

The same contrasting behaviour with different combinations can be seen even more strikingly with mice or rats of different strains joined parabiotically. This is usually an unstable situation and the commonest result is for one partner to develop an immunological ascendancy over the other. If they are then separated the ascendant one will survive; the other will die of a graft-versus-host reaction, presumably of a highly complex pathogenesis. On occasion, however, both partners will survive and the combination remain viable indefinitely.

In these two related conditions, the tolerated chimerism without runt disease and the mutually tolerated parabiosis, one must postulate a double process by which both the donor immunocytes active against host antigens and host immunocytes active against donor antigens are eliminated. Such a process is of course not always successful. When the double elimination does take place the process is probably analogous to the unilateral tolerance obtainable in adult animals by the continuing intravenous infusion of antigen. Despite a number of theoretical formulations calling for the existence of 'tolerant cells' and one or two claims that they have been experimentally demonstrated, the established experimental results are compatible with the straightforward interpretation that an animal or a population of immunocytes is tolerant because it *lacks* immunocytes adequately reactive against the tolerated antigen.

The role of the thymus

In chapter 3 the 'censorship' role of the thymus in preventing the development of immunocytes carrying patterns reactive against accessible self-antigens was postulated. If this is true, the thymus must also play a significant part in the development of neonatal experimental tolerance. The available evidence does in fact support such an approach. It is well known that when antigen is administered intravenously to adult animals or even to laboratory rodents more than a week or two old, very little antigen lodges in the thymus and practically none in the cortical zone. A number of authors have in fact spoken of a 'blood-thymus barrier'.

In neonatal rabbits, rats and mice it has now been shown that antigen labelled with radioisotope or fluorescent dye can pass freely into the substance of the thymic cortex. If, as we contend, to produce tolerance antigen must react perhaps more than once with *all* immunocytes in the body which bear an appropriate pattern, the chief advantages of using the neonate are, first, because the number of cells of any one pattern must be small, and second, because all immunocytes, particularly those newly differentiated in the thymus, are accessible to adequate concentrations.

Where the matter has been specifically studied, most animals which are fully tolerant to homografts have been found to be thymic chimeras. We should be on safe ground in postulating that tolerance to homograft needs for its establishment the development of persisting lymphoid cell chimerism involving the thymus. If this is the case, the effectiveness of the tolerance induced will presumably depend (a) on the relative proportion of donor cells present in the thymus and their continual reinforcement by stem cells of donor origin from the bone-marrow or elsewhere, and (b) on the concentration of the relevant antigens being liberated or otherwise made available within the thymus.

UNRESPONSIVENESS ASSOCIATED WITH LYMPHOCYTE DELETION

Drainage of the thoracic duct

One of the most unequivocal of immunological experiments is to deplete a rat of lymphocytes by chronic drainage of the thoracic duct. With this technique, Gowans not only established the mobility of the lymphocyte as between circulation and lymphoid tissue in the rat but showed that, with an adequate degree of depletion, power was lost to produce a primary antibody response to a normally effective dose of sheep red cell antigen or to reject a homograft from an animal differing only by minor histocompatibility antigens. These capacities could be restored by infusion of adequate numbers of lymphocytes from normal rats.

There were, however, considerable limitations to this approach. If a rat had been previously immunized with sheep red cells and was then heavily depleted of lymphocytes, it was still capable of giving a secondary-type antibody response to a new antigenic challenge. When a depleted rat was tested with a skin homograft from a rat with a major histocompatibility difference, the graft was rejected virtually as rapidly as from an undepleted rat of the same stock.

It is probable that at least part of the immunosuppressive effect of X-irradiation or corticosteroid administration is referable simply to the associated destruction of lymphocytes.

Recapitulation of lymphocytic function

The lymphocyte is unique among body cells in its susceptibility to destruction by X-irradiation and cytotoxic drugs and both types of agent have been very extensively used in immunological investigation. Before summarizing the results of this work it is worth while restating briefly our earlier conclusions on the natural history of the lymphocyte in mammals. Under the morphological guise of the small lymphocyte there is a wide range of cells of varied potentialities, but all can be regarded as essentially mobile carriers of information. There are probably some 'lymphocytes' that have no concern with immunology, but from the immunological standpoint we can be reasonably certain that circulating lymphocytes include (*a*) stem cells of bone-marrow origin, (*b*) progenitor immunocytes as yet without experience of specific contact and (*c*) committed immunocytes with potentialities to take part in delayed hypersensitivity reactions or to produce antibody.

Only immunocytes in the small lymphocyte form are immediately relevant here. They are serving as carriers of information and each will be stimulated to function and sometimes to proliferation only when it meets the appropriate circumstance—usually antigen contact—calling for its specialized function. To make use of such a generalized mechanism of information transport there are three basic requirements. There must be a constant production of many cells of many types; the cells must be freely mobile, freely mixing and widely dispersed through the body and, finally, in order to allow a fully flexible response to transient needs and therefore a continuing rejuvenation of the population, there needs to be a high rate of destruction. This high turnover probably serves another important purpose. When there is need for proliferation of one functional type of cell there is a parallel requirement that the necessary building blocks for nucleic acid and protein synthesis should be accessible. As many have pointed out for other reasons, the lymphocyte (and the other leucocytes) can serve on autolysis as a very effective mobile store of nucleotide and amino acid.

Lymphocyte deletion by irradiation and drugs

The high vulnerability of the lymphocyte is essential to its proper functioning. At the physiological level it is vulnerable to an increase in concentration of adrenal corticosteroids and to contact with specific antigen. It is probably of the essence of the problem that, under different circumstances, hydrocortisone is essential for antibody production and specific antigenic contact provokes proliferation and antibody production. As well as by such physiological agents, lymphocyte levels can be lowered by a wide range of damaging stimuli—from acute infection to X-irradiation or the injection of toxic materials. It is very frequently an open question whether the action of the noxious agent is directly on the lymphocytes or is mediated by the liberation of corticosteroids.

When an animal is heavily but sublethally irradiated and given an immunizing injection approximately 24 hours later, there is often complete failure of antibody response. If very large doses of antigen are given, tolerance may be induced that is specific for the antigen. To obtain unequivocal results, the quantitative conditions seem to be critical. Usually there is a definite reduction in antibody response with a prolongation of the period during which Ig M antibody persists and sometimes loss of 'memory'. Irradiation two to three days *after* the immunizing injection will generally increase the antibody titre obtained and there is little or no effect on the secondary response in a primed animal. With some experimental models X-irradiation four or five weeks after the primary immunization will prevent the development of 'memory'.

In transplantation studies, the simplest means of producing tolerance in adult mice is to give mice of strain A a lethal dose of irradiation and to save them by intravenous injection of bonemarrow cells from strain B. Such mice will accept skin homografts of B and retain them indefinitely. In some instances it is reported that these chimeras will reject a syngeneic (A) graft but in other combinations the normal tolerance to the isologous skin graft is retained as well as the acquired tolerance.

What are essentially very similar results are obtained with immunosuppressive drugs such as 6-mercaptopurine, azothioprine ('Imuran'), and cyclophosphamide. It is easy enough to diminish antibody production, particularly if the drug is continued at the highest tolerated dose over the period of immunization, but persisting specific tolerance requires strict conditions depending on the nature of the antigen and the species of animal as well as the type and dosage of immunosuppressive drug. All cytotoxic drugs of this sort have a strong lympholytic effect, particularly evident in the thymus.

Another method of inducing tolerance (which has not been extensively studied) is to induce a temporary pyridoxine deficiency either by dietary restriction or by administration of deoxypyridoxine. Under these circumstances, administration of a dose of allogeneic spleen cells can induce specific tolerance which persists after the animal is returned to a complete diet.

THE REQUIREMENTS FOR TISSUE AND ORGAN TRANSPLANTATION

From the human and medical point of view, an important current objective in immunology is to achieve effective and long-lasting transplantation of a healthy human organ, usually a kidney, to replace organs functionally destroyed by disease or injury. In the early 1950s surgical technique had advanced to the level where effective junction of arteries, veins and ureter could be done with confidence, blood dialysis by 'artificial kidney' was developing well and a number of kidney transplants were attempted. The results were as would be expected—some initial kidney function followed by immunological rejection. In 1954 an opportunity arose to transplant a kidney donated by an identical twin of the patient. Again, as might also have been expected, the operation was successful and the patient survived for several years.

The problem was clearly to find a means by which immune tolerance could be induced toward the foreign tissue or, alternatively, to find donors who, from the point of view of relevant histocompatibility antigens, were the equivalent of an identical twin of the proposed recipient. The current partial solution to the problem is the use of immunosuppressive drugs of which a derivative of 6-mercaptopurine, azothioprine (or 'Imuran') is the one that has so far proved the most effective.

Research on kidney transplantation has been intensive and widespread but few of the results have much bearing on the general problems of tolerance. Since the use of azothioprine with or without ancillary drugs including corticosteroids and actinomycin D, the proportion of patients surviving one year or more has been rising in a gratifying fashion. This is probably due to an increasing competence of surgical technique and biochemical control plus empirical experience in the handling of immunosuppressive drugs to deal with crises of rejection. There are still very few individuals bearing a transplanted kidney who have been able to maintain normal kidney function without the continuing use of immunosuppressives. Even where there has been a complete technical and immunological success with transplantation from an identical twin donor, the long-term results have not been happy. At least five recipients have died, after successful transplantation, from glomerulonephritis of much the same type as their original disease. Here the problem goes beyond the physiological and must be discussed with autoimmune disease.

The action of 6-mercaptopurine

The first immunosuppressive drug to attract the attention of experimenters was 6-mercaptopurine (6-MP) whose action was reported by Schwartz and Dameshek in 1959. More laboratory work has been reported with this drug than with any other and, as indicated above, its derivative azothioprine, commonly used in human transplantations, has a similar or identical activity but is less toxic in man.

In order to obtain suppression of antibody production and continuing tolerance to a given antigen by the use of 6-MP, several requirements must be fulfilled. In the first place the dose of the drug must be large and close to the toxic level for the species being used. The drug must be continued for some days after the injection of antigen and good results are not obtained unless large doses of antigen are given. The standard experimental animal has been the rabbit but mice can also be used; guinea-pigs do not develop tolerance. The tolerance, after such treatment, is specific and can be demonstrated either in relation to antibody production or homograft rejection. The secondary response in rabbits previously immunized can also be blocked by 6-MP with specific tolerance to a third immunization.

The findings are most readily brought together on the assumption that 6-MP, a mitotic poison, acts more or less selectively on immunocytes stimulated to proliferate by specific antigenic contact, destroying such cells and so eliminating or greatly reducing the size of the clones involved. As in all situations inducing toler-

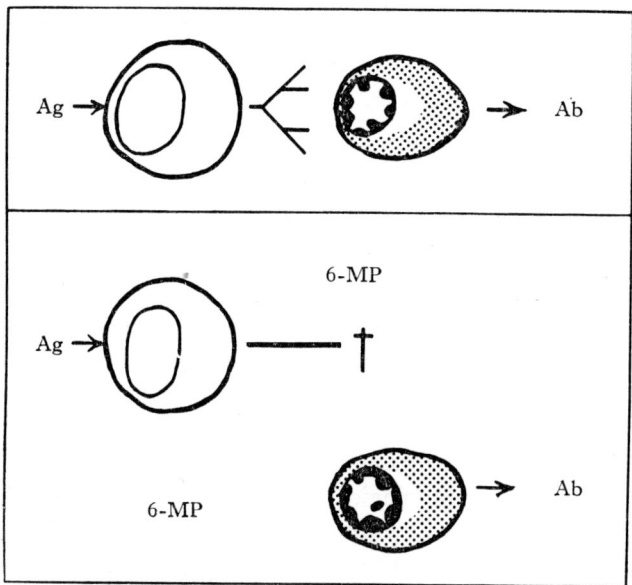

Fig. 24. To illustrate the antimitotic effect of 6-mercaptopurine on a stimulated immunocyte and its lack of action on mature plasma cells.

ance, it is necessary that *all* reactive immunocytes must be exposed simultaneously to antigen and mitotic poison. This is the explanation for the need of high concentrations of both antigen and drug persisting over some days.

It is reported that if 6-MP is given to rabbits for a week and 5 days later a dose of antigen (bovine γ-globulin), there is a strongly marked *increase* in the response compared to that in untreated rabbits. This is reasonably ascribed to secondary effects from the destruction of proliferating immunocytes reacting to 'normal' antigens at the time of treatment. This provides an increased

Immunological unresponsiveness

Lebensraum for stimulated immunocytes to proliferate and perhaps a higher local concentration of products of nucleic acid and protein breakdown which will facilitate synthetic activities in proliferating cells.

Of other drugs with immunosuppressive action, cyclophosphamide, a modified nitrogen mustard (and, again, a mitotic poison) is the most interesting. In guinea-pigs it is an effective agent in producing specific unresponsiveness to proteins and hapten-protein conjugates. In mice there is a strong immunosuppressive effect but at least, with bacterial antigens, no indication of subsequent tolerance.

GENERAL COMMENTS ON UNRESPONSIVENESS AND TOLERANCE

A re-examination of the available experimental material bearing on tolerance seems to reinforce the basic postulate of clonal selection theory: that immune pattern is of genetic origin arising by a random process and that the development of natural tolerance or experimentally produced unresponsiveness is due to the complete or partial elimination of cell lines carrying patterns reactive with the antigenic determinants concerned.

Everything in immunological phenomena is soft-edged. There are no clear-cut absolutes—whether or not a given reaction occurs when cell meets antigen can only be expressed as a probability whose magnitude depends not only on factors that in principle might be expressed definitively, such as the structure of the antigenic determinant and its concentration in the environment of the cell concerned, but on many others that are virtually as complex at a cellular level as the genetic and ecological factors which determine the course of evolution at the macro-level.

In the most general terms, for effective inhibition of capacity to respond to a specific antigen, a situation must arise or be contrived by which sufficient antigen can make effective contact with *all* specifically reactive immunocytes which can have descendants. This means that all cells must either be set into irreversible antibody production as plasma cells or be inhibited or destroyed. Since there is good evidence that lymphocytes may remain inert but potentially capable of mitosis for long periods (several years in man) this may well require that antigen remains present for a long time in order to catch some of the cells in a vulnerable phase.

On the other hand, antibody production can theoretically result from contact of a single immunocyte with antigen. There are, in fact, several observations to suggest that populations of antibody molecules may be derived from a very small number of progenitor cells. In the following chapter the more definite evidence in regard to the origin of some pathological antibodies from a single clone will be discussed. The fact that a major population of antibody molecules may be produced by a single clone, and therefore in the last analysis from a single cell, does not of course mean that the appearance of an immunocyte with pattern a and the existence of antigen A in the body will necessarily result in the production of anti-A antibody in demonstrable amount. A somewhat similar evolutionary situation arises when a mutant strain of a pathogenic micro-organism arises. It is not enough that the new strain should have qualities which would ensure the survival and wide dissemination of the strain if it ever became well established in a population of the susceptible species. It must also survive a thousand possibilities of extermination before it can succeed in that initial establishment of a viable 'beach-head' in the host species.

An indication of the importance of such factors in immunology can be drawn from the almost universal use of Freund's adjuvant to ensure a satisfactory antibody response. Whenever a group of rabbits or mice are injected with any 'rather poor' antigen, bovine serum albumin for instance, a considerable proportion of the animals will give feeble or negative responses. If an exactly equivalent group is given the same antigen with adjuvant of a number of types, a significantly larger proportion will give satisfactory antibody responses and the mean titre will be higher. If one can judge from the physical heterogeneity of all antibody populations that have been studied, in contrast to the homogeneity of almost all myeloma proteins from a single patient, antibody production usually occurs only when a fairly commonly occurring set of immune patterns can react to varying degrees with the antigenic determinant in question.

11 The integration and deployment of immune responses

It is an essential background to this book that experimental immunology, like any other special branch of biology, is justified (a) by providing material that can be integrated into the developing picture of the nature of living function in its evolutionary setting and (b) by providing information relevant to experienced human needs. The great majority of currently reported experiments concern highly artificial situations devised to supply valid information about individual facets of the natural phenomena. In many instances it would be more correct to say that the experiments are concerned with individual facets of laboratory phenomena encountered at one, two or more removes from any of the natural, that is, evolutionarily significant phenomena. It is therefore salutary to try to integrate the information obtained from the laboratories into an interpretation of the natural phenomena of defence or, as I would prefer, of the maintenance of bodily integrity.

Even for the purposes of such a discussion the situation must be simplified and three conditions only need be dealt with.

The first is a generalized infectious disease transmitted by a mosquito-borne virus—a contingency which must certainly have been relevant to the evolution of mammals and birds since their first appearance. Yellow fever can be taken as a prototype.

The second has been equally universal throughout the history of vertebrates—superficial, non-lethal trauma involving haemorrhage, exposure of normally sheltered tissues and infection by environmental micro-organisms. The third example, haemolytic disease of the newborn, represents an immunological accident whose more or less frequent occurrence is an inevitable consequence of the process of placental mammalian reproduction. It can be shown with reasonable certainty to have had an important influence on human population genetics.

The final example is an examination of the phenomena of delayed hypersensitivity from an unorthodox angle. The view adopted is that both delayed hypersensitivity reactions and the rejection of skin homografts are laboratory phenomena based on the natural processes of immunological surveillance by which any groups of cells with aberrant surface antigens can be removed from the body.

HUMAN ARBOVIRUS INFECTION

The process of infection in a nonimmune individual is initiated by the injection of a small amount of virus in the mosquito's salivary fluid into the circulation. Virus particles are taken up by macrophages, particularly by the Kupffer's cells of the liver. The ability of the virus to multiply in these cells of its primary lodgment is probably a crucial step in the process. In mice it has been shown that inherited resistance of a mouse strain to one group of arboviruses could be correlated with failure of the virus to proliferate in tissue culture of macrophages of the resistant line in contrast to those from susceptible mouse strains. Once significant numbers of virus particles are being liberated from primarily infected cells, a rising viraemia will ensure infection of all susceptible cells in direct contact with the blood and, from these, secondary infection of other susceptible cells such as those of the liver in the case of yellow fever.

Large amounts of particulate and soluble antigens are present and, if the infection is to be overcome, any immunocytes capable of responding to the antigens will be stimulated to proliferate and produce antibody. This is initially of M type, but if animal experiments give an appropriate guide there is a rapid appearance of G- and probably A-type antibodies. Since it is easy to show that a mixture of virus with serum containing antibody has greatly reduced infectivity for the susceptible test system, whether this be mouse, chick embryo or tissue culture, it is easy to think of the process as a simple neutralization. Analysis of the situation, however, indicates that the effect of antibody must be a complex one interfering with one or more of the processes by which infection of the cell and viral proliferation occurs. Whatever the process, recovery from infection is associated with the appearance of 'neutralizing' antibody and substantial immunity.

The most characteristic feature of immunity to yellow fever in man is its extremely long duration, not only in the sense of immunity against symptomatic reinfection, but equally of very long (more than fifty years) persistence of measurable antibody in the blood despite residence in areas quite free of the virus. This has the implication that a large population of immunocytes developed during the infection including an exceptionally large number of memory cells. This in its turn implies that despite relatively large concentrations of viral antigen the concentration was not great enough (in recovering patients) to produce unresponsiveness. It is highly probable in fact that the concentration of antigen per kilogram was far smaller than the concentration of bland antigens needed to produce unresponsiveness in laboratory animals.

A second implication of interest from the theoretical angle is that in immunized individuals living in non-endemic areas there must be recurrent or continuous nonspecific stimulation of immunocytes to produce plasma cell derivatives which will maintain a constant or very slowly falling level of circulating G-type antibody. At one stage this was often ascribed to the indefinite persistence of antigen-producing virus in the body, a hypothesis which nowadays appears neither necessary nor credible.

There are still many points to be worked out in regard to how the presence of an immune response destroys the activity of virus and allows its elimination from the infected organism. Work that has been done with standard G-type antibody shows that union of antibody with virus receptors is reversible and is not in itself lethal to the virus. In view of the much firmer attachment of M-type antibody, each molecule of which has twelve potential combining sites, it is conceivable that M-type viral antibody may produce an essentially irreversible union which with subsequent action of complement might be effectively lethal for the virus. The 'neutralizing' activity of G antibody presumably depends on impeding attachment of the virion to any necessary cell receptors and distorting the initial intracellular changes. Simple thermal inactivation and the action of intracellular proteases and nucleases would then return the viral components to the metabolic pool. Damaged cells would be dealt with just as those damaged by trauma.

Workers with arboviruses have uncovered several immunological phenomena of interest concerned with matters other than the quelling of an established infection. From the practical point of view the most important is the long-lasting immunity that follows either a natural infection or appropriate vaccination, usually with an attenuated living virus. There is no reason to believe that the mechanism of this protective action is other than what is seen in the closing stages of primary infection, rendered much more effective by the fact that the whole process can be brought to bear on the infection at its earliest stage.

The main epidemiological feature of yellow fever in the days before its mode of transmission was known was its concentration of attack, very frequently lethal, on the newcomer while the indigene went unscathed. Every European army brought to the West Indies in the Napoleonic wars suffered disastrously. Men and women who had been born and raised in the endemic area were resistant, irrespective of their skin colour. For obvious reasons none of the regions studied for the distribution of yellow fever antibody when techniques became available between 1930 and 1940 were still in the hyperendemic state of West Indian cities in the eighteenth and nineteenth centuries. The results of these surveys, however, allow a reasonable interpretation of the former conditions. Infection-carrying mosquitoes were almost constantly present and children would be infected at an early age. In many there would be enough maternal antibody still in circulation to allow opsonization of the virus and a more effective immune response. Even in wholly unprotected children, however, a primary attack was milder than in an adult infected by the same strain; just as is known to be the case with polio-virus infection.

In yellow fever then—taken as a model of severe virus infection —the biological significance of the immune mechanism must be related not only to the capacity of a primary infection to be followed by resistance to the disease but equally to the fact that first infections in childhood are on the average much less likely to be lethal than those experienced for the first time in adult life.

It may be wise to stress that whether or not a primary infection with a given virus is lethal is much more related to metabolic and genetic factors than to the existence of the mechanism of adaptive immunity. The classically lethal virus disease is myxomatosis of rabbits, which in a virgin population will kill about 99·7 per cent of animals infected. Even with such a strain of virus, however, a proportion of rabbits will recover if they are maintained in a hot environment. Under conditions of the natural spread of myxomatosis in Australia during the 1950s there was a high survival premium on any development of genetically based resistance. Within ten years there was a highly significant increased proportion of survivors, given a standard inoculum of virus and a recrudescence of rabbit numbers in the field.

The evolutionary significance of adaptive immunity in this general field is presumably related to the possibility of transfer of maternal immunity and to a less extent the maintenance of post-infection immunity.

TRAUMA AND LOCAL INFECTION

Twenty years ago there was much interest in the question as to whether hypersensitivity as expressed in the course of tuberculosis infection was relevant to the process by which infection was overcome. No decision on the point was ever reached, and current interest in delayed hypersensitivity is almost wholly at the experimental level, with the significance of the cytological changes in the site of the reaction the most frequent theme for study. Teleological or evolutionary considerations are out of fashion.

To introduce a discussion of the integration and effect of immunological reactions involving changes in the micro-circulation and movement of cells from the blood into tissues, one must have some natural phenomenon as defined above to maintain contact with biological realities. Even a very superficial consideration of significant evolutionary conditions makes one choice obvious—non-lethal trauma. In the wild, any serious trauma involving broken limb bones or severe haemorrhage is necessarily lethal through leaving the victim defenceless against predators. Minor trauma from accident or attack is frequent and the process of haemostasis, minimization of infection and repair is rapid and effective. The effective co-ordination of these three processes must have been a major consideration for survival and, if there is an evolutionary angle to immunological reactions involving blood vessels and cell migration, this is where it will be found.

It is a very interesting surgical principle that in the immediate neighbourhood of sites particularly prone to minor trauma such as the teeth, the anus and the skin generally, surgical procedures can be successfully carried through with a minimal degree of aseptic care. Any opening of the cranial cavity, peritoneum or major joint cavities—regions exposed only by lethal trauma in nature—must be made with far greater circumspection.

Many non-immunological factors are concerned in such local defence. It may be almost wholly a mobilization of nonspecific defence in the form of polymorphonuclears and monocytes assisted by responsive action of the micro-circulation in the area. Modern approaches to the nature of delayed hypersensitivity are more sophisticated than they were (see pp. 245–54) but as one who many years ago was intensely interested in staphylococcal infections, I still feel that one aspect of delayed hypersensitivity may be concerned with the facilitation of defence against traumatic entry of common saprophytes—semi-pathogens on the skin or in the body cavity. It is of the essence of my picture of the evolution of immunity that on top of a nonspecific capacity to resist invasion by pathogens which has been necessary since many-celled animals first arose, there developed a system of internal surveillance to recognize much finer differences between self and not-self. The two systems developed together to evolve into the complex and highly effective defence system of the mammal in which the mechanisms of adaptive immunity can be applied to increase the effectiveness of the older system.

There is a certain primitiveness about delayed hypersensitivity and it may have been in relation to surface infections, internal and external, that adaptive immunity was first linked to nonspecific defence processes. *Staphylococcus aureus* infection in man can be used as an example. The staphylococcus is a robust and ubiquitous potential pathogen. If one follows the course of a particular staphylococcal antibody (α-antitoxin) at various ages, the curve falls to a minimum at 2–3 months and is rising at 1 year, average titres reaching a level of about 20 which is maintained for the rest of life. Infection clearly begins very early. It is also on record that young infants show no skin reaction to staphylococcal filtrates but increasing proportions react with age.

In many ways these staphylococcal findings belong to an earlier age of immunology but they suggest that low-grade exposure to bacterial products could gradually build up populations of immunocytes which could play a part in ensuring that entry of such bacteria through trauma is more rapidly and effectively contained. In part, this increased effectiveness may be associated with an accelerated accumulation of lymphocytes and monocytes, following the first impact of polymorphonuclear leucocytes, and mediated by what is essentially the mechanism of delayed hypersensitivity.

There is much to be said for Spector's point of view that whenever local irritation induces increased capillary or venular dilatation there is an escape of all types of cell into the tissues along with fluid from the plasma. In general, such cells are rapidly removed by lymph drainage unless there is a positive reason for keeping them *in situ*, such as:

(*a*) the presence of a chemotactic substance attracting leucocytes toward it;

(*b*) the existence in the tissues of an antigen which can stimulate the cell in question to become 'sticky';

(*c*) endotoxins or similar agents causing cell death.

The second of these is the one in which we are chiefly interested and it will be discussed in a later section where we are dealing directly with the significance of delayed hypersensitivity. Here we need only make the point that if the delayed hypersensitivity reaction has any direct teleological relation to infection it is to allow accelerated movement of functionally important cells from blood to tissues. If there is associated circulating antibody this also will pass more readily to the site of infection.

Before leaving the topic it is perhaps advisable to mention the very familiar phenomenon of accelerated and immune reactions to jennerian vaccination against smallpox. Here is a perfectly typical delayed hypersensitivity reaction preceding a mild or abortive infectious lesion which rapidly fades.

This approach to the nature of delayed hypersensitivity via traumatic infections is admittedly very incomplete. At most it is only of secondary importance and it may be that adaptive immunity has been of no real evolutionary significance at this level.

Where local trauma has been relevant to the course of

mammalian (or vertebrate) evolution has been in the field of haemostasis and repair. These fall outside the scope of this book, but it is relevant to discuss the nature of micro-circulatory adjustments both in relation to traumatic damage and to various aspects of hypersensitive reactions.

Changes in the micro-circulation related to immune reactions

An important aspect of many immune processes is seen in the part played by the vascular system in the phenomena of inflammation, acute and delayed hypersensitivity, passive cutaneous anaphylaxis, and the various local manifestations of allergic and autoimmune disease. In general the change from normal involves capillary or venular dilatation and increased permeability, surface changes in endothelial cells leading to stickiness for leucocytes, and migration from the vessel into the tissues by polymorphonuclears, monocytes and lymphocytes. A feature of special interest to the immunologist is that these reactions are to a considerable extent inhibited or reversed by appropriate concentrations of hydrocortisone or equivalent drugs.

There is no unanimity in regard to the detailed mechanism of these inflammatory and related responses but all are agreed about the importance of histamine in its initiation. One gathers, in fact, that in recent years there has been a considerable return to the classical views of Lewis on the importance of H-substance, histamine. In the body the main and perhaps only source of readily liberated histamine is the mast cells. The histamine is apparently held in some form of physical association with the heparin granules of the mast cells and is liberated by a variety of pharmacological agents and by appropriate antigen–antibody reactions involving the mast cell surface. No function of the mast cell other than the liberation of histamine, and in certain species other pharmacologically potent amines, is clearly established. One must therefore regard the widely distributed mast cells of the body as having primarily an emergency function to aid in the initiation of the local tissue conditions needed to deal with injury or infection.

In health the outstanding character of the micro-circulation from terminal arterioles to postcapillary venules is its adjustment of blood flow to local needs. This adjustment is necessarily a local one and is not seriously influenced by removal of nervous or systemic hormonal control. Schayer has postulated that histamine is also the basis of this local control largely on the basis of the distribution and changes in activity of the enzyme histidine decarboxylase.

Since the postulated action of intrinsically produced histamine is not readily inhibited by antihistamines the view is by no means universally accepted. It seems, however, that an intrinsic dilator with the general properties of histamine is needed to account for the natural processes and until a more satisfactory candidate appears it is reasonable to accept the histamine hypothesis.

On this view, vascular endothelium contains inducible histidine carboxylase capable of producing and building up concentrations of histamine as called for. This results in opening of precapillary sphincters and dilatation of postcapillary venules with partial opening of intercellular spaces between endothelial cells. Such action is antagonized by circulating catecholamines and glucocorticoids, both adrenal products, and when the local need is met these will lead to the gradual closing down of the local circulation to normal level. In traumatic and inflammatory situations the local situation is pushed beyond the 'normal' reversible state by the accumulation of active products of gross cell damage—bradykinin and other peptides, lysolecithin, and a variety of proteases and other enzymes. From the point of view of theoretical immunology these later changes are irrelevant.

DIFFICULTIES OF THE MATERNAL–FOETAL RELATIONSHIP

In seeking examples of immune phenomena which are natural in the sense of having possible significance in the evolution of the immune mechanism, the special problems of pregnancy come to mind. One of the major problems confronting the development of placental mammals must have been the necessity to render compatible the already established requirement that in nature there should always be histocompatibility differences between individuals of the same species including therefore, and perhaps especially, differences between mother and offspring, and the need for nutrition of the embryo from the mother's circulation. Clearly, in the placental mammals, foetus and the foetal components of the placenta represent a tolerated homograft in the uterine tissues of the mother.

There are interesting aspects of the function of the intermediate layer between foetal and maternal tissues and of the special immunological character of maternal tumours (chorioncarcinomata) derived from foetal cells, but the phenomenon of haemolytic disease of the newborn is a much better worked out example of immunological principles in action.

During pregnancy the plasma proteins of the mother, with some exceptions including Ig M, pass into the foetal circulation. Many of these proteins, including Ig G, will have antigenic differences from those of the foetus but for reasons discussed in chapter 10, the foetus makes no response against them. After birth the foreign proteins disappear gradually and tolerance persists for a variable period. Circulating maternal cells do not normally enter the foetal circulation, though there have been some rare cases of generalized disease in newborn infants which have been ascribed to a 'graft-versus-host' activity of maternal immunocytes which entered the foetal circulation *in utero*. There has even been a suggestion that the Burkitt lymphoma in African children may have such an origin.

Haemolytic disease of the newborn
In what is popularly called 'Rh disease', the important happening is a leak of foetal blood into the maternal circulation. This is an accident that could conceivably occur at any stage of pregnancy, but detailed studies (based on the possibility of distinguishing red cells which contain foetal haemoglobin from those which contain haemoglobin of standard adult type) have shown that it is far commoner at the time of delivery. Significant amounts of foetal blood enter the maternal circulation in about 10 per cent of births and if conditions are appropriate the mother may produce antibody against any antigen in the foetal cells which she does not possess.

Among the very large numbers of genetically based differences in the antigenic qualities of red blood cells the only one of major practical importance is that between Rh+ and Rh− or more precisely between the possession of antigen D as against d. When a woman genetically d/d is impregnated by a D/D man, her child will have both d and D antigens on its red cells. If the husband is D/d, half the children will be D/d, half d/d. The entry of D/d (or D/D) blood into a d/d individual is liable to immunize and result in the production of anti-D, initially Ig M and later Ig G. In addition, a mother so immunized will almost certainly develop clones of memory cells to be stimulated by any renewed contact with antigen D.

If she again becomes pregnant with a D/d foetus and her level of anti-D is high enough this antibody, with all other Ig G antibodies, will enter the foetal circulation. A dangerous haemolytic process develops which, in addition to causing severe anaemia, may have grossly damaging effects on the brain. The problems of this disease and its treatment by exchange transfusion immediately after or even before birth are now well known. Current interest in the possibility of the prevention of Rh disease, however, provides a story of much more interest for immunological theory.

The prevention of Rh disease

It has been known for some time that only a small minority of pregnancies where the mother is d/d and the foetus D/d are followed by haemolytic disease. From what has been said it cannot happen with the first pregnancy unless the mother had inadvertently been transfused previously with the Rh+ blood. In general, with each successive pregnancy the likelihood of disease increases, for obvious reasons, but there are still many who do not suffer.

Some years ago it was recognized that when the ABO blood group of the mother was incompatible with that of the foetus D/d cells failed to immunize. If we have an Rh− O mother and an Rh+ A father and the d/D, AO blood of the foetus enters her circulation during delivery, the cells will be immediately opsonized by her anti-A, phagocytozed, and removed briskly from the circulation. No anti-D will be produced. If, however, the foetal cells were d/D,O they would circulate for a long time and find opportunity to stimulate immunocytes of appropriate pattern and more important to repeat the stimulation of any previously committed cells.

This phenomenon plus the progressive recognition of the power of Ig G antibody to block specifically the primary response to the corresponding antigen led Finn and others to suggest a means of eliminating Rh disease. If an adequate dose of anti-D can be given to a vulnerable mother who has just borne a D/d baby, the foetal red cells will be opsonized and removed from harm's way and no immunization should result. Anti-D can be obtained in the form of human Ig G prepared from a person immunized by pregnancy or transfusion and progress reports of its efficacy are highly favourable. For obvious reasons, strictly limited quantities of anti-D are available and its administration is only justified when proper blood tests of baby and mother show the infant's blood to be D/d and ABO compatible with the mother. The possibility of producing virtually unlimited amounts of anti-D by immunizing Rh – *men* with Rh + blood is already being explored.

Selective effects of blood group incompatibility
It is clear that these maternal–foetal differences should have some selective effect on the proportion of individuals with the various blood group antigens. There are very striking racial differences in regard to the proportion of Rh combinations, but it is not known to what extent these differences depend on the selective effect of haemolytic disease. Theoretically the effect of the disease should be to lead to the extinction of D or d, whichever was initially the rarer, apart from any reappearance by mutation. In this connection it is of interest that of the six genes (antigens) C D E c d e, D:d is the only pair which shows 100:0 ratio in any human groups. No individuals with d genes are recorded among South Chinese

TABLE 5. *Frequency of Rh genes in three races* (%)

	C	c	D	d	E	e
English	43	57	59	41	16	84
Australian Aboriginal	71	29	87	13	22	78
South Chinese	76	24	100	0	20	80

Derived from G. A. Harrison, J. S. Weiner, J. M. Tanner and N. A. Barnicot (1964). *Human Biology*, p. 270. Oxford: Clarendon Press.

and New Caledonians, while in Australian Aborigines it is found only in the combination C d e. The absence of d in the South Chinese is at least suggestive of the action of what may be called 'immunogenetic selection'.

The only other area where immune factors may be important in selective survival of human genotypes concerns the ABO group. Haemolytic disease due to ABO differences is very rare but can occur, for example, when an O mother has an AO or BO infant. This is too rare to be significant in modifying blood-group frequencies. There is, however, statistical evidence that there may be a considerable prenatal loss associated with ABO incompatibility particularly when a group O mother has a group A child.

DELAYED HYPERSENSITIVITY

The tuberculin reaction

The phenomenon of delayed hypersensitivity was first induced in the course of Koch's experiments with tuberculin, and the Mantoux reaction in human beings infected with the tubercle bacillus is still the classical example of a delayed hypersensitivity reaction. Equivalent reactions are observed in experimentally infected guinea-pigs and other animals, so that there has been abundant opportunity to study the significance of the reaction. The essential features of a delayed hypersensitivity reaction in the skin of man or guinea-pig are its slow appearance and persistence beyond 24 hours. In man, a positive Mantoux reaction takes the form of a patch of erythema rather dull red in colour with moderate swelling and slight local tenderness. The reaction reaches a peak between 24 and 48 hours and fades slowly. The guinea-pig reaction is similar in all essentials.

The most generally accepted interpretation of what happens is probably that of Spector. At a rather superficial level the process can be described as follows. The deposition of the tuberculin antigen in the tissues produces minor endothelial damage allowing movement of polymorphonuclear cells, monocytes and lymphocytes from the capillaries into the tissue. When a sensitized cell, presumably a lymphocyte, reacts with the antigen a variety of pharmacologically active agents are produced. These have two important effects: fixation of the lymphocyte in the area in contrast to the speed with which other cells, notably the polymorphonuclears, are removed by the lymph flow, and fixation of other non-sensitized mononuclear cells in the region and variable further degrees of damage to the capillary endothelium. This secondary increase in permeability leads to the entry and fixation in the tissue of many more mononuclear cells, sensitized and non-sensitized, and the reaction builds up to its typical form.

It was obvious from the beginning that the reaction, whether invoked locally or generally, was harmful to the infected human patient or experimental guinea-pig. On the ground that any bodily reaction to a natural hazard is likely to be basically advantageous in dealing with the emergency, there has been a constant effort and debate to find some 'useful' function for the tuberculin reaction. The overall results have not been enlightening. Undoubtedly, there is a significant degree of postinfective immunity in tuberculosis but there are many antigens concerned, with very little indication as to which are significant for immunity.

Neither is there any real indication that infections by acid-fast bacilli played any significant role in mammalian evolution or that the manifestations of delayed hypersensitivity in tuberculosis are of any relevance to the outcome of the infection. If neither tuberculosis nor superficial trauma have been responsible for the evolution of delayed hypersensitivity we are almost forced to look at the possibility that non-infective processes must have been concerned.

The range and character of delayed hypersensitivity reactions

It seems worth exploring the hypothesis that the special characteristics of delayed hypersensitivity have arisen as part of a process which has been evolved to deal with body antigens modified either by environmental agents or by somatic mutation. In developing the hypothesis we shall necessarily equate homograft immunity with delayed hypersensitivity, an opinion which appears to be acceptable to most immunologists.

On this basis, delayed hypersensitivity-type reactions include, or are relevant to, the following phenomena:

(*a*) Sensitivity to tuberculin, coccidioidin and other reagents associated with subacute infectious processes. There is direct evidence of delayed hypersensitivity in two virus infections, vaccinia and lymphogranuloma venereum, and in all probability other viral infections could be added.

(b) Skin hypersensitivity produced by reactive chemicals such as dinitrofluorobenzene and picryl, with poison ivy as a 'natural' agent of similar type.

(c) Experimental allergic encephalomyelitis may well be only the best-known example of a common process by which autoimmune damage to inaccessible organs may be produced. The lesion closely resembles a delayed hypersensitivity skin reaction in its cellular character.

(d) It is convenient to mention here three examples of immune processes related in one way or another to malignant change. These will be considered in chapter 13, but it is essential for the understanding of delayed hypersensitivity that they should be kept in mind:

(i) There are several instances in which virus-infected cells provoke a response of immunological character—either an inactivation of the modified cells or an inflammatory change based on the altered tissue—polyoma virus infection in young animals and Rous virus infection of neonatal rats may be cited.

(ii) Tumours produced in mice by methylcholanthrene and some other carcinogenic hydrocarbons are antigenic, and by suitable manipulations syngeneic mice can be immunized specifically against any such strain.

(iii) Evidence from human pathology suggests that many initiated tumours are destroyed, presumably by immunological means, before they become clinically evident.

(e) Experimental homograft immunity is mediated by delayed hypersensitivity-like activity.

There is a general consensus of opinion that delayed hypersensitivity reactions are mediated by cells, not by circulating antibody. The actual lesion seen in a test intradermal reaction is assumed to be the result of a damaging action of the antigen on sensitive lymphocytes with the release of material capable of affecting adjacent cells more or less harmfully. The sensitive cells may be specific immunocytes with appropriate receptors or, less probably, cells passively sensitized by attachment of cytophilic antibody.

The actual antigen and antigenic determinants are known in only a few of these conditions. It is possibly significant, however, that wherever they are known there is good reason for believing that the antigen is of host origin, modified either by the union of a haptene or as a result of somatic mutation or its equivalent.

Tuberculoprotein has a lower molecular weight than typical antigens while the encephalitogenic protein involved in experimental allergic encephalitis appears to be a polypeptide of mol. wt around 5,000. The effective antigen in both cases could well be a compound with a host component. Skin-reactive chemicals and certain drugs must combine with host protein to induce their immunological action. The intrusion of a virus genome into the genetic system of infected but resistant cells could be expected in one way or another to allow or enforce the synthesis of modified host proteins. The changes resulting from somatic mutation are probably of very similar character to the changes in histocompatibility antigens that become manifest when pure line strains of mice are developed and split into further sublines.

There are several reasons for considering the immunocytes concerned in these delayed hypersensitivity reactions as differing in some significant fashion from standard immunocytes. *In vitro* reaction of human lymphocytes with antigens to give blast transformation and mitosis is seen only in relation to delayed hypersensitivity. This holds also for the production by cell–antigen interaction of agents inhibiting macrophage migration *in vitro*, using guinea-pig material. Demonstration of specific antibody (or receptor) by immunofluorescence in small lymphocytes also has been successful only in relation to active delayed hypersensitivity. There is therefore considerable justification for exploring Raffel's suggestion that the antigenic stimulus is applied in some abnormal fashion and results in 'differentiation of a multipotential immunocompetent stem cell along a pathway which it ordinarily does not take in response to primary antigenic stimulation'. In line, however, with the point of view we have adopted, the phrase 'multipotential immunocompetent stem cell' would be replaced with 'progenitor immunocyte'.

The special quality of delayed hypersensitivity immunocytes

There are two main suggestions as to the nature of the difference. The first is that the receptors concerned are of high avidity for the antigenic determinant and that delayed hypersensitivity develops when conditions favour the stimulation and proliferation of immunocytes carrying combining sites of high avidity.

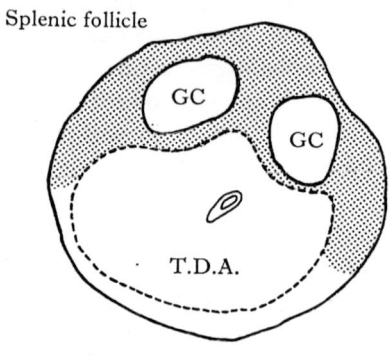

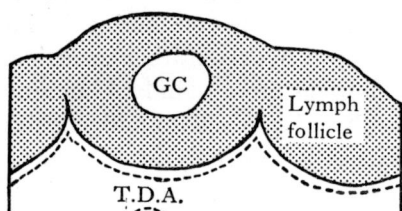

Fig. 25. Schematic diagrams of a splenic follicle and a portion of a lymph node to show the location of the thymus-dependent area (T.D.A.). GC = germinal centre.

The second (which may not exclude the first) is that the sensitizing antigenic determinants include an autologous component, and the stimulus to the immunocyte is of a different quality. Combining suggestions from a number of sources, we may consider the possibility that any antigen which is going to provoke delayed hypersensitivity must be held in some significant relationship to the lipoprotein histocompatibility antigens on the surface of some appropriate cell. *A priori* one would consider the dendritic phagocytic cells of the lymph follicles to be the most likely, but recent experimental work on sensitization by simple chemicals indicates the primary involvement in lymph nodes of the 'paracortical' or 'thymus-dependent areas' where such cells are not normally seen. There is a real possibility that the effective antigen may reach the lymph nodes in the surface of mobile wandering cells, lymphocytes or monocytes, from the area to which the chemical is applied.

Whatever the cells involved, the association of the antigenic determinant with the lipoprotein histocompatibility antigens would allow an entirely different type of presentation of antigenic determinant from that characteristic of ordinary antigens. The latter are, by hypothesis, held on the dendritic phagocytic cell surface in association perhaps with normal opsonin, perhaps with some form of RNA. The immunocytes capable of making effective stimulatory contact with the delayed hypersensitivity-type of antigen might well be characterized by some special quality, such as the need for high avidity toward the antigenic determinant and perhaps for a certain stable component within the different combining sites to facilitate union with antigenic determinants of this special type (see p. 140). If the surveillance function has the biological importance ascribed to it in chapter 13 it is even possible (or probable) that a subpopulation of immunocytes—equivalent to the subpopulations A, G, M and D—may exist, specially adapted by evolution to mediate the surveillance function.

It would be quite in line with biological principles if such a subpopulation had been differentiated evolutionarily to deal with contingencies arising through the production of abnormal body components. On this view the curious pathology of tuberculosis and leprosy may be very largely due to the fact that such infections were not significant factors in evolution and the response we see is, as it were, the best that could be done with available mechanisms. In 1950 I wrote about

> a principle of very great importance in pathology—and there is an exact analogue of this principle in social history. It is that when a bodily mechanism has been evolved to favour survival it can be expected to function satisfactorily only in dealing with the standard

common and significant type of situation which was (indirectly) responsible for its evolution. Once the mechanism has been established, however, it will be called into action by other more or less relevant situations to give responses which may be ineffective or positively harmful in dealing with the unusual situation.

Delayed hypersensitivity in relation to infection

For many years there has been great interest in the relationship of hypersensitivity to immunity against tuberculosis and other bacterial or mycotic infections with more or less similar sensitizing proclivity. The experimental approach has been largely concerned with providing conditions which will allow effective immunization of animals against lethal or symptomatic infection and with the study of the capacity of macrophages to deal with ingested bacteria under various conditions.

The essential features stressed in Mackaness's recent review are that both protective immunity and the production of delayed hypersensitivity in mice against the 'facultative intracellular parasites' *Brucella abortus*, *Listeria monocytogenes* and *Salmonella typhimurium* can be produced only when there is infection by living bacteria. The delayed hypersensitivity is specific; resistance against death from infection is nonspecific, being associated with resistance against bacteria other than those used for immunization.

This has an interesting relevance to the hypothesis we are considering. It seems highly probable that non-lethal infection of cells would result in bacterial antigenic determinants accumulating to some extent in the lipoprotein surface of the macrophages involved. This would allow presentation of the bacterial immunogen to appropriate immunocytes in the fashion postulated as necessary for the induction of delayed hypersensitivity.

If this does represent the sensitizing situation it has obvious relevance to the nonspecificity of the resistance as tested by intraperitoneal challenge with heterologous bacteria. When the other strain of bacteria is inoculated there will be a movement into the peritoneal cavity of lymphocytes and monocytes from local sources and from the blood. These will include both specifically sensitive immunocytes and cells carrying surface bacterial antigen from past infection as well as other lymphocytes and monocytes with no specific qualities of either sort.

If, like most contemporary immunologists, we eliminate any active sensitization of monocytes, their increased capacity to deal with infection must result from activation by products of antigen–sensitive cell contact—a concept for which there is direct experimental evidence, and which is colloquially known in technical circles as the 'innocent bystander' effect. It follows, therefore, that when the heterologous bacterium is inoculated there is, by hypothesis, an almost equivalent opportunity for macrophage activation by interaction of the persisting homologous antigen and sensitive cells. The activated cells, perhaps by reason of increased lysosome production and activity, thus become available for ingestion and destruction of the organism against which the animal was *not* immunized.

Processes of this general character do not in any way interfere with the ability of the animal to produce circulating antibody of various types, including cytophilic antibody which has a special propensity for attachment to macrophages.

The surveillance function

A discussion of the more specific aspects of this interpretation of delayed hypersensitivity in relation to surveillance and homograft immunity will be deferred until chapter 13. It is desirable, however, to elaborate one aspect because of its relevance to the understanding of autoimmune disease; namely, the nature of immune cytotoxic effects whether by antibody or by immunocytes.

If our general interpretation is correct the significance of the subpopulation of immunocytes concerned in delayed hypersensitivity reactions is to be sought in their surveillance function. They have been evolved to 'seek and destroy' aberrant cells carrying the antigenic determinant to which they are attuned.

At the experimental level there have been extensive studies of the damaging effect of specifically immune cells, obtained either from lymphoid tissue or in the form of a peritoneal exudate, against target cells. For reasons of technical convenience, malignant cells have usually been used as target. *In vitro* with a suitable pair of cell suspensions, the usual picture is for the immune cells to clump around the target cells which then show various degrees of vacuolation and disintegration. In some situations but not in others the immune cells are also damaged. The specific action of spleen cells or peritoneal exudate cells may also be demonstrated by *in vivo* experiments in which graded mixtures of immune cells and target cells are injected into an animal in which the neoplastic target cells can produce ascites or solid tumours.

The process by which the damage is produced does not seem to have been studied directly. It seems reasonable, however, to assume that the immune cell carries on its surface either fixed cytophilic antibody or its own characteristic receptor with the equivalent specificity. Union of this with the antigenic determinant on the other cell, and presumably a gradual increase in the number of such unions, will be expected to produce locally increased permeability with damage to the cell surface and lysosome breakdown. The possibility is very high that the proximity to a specific union between cells may result in a nonspecific increase in stickiness and reactivity of adjacent intrinsically non-sensitized immunocytes.

On the basis of this general approach the natural function of the sensitized immunocyte is to recognize cells which by mutation, damage or viral action have developed aberrant antigenic determinants as well as their normal surface antigens. When recognized they must be destroyed and eliminated. In the normal healthy animal the function would be recognizable only by the transient appearance of a few lymphocytes and a macrophage or two. It may be none the less important for having such insignificant manifestations.

Aggressiveness of immunocytes

In various sections of this book I have discussed phenomena in immunologically modified animals in which passage of cells takes place from the blood to the tissues of a region where antigens or antigenic determinants were present. These include the standard ways by which delayed hypersensitivity reactions are demonstrated experimentally, positive reactions from simple application of sensitizing chemicals to the skin, the paralysing response in experimental allergic encephalomyelitis and the phenomena of autoimmune disease of specific organs. The mechanism of a straightforward test for delayed hypersensitivity has already been discussed in terms of Spector's interpretation. This, however, is quite inadequate to account for the phenomena of experimental allergic encephalomyelitis and it seems likely that in addition to the passive mechanism postulated by Spector for the entry of mononuclear cells from the blood there is another more active process. In some way it appears that small numbers of sensitized cells can be held in capillaries adjacent to a source of antigen and then pass into the tissue spaces. Once this has happened the pharmacological results of immunocyte-target cell or immunocyte–antigen contact will ensure the nonspecific entry of normal mononuclear cells, both monocytes and lymphocytes. The initial entry, however, appears to call for a special quality which can be called aggressiveness in the immunocytes concerned.

Aggressiveness is manifested against tissue antigens or their experimental analogues. It is specially characteristic when sensitization is by the use of antigen in Freund's complete adjuvant. It appears to be annulled with considerable regularity by circulating antibody, probably always Ig G, of the same specificity. There seems, therefore, to be another special quality of the immunocytes concerned with delayed hypersensitivity and related conditions which makes them specially prone to adhere to local endothelium carrying antigenic determinants, to pass into the tissues and perhaps undergo there lethal damage which allows changes leading to nonspecific entry of other lymphocytes and monocytes.

A hypothesis of the cellular basis of delayed hypersensitivity
None of the current hypotheses of delayed hypersensitivity is at the same time reasonably illuminating in regard to the experimental and clinical facts and consistent with the general clonal selection outlook. It is clear that any theoretical treatment must be wide enough to cover the other immunological phenomena which have been mentioned above as related to delayed hypersensitivity particularly contact sensitivity, homograft rejection and immunological surveillance. An attempt has therefore been made to summarize the situation in terms of a broad theoretical approach in the following terms.

The immunocytes concerned are derived from the thymus, and lodge primarily in the paracortical area of the lymph nodes. This is also the region where lymphocytes entering the node from the afferent lymphatics lodge. The delayed hypersensitivity lymphocytes represent a class of immunocyte analogous to but distinct from the classes producing G, M, A and D immunoglobulins. The uncommitted cell is reactive only to its corresponding antigenic determinant when this is incorporated in a special relation to the lipoprotein surface of another cell. On stimulation, change to the lymphoblast form occurs with subsequent active proliferation to committed lymphocytes. Secondary nonspecific proliferation of adjacent immunocytes is also probable, giving rise to a considerable population of recently 'born' lymphocytes which pass to the circulation. The committed delayed hypersensitivity immunocytes can react with the corresponding antigenic determinant when it is incorporated in a cell surface or free. In the first instance the result is to activate the metabolism of the immunocyte and produce some damage to the target cell. This will result in release of kinins, etc. and, in the case of capillary endothelium, opportunity to move into the tissues where the antigen is present.

As a secondary development of this point of view we need to look at the mechanism of immunological surveillance to be discussed in chapter 13. The primary assumption must be that histocompatibility antigens of tissue cells are labile and transferable to other cells, notably to any wandering lymphocytes in the area. Lymphocytes reaching the paracortical areas of the draining lymph node will therefore be carrying a sample of any aberrant surface antigens present in the tissues. Aggressive delayed hypersensitivity immunocytes of appropriate type will be able to proliferate and eventually deal with the focus of aberrant cells.

One of the outstanding conundrums of immunology is the nature of Lawrence's 'transfer factor' by which human leucocytes from a tuberculin-positive individual can confer a long-lasting reactivity on an initially non-reactive recipient. It would be inappropriate to elaborate this theme here beyond mentioning the possibility that the phenomenon may be based on the capacity of antigen incorporated in the cell surface to be passed on from one cell to another.

12 Autoimmune disease as a breakdown in immunological homeostasis

There are few people who at one time or another in their lives are not subject to some pathological manifestation of the immune mechanism. It is a highly complex mechanism of great significance for survival and in the course of evolution it has necessarily developed a series of controls, of homeostatic processes, to ensure that the potentially destructive reactions of the immunocytes are directed toward proper targets. The old analogy of the immune processes to national defence in fact takes on a modern flavour if we look on the whole function as a fail-safe system ringed around with controls to ensure that action against the 'enemy' does not damage the resources of the organism, whether that organism be a political one or a mammalian body.

The earlier approach to autoimmune disease was to look upon it simply as a failure of natural tolerance to develop. With the immense activity in the field of immunopathology during the last decade the approach at the theoretical level must be greatly broadened. Our approach now must be to consider each pathological condition or set of symptoms as a manifestation of some breakdown in one or more of the normal controls. Each disease and probably each individual example of autoimmune disease will have its own individual features. It is quite unjustifiable to seek a single formula to cover the nature of all autoimmune disease.

In immunopathology we are concerned, as in every other field of pathology, with environmental and genetic factors but here, more than in other fields, we must add a third qualitatively distinct set of factors—somatic mutation—which includes processes which might equally be called irreversible anomalies of differentiation. The working rule will be accepted that somatic mutation may take quite a similar form to mutation in germinal cells and that in any given immunocyte, somatic mutation will take place against a background of the genetic endowment of the cell. The influence of any mutational event occurring after the first division of the fertilized ovum will be expressed in relation to the other genetically controlled activities of the cell. The possibility that has arisen from results in tissue culture studies, that recombination and segregation may take place between somatic cells, has been referred to earlier (p. 200). There is as yet no evidence that this has any significance in relation to autoimmune disease but the possibility should be kept in mind.

At the environmental level we have first to recognize that it is a prime function of the immune mechanism to deal effectively with every type of 'natural' occurrence that introduces foreign material into the body. Immunologically speaking, local and general infections by micro-organisms are natural hazards providing stimuli to normal defence activities. The environmental agents relevant as such to immunopathology are of two groups:

(a) unnaturally reactive substances produced either by synthetic processes—dinitrofluorobenzene, picryl, etc., or evolved as specialized protective mechanisms by plant or animals, poison ivy being the classical example;

(b) potentially invasive micro-organisms which, apparently for wholly accidental reasons, carry antigenic determinants cross-reactive with potential antigenic determinants in certain organs of the susceptible individual. Streptococcal antigens in their relation to rheumatic fever and acute nephritis are the standard prototypes in this group.

There are of course antigens, pollens for instance, which are traditionally associated with allergic complaints but these represent an environmental impact common to everyone. Internal factors, genetic or somagenetic,* are responsible for the differences in response between allergic and normal subjects.

Autoimmune disease can be defined as a condition in which

* 'Somagenetic'—In the course of writing this book it became clear that on many occasions one would have to differentiate between cell characteristics genetically determined in the usual sense and others that had arisen subsequent to the initial development of the fertilized ovum by somatic mutation. The actual genotype and its phenotypic expression of any given cell will be influenced by both. In the interests of clarity the word 'genetic' and its derivatives will be used in its normal sense. For inheritable changes arising by somatic mutation, the word 'somagenetic' will be used with, in many places, the additional implication of recognizing that any change or character labelled 'somagenetic' is expressed on a background of the whole genotype of the cell.

structural or functional damage is produced by the reaction of immunocytes or antibodies with normal components of the body. This is wide enough to cover an extensive range of minor and major illnesses and disabilities. It will be best to sort out from these a small number of clinical patterns each of which seems to consist of a constellation of related conditions. It is of the essence of our approach to immunity that no two cases of autoimmune disease should be the same, but as long as this heterogeneity and the necessary existence of mixed and intermediate forms is borne in mind, classification into groups can be helpful.

The approach adopted is to consider first, three general autoimmune diseases: acquired (autoimmune) haemolytic anaemia (AHA), systemic lupus erythematosus (SLE) and rheumatoid arthritis (RA). Here we have three important sets of target antigens, respectively the red cell surface, nuclear and cytoplasmic constituents common to many cell types and, for RA, γ-globulin, all of which are readily accessible antigens in the sense of being available in adequate concentration in lymphoid tissues.

In a second group we have the organ-specific autoimmune diseases of which thyroid disease, as the most closely studied example, and myasthenia gravis, because of its relation to the thymus, are chosen for discussion. These are conventionally regarded as involving inaccessible antigens which are either absent from lymph and blood circulations or present in insignificant amounts. More information is required in regard to the amount of recognizable antigen liberated into lymph and blood from different tissues and at different stages of development. Current work suggests that the accessibility of such tissue antigens varies from one organ to another and according to the age of the animal. It is probable that the convenient division into accessible and inaccessible antigens is by no means sharp and may eventually be discarded.

Finally, it is necessary to consider the two groups of conditions mentioned earlier in which unusual immune responses to antigens from the environment inadvertently, as it were, give rise to damaging results. The examples to be taken are rheumatic fever and rheumatic carditis and the drug purpuras and haemolytic anaemias.

The application of the principles of clonal selection theory, particularly as they have been developed in relation to normal and experimentally produced immune tolerance, is best done in relation to the specific qualities of the separate autoimmune diseases. Throughout the central theme is the emergence of 'forbidden clones' of pathogenic immunocytes and the various ways by which these can arise and find ways of escaping the normal controls.

AUTOIMMUNE HAEMOLYTIC ANAEMIA

Red blood cells have been favourite objects for immunological experimentation since the days of Ehrlich and Bordet, and as a basis for the discussion of autoimmune disease there is no better starting point than the disease in which a patient's own red cells are destroyed immunologically.

There are almost as many variants, minor and major, in the manifestations of autoimmune haemolytic anaemia (AHA) as there are patients with the disease. If we neglect minor points and concentrate on a 'standard' case of 'warm-antibody type' acquired haemolytic anaemia, there are several statements that can be made which bear directly on the general character of autoimmune disease.

(*a*) The destruction of the patient's red blood cells is not due to any abnormality in the red cells. If a healthy donor provides compatible cells for transfusion into a patient's veins, these are destroyed at the same abnormally rapid rate as the patient's own red cells.

(*b*) The destruction takes place for the most part in the spleen but is due primarily to the presence of antibody attached to the surface of circulating red cells.

(*c*) The antibody is of 7S (Ig G) type and is characteristically incomplete, that is, it does not cause direct agglutination of normal red cells in saline nor haemolysis when complement is also present. It is detected by the use of antiglobulin sera in the direct Coombs test.

(*d*) In some 75 per cent of cases the antibody eluted from coated red cells can be shown to contain only one type of light chain antigen. This is the best evidence available that such antibody is of monoclonal origin.

(e) With only 10 per cent or less of exceptions the antibody is 'nonspecific', reacting with all types of human cells and not corresponding to any of the antigenic determinants defined by blood-group studies with natural or immune isoantibodies.

To these should be added two other statements in regard to other types of autoimmune haemolytic anaemia:

(f) In the cold-antibody type of human haemolytic anaemia the antibody is an Ig M globulin which does not attach to the target cells at 37 degrees, but at room temperature shows high titre agglutinating and often haemolytic activity.

(g) In the NZB mouse strain there is a model with virtually all the fundamental qualities of the warm-type human disease. Here the development of the disease between 3 and 9 months of age is a regular occurrence and appears to be a definite inheritable quality.

The origin of pathogenic clones

If these qualities are accepted as typical of autoimmune haemolytic anaemia, any discussion of its aetiology in terms of the general clonal selection approach to immunity must start with point (d), the evidence that the antibody present in most patients is monoclonal in type. It is now generally accepted on precisely similar evidence that most cases of multiple myelomatosis are monoclonal and arise by the proliferation of a single pathogenic stem cell. Our contention, then, will be that AHA arises by the appearance through somatic mutation of a single immunocyte with the capacity to react by proliferation and antibody production when it makes effective contact with the nonspecific red cell antigen always present in the circulation, and to give rise to a continuing sequence of memory cells of the same quality. This formulation does not mean that the appearance of a progenitor cell of the right quality to produce AHA is a single unique episode. In both human patients and NZB mice it is probable that many such cells appear. The essential point is that of these it is only a rare individual cell that can escape all the controls and random obstacles and go on to establish a persisting clone with disease-producing capacity (fig. 26).

Acceptance of this hypothesis has the virtue that it immediately calls for discussion of many other questions. It has been emphas-

Autoimmune disease

ized, for instance, that clinical and immunological details vary widely from one case of the disease to another. A proportion, for instance, show a specific antibody most commonly directed against the Rh antigen e; some show active haemagglutination. This variability is a characteristic marker of somatic mutation. It is seen

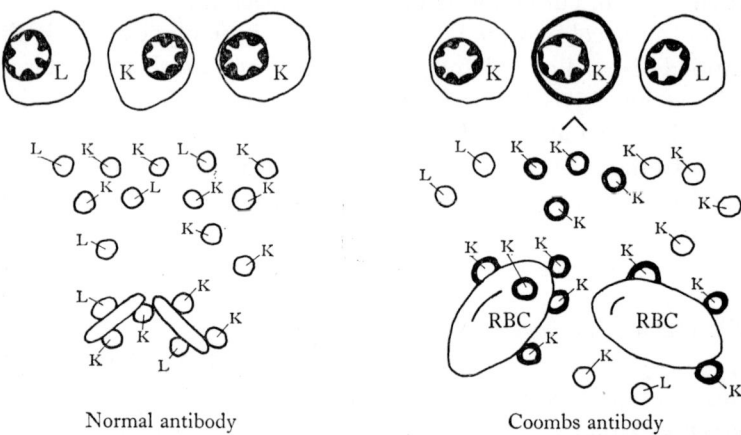

Fig. 26. To illustrate the concept of autoimmune Coombs antibody as the product of a single clone in contrast to the heterogeneity of normal antibody.

even more clearly in multiple myelomatosis where virtually every case produces a single myeloma protein demonstrably different from that in any other patient. On our basic understanding of immune pattern there must regularly arise immunocytes carrying patterns that can react with one or other of the antigenic determinants of the individual's red cells. In the normal individual, none of these develops into an active antibody-producing clone. The primary aetiological question is to understand what allows a cell with such reactivity to do so in the individual developing autoimmune haemolytic anaemia.

The monoclonal character virtually forces us to look primarily for abnormality in the cell line. If the fault were in the internal environment, one would expect cells of varied character to escape control and produce antibody as varied in quality as that arising physiologically. The cell which is predestined to initiate the disease must differ genetically or somagenetically from its congeners. In the NZB mice with certainty, and by implication in human patients, there must be a genetic component. It is significant that in Dacie's series of cases of warm-type AHA, 9 out of 129 were associated with other autoimmune disease, six of them with SLE. It is at least evident that somatic mutation is more effective on some genetic backgrounds than others.

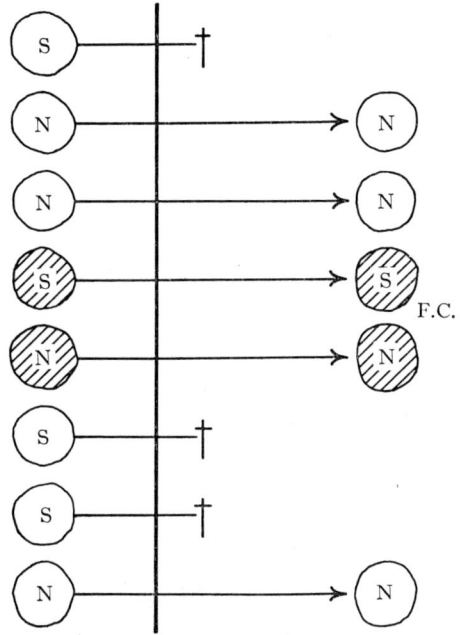

Fig. 27. The role of the thymus in relation to autoimmune disease.
Newly differentiated immunocytes capable of reacting with 'self' antigens (S) are normally destroyed on contact with the antigen in the thymus.
Non-reactive cells (N) escape as do S cells which have become resistant to the censorship function (shown by hatching) and can give rise to forbidden clones (F.C.).

Once the necessary somagenetic configuration has appeared it must, as it were, run the gauntlet of the controls provided by nature to prevent such cells from prospering. Red cells are ubiquitous and many of their antigens are shared with other cells. Whether the primary elimination of self-reactive immunocytes takes place in the thymus or elsewhere we must postulate that all the relevant antigenic determinants are present in the environment where differentiation to immunocyte takes place. Newly differentiated immunocytes reactive with antigenic determinants of the red cell surface would therefore normally be destroyed. The most probable somagenetic change responsible for the 'forbidden' quality is one which confers resistance or partial resistance to destruction when the newly differentiated immunocyte makes contact with its corresponding antigen in a thymic or equivalent environment. In previous discussions this has been taken as the basic abnormality leading to the development of a forbidden clone and the initiation of autoimmune disease (fig. 27).

Avidity and incompleteness

There are, however, other requirements to be met, notably the incomplete character of the antibody produced. There are many differences between 'warm' and 'cold' types of haemolytic anaemia, but both have in common that the operative antibody is not overtly destructive *in vivo*. Since human beings can produce fully active immune antibody against foreign red cells, one must postulate some additional type of control which allows incomplete (that is, low-avidity antibody-producing) cells to flourish but not those capable of producing high-avidity antibody. There are two possibilities. The immunocyte with a highly avid receptor (and producing correspondingly avid antibody) may be overwhelmed by the impact of the abundant and readily accessible antigenic determinant. Except under quite exceptional circumstances, no somagenetic change is adequate to allow a fully avid immunocyte clone to escape destruction by antigen. The alternative is that immunocytes of high avidity that could escape the primary censorship and become committed cells could still fail to become an established clone if antigenic contact produced proliferation and antibody production but failed to allow any production of memory-cell descendants from such a cell. Unless memory cells *are* produced there is no possibility of antibody concentrations or immunocyte populations rising to a level which could be effectively pathogenic.

In line with the general Darwinian approach, one pictures within the population of immunocytes a vast repertoire of immune patterns arising within the labile segments of the somatic genome, but there is also scope for a lower level of somatic mutation in other regions of the genome. Following Burch's general approach it may well be that more than one independent mutation may be necessary before a cell has all the necessary qualities which will allow it to emerge as the progenitor of a pathogenic 'forbidden' clone. Such changes could be either genetic or somagenetic. For instance, when three independent mutations are needed to produce the necessary quality of resistance to homeostatic processes, if one or two are pre-existent as a result of genetic change the chance of the appropriate state being reached by somatic mutation will be increased correspondingly. In one way and another we must picture cells with an extreme variety of individual qualities, a proportion of which, depending largely on the genotype of the individual, will have a greater than normal chance of circumventing controls and giving rise to a pathogenic clone. As in equivalent evolutionary or epidemiological problems there are no absolutes, only varying probabilities, that a clone of cells, a new subspecies of mammal or a particular strain of micro-organism will develop to an effectively established population.

SYSTEMIC LUPUS ERYTHEMATOSUS

SLE is the prototype of severe autoimmune disease involving a variety of tissues and associated with a wide range of abnormal antibodies in the circulation. It shows two theoretically important features lacking in AHA, a high concentration on the female and a characteristic age-specific incidence of the disease. Although the evidence is still incomplete and uncritical there is also a stronger indication of the part played by genetic factors than in AHA. There is further indication of the importance of the genotype in the existence of a mouse strain F_1 NZB × NZW which manifests with great regularity the essential features of SLE.

In the human disease there is a wide variation of symptoms and signs depending on the tissues predominantly attacked. The kidney is almost regularly involved and kidney failure is the usual cause of death. In the hybrid mice *all* deaths, except for accident, are due to kidney disease and life expectation is greatly reduced.

The antibodies of systemic lupus erythematosus

In the features relevant to theoretical immunology the most important difference from AHA is probably the large number of different antibodies that can be found in a single patient's serum and their apparent concentration on antigenic determinants in DNA and other nuclear components. In looking over case histories of young women who develop SLE, there is an insistent suggestion of a preceding period of minor ill-health with a rather sudden onset of multiple symptoms that lead to the diagnosis. It is common for an emotional experience, an infection, administration of a drug or something else to be credited with triggering the onset.

Although there have been some very refined studies of the antibodies in a few individual sera, most serological work has been limited to following the LE cell test or the demonstration of antinuclear factor by immunofluorescence techniques. I am not aware of any careful study of sera taken before and during the development of the clinical condition. This would be of especial value in helping to clarify the pathogenesis of the disease. The simultaneous appearance (if it occurs) of a wide range of forbidden antibodies suggests the sudden collapse of a type of control not yet formulated.

In the full-blown case of SLE there is hypergammaglobulinaemia with auto-antibodies reacting with both nuclear and cytoplasmic cellular constituents. Kidney lesions are almost constant and of a type suggesting damage by soluble antigen–antibody complexes. Detailed study of sera with DNA and nucleotide combinations points to the existence of multiple antibodies. There is no substantial evidence that these antibodies are intrinsically pathogenic except in so far as soluble complexes with antigen in the circulating blood may be responsible for the kidney lesions. Current studies on the antibodies that can be released from SLE kidneys obtained at autopsy indicate that antibody specifically directed against components of the glomerular basement membrane is also present. As usual there are doubts as to how far such antibody is responsible for the actual lesion observed.

The pathogenesis of the disease

In an attempt to picture the pathogenesis of SLE, one is compelled to assume an important genotypic abnormality, possibly, as Burch suggests, involving the X chromosome. It is reasonable that these genetic changes should make it easier for somagenetic change to increase resistance of a proportion of immunocytes to the destructive effect of contact with antigenic determinants of body constituents present in the thymus. SLE, however, differs sharply from any other autoimmune disease in the multiplicity of 'forbidden' immune patterns which emerge, and some explanation of this is called for. It seems as if there is at some point a massive breakdown in the control function, and an exceptional opportunity for immunocytes to be stimulated by products of nuclear autolysis.

A good case can be made for believing that this breakdown of homeostasis may be a result of the thymus becoming a target organ for the autoimmune process. At a certain stage of this attack the censorship function is lost or weakened so that there can be actual stimulation by antigens present in the thymus of any appropriate newly differentiated cells. All workers are agreed that the most striking metabolic activity of the thymus is the rapid proliferation of lymphocytes with a high nucleocytoplasmic ratio and their almost as rapid breakdown and presumed re-utilization as building blocks for the newly synthesizing cells. There must therefore be a high concentration of nuclear fragments and antigenic determinants of every sort. In the normal individual this merely ensures the elimination of all newly differentiated immunocytes capable of reacting with nuclear material. If, in the individual predisposed genetically to SLE, a relatively large proportion of immunocytes take on resistance of this type, then it will be particularly those cells reactive with nuclear determinants of various types which will emerge, since there is a higher concentration of these than of any other 'self-antigens' in the thymus. A process of this type would almost certainly give rise to germinal centres in the thymus in early SLE. It would also inevitably produce an intolerably unstable situation in the thymus, that could well lead to the disappearance of cortex and increase in epithelial cells that is in fact observed in the thymus even of untreated SLE.

Within this hypothetical frame there is scope for introducing other factors that might be concerned in determining when the disease is initiated. The balance between destruction and stimulation of cells carrying receptors of appropriate pattern within the thymus would be a very delicate one, and quite minor stress episodes with increased cellular destruction in the thymus could swing it toward the conditions allowing increased emergence of pathogenic clones. There is no suggestion that SLE is a monoclonal disease. Detailed serological study points to the involvement of many distinct clones of pathogenic immunocytes. No procedure exactly comparable to the elution of antibody from Coombs-positive cells in anti-nuclear factor is possible but it has been shown that ANF may be present in both G and M immunoglobulins and that each type contains light chains of both κ and λ specificity.

RHEUMATOID ARTHRITIS

Rheumatoid arthritis (RA) may well be the commonest of autoimmune diseases. Burch calculates that approximately 50 per cent of the populations in northern Europe are genetically susceptible and that, in women, most of that 50 per cent will show clinical signs if they live long enough.

The only fully established serological change associated with RA is the presence of rheumatoid factor, an M-type immunoglobulin strongly reactive with partially denatured immunoglobulins of human and, to a lesser extent, other mammalian origin. There is, as in every other well-studied autoimmune disease, a great heterogeneity of detail at both clinical and immunological levels, and an attempt to present a unitary picture of the pathogenesis is perhaps premature. Nevertheless there is nothing equivocal about the information that has been obtained serologically nor does there seem to be any reason to doubt that interaction between partially denatured immunoglobulin acting as antigen and corresponding antibodies or immunocytes plays a significant part in the pathogenesis of RA.

Immunoglobulin as antigen

The control of the antigenic potentialities of immunoglobulins is probably the most subtle of all the problems of immunological homeostasis in the body. The primary function of an antibody is to lay down on the surface of a foreign particle a coating of immunologically inert protein which is nevertheless effective in facilitating the phagocytosis of the foreign particle. When an antibody molecule is firmly attached to an antigen particle or surface it will undergo a variable degree of molecular distortion which may either result in the appearance of a new antigenic determinant or render an existing one more accessible. The standard approach to the antigenic differentiation of human Ig G has been to examine the capacity of human sera from suitable donors to agglutinate red cells coated with incomplete Rh antibody which acts as the antigen in the system. In this way a means has become available for categorizing the Ig G of the person who provided the Rh-antiserum. The tests can be elaborated in various ways by the use of cross-absorption and inhibition experiments to allow an easy classification of any human Ig G. The details have been of very great interest in regard to the genetic aspects of immunoglobulin production but are of no particular relevance to the pathogenesis of RA. The essential feature is that there are antigenic determinants by which individuals differ in the structure of either heavy chain (Gm factors) or light chain (Inv factors) of Ig G. Most rheumatoid factor antiglobulins are in antibodies not reacting with the patient's own immunoglobulin but some have also the quality of auto-antibodies.

Anti-γ-globulins are not unique to RA patients. If a Gm(a+) mother gives birth to a Gm(a−) child, her Ig G will be present in the child's circulation for some months after birth. A proportion of such children produce indefinitely antibody reactive with Gm(a+)-coated cells. In general, about 1 per cent of normal human sera can agglutinate one or other type of coated red cell. Such antisera always lack the factor they react with; in other words the antibodies are isoantibodies, not auto-antibodies.

Another finding which may be relevant to the pathogenesis of rheumatoid fever is the regular appearance of rheumatoid factor in cases of subacute bacterial endocarditis. Here there is a constant production and liberation into the bloodstream of bacteria from the damaged heart valves. Antibodies against the bacteria are also being produced and antibody-coated bacteria are therefore constantly being taken up by macrophages. The antiglobulin produced is an auto-antibody with most of the qualities of rheumatoid factor but, unlike the antiglobulin in an RA patient, it disappears when the infection is effectively removed by antibacterial therapy.

There is no evidence that rheumatoid factor as such has any pathogenic effect whatever and a good deal to suggest that it may have a protective effect against symptomatic expression of the genetic and immunological weakness.

The pathogenesis of the disease

The pathological evidence that a part is played by immune processes related to the immunoglobulins has been obtained by the use of immunofluorescence studies of synovia from infected joints and draining lymph nodes. Many plasma cells in this situation are producing anti-human γ-globulin; there are phagocytic 'RA' cells which appear to contain complexed globulin, presumably antigen–antibody complexes, and there is an abnormally low amount of complement in the synovial fluid. Although persons can have a high titre of rheumatoid factor in their circulating blood without symptoms, it is interesting that several of the rare complications of RA in which cellular infiltrates are conspicuous are always accompanied by a high rheumatoid factor titre. These include subcutaneous nodules, Felty's syndrome of splenomegaly and generalized vascular disease.

In attempting an interpretation of RA in terms of the general approach we are using, we must consider first the almost constant presence within the body of partially denatured immunoglobulins. Harmless casual infection of the bloodstream is an everyday occurrence and more overt local or general infections will at frequent intervals be dealt with by processes in which fixation of antibody on micro-organisms or their products will result in its partial denaturation. In one way or another it is a necessity for survival that such material should not be antigenic. The actual way in which this form of natural tolerance develops is unknown. It may be that sufficient of the antigenic determinants are present on native circulating immunoglobulins to ensure that reactive immunocytes are destroyed soon after they differentiate. The anomaly in the potential rheumatoid individual would be, as in other autoimmune conditions, the emergence of mutants abnormally resistant to destruction by antigenic contact. All antiglobulins produced in man by any of the ways that have been mentioned are macroglobulins (Ig M) and as such are not significantly supported by the appearance of 'memory cells'. Normally, therefore, any reactive clone that emerged to produce rheumatoid factor would fade out fairly rapidly, just as happens when a patient with subacute bacterial endocarditis eliminates his infection. The anomaly in RA could well be a capacity for antibody-producing cells to go on proliferating, once specific stimulation has occurred for a longer period than normal. Such delayed maturation of committed immunocytes in which Ig M antibody fails to be replaced as normally by Ig G antibody is frequently seen experimentally when X-irradiation or immunosuppressive drugs are used. A pathological and persistent failure of maturation is the most direct interpretation of Waldenström's macroglobulinaemia, and in this connection it is of great interest that in some cases of macroglobulinaemia the abnormal immunoglobulin M has the reactivity of an antiglobulin.

So far we have been concerned only with the appearance of the abnormal antibody. Its presence implies proliferation of abnormal immunocytes and in all probability the symptoms and lesions of RA represent the cytopathic activities of immunocytes plus secondary changes. A certain 'aggressiveness' can be postulated as differentiating the antiglobulin immunocytes in the rheumatoid patient from those in the person with rheumatoid factor but no symptoms. The nature of this aggressiveness is unknown, but it can probably be equated with the similar increase in the cellular pathogenicity of immunocytes that is associated with the use of Freund's complete adjuvant. It is significant that a subacute arthritis can be produced in rats by injection of F.C.A. alone.

The abnormality in persons subject to RA is primarily genetic, allowing the appearance of somatic mutant cells which, in one way or another, have developed a capacity to enter tissues and react damagingly with any Ig G in some partially denatured form that may be present there. The joints are sites of election for serum sickness reactions and for the manifestation of postfebrile synovitis as seen in rubella and other infections. It is apparently a common site for the local fixation of antigen–antibody complexes. When this occurs the joint is in essentially the same position as any other local target organ. The specific antigen, in this case partially denatured γ-globulin, is in the tissue and with the entry of an immunocyte with the needed aggressive quality, reaction with the antigen will allow further damage and greater opportunity for both immunocytes and antibody to reach the area. It is reasonable to consider Kunkel's suggestion that there may be a special type of pathogenic antibody, perhaps of abnormally high avidity, which is more likely to fix complement and mediate cell damage. Entry and accumulation of lymphoid cells (including plasma cells) is a feature, however, and it seems best to think of both immunocyte and its corresponding antibody as playing parts in the pathogenic process. The main result will be the inauguration of a vicious circle with fixation of globulin-antibody which, by local denaturation, becomes globulin-antigen.

If, as is the case in many analogous situations, contact of some types of antibody with cell-bound antigen is much less damaging than specific immunocyte contact, the presence of high levels of antibody may be beneficial to the patient by rendering antigen unavailable to react with immunocytes. In congenital agammaglobulinaemia, arthritis of rheumatoid type is common in the absence of rheumatoid factor or of more than minimal amounts of other immunoglobulins.

The variability in age and sex incidence, in intensity of the disease and in the occurrence of spontaneous, or drug-induced remissions of the disease, is in line with the factors concerned in the pathogenesis of RA. At the genetic level we may adopt Burch's formulation that susceptibles are homozygous at an autosomal locus and in addition must undergo one, two or more sequential mutations on the X chromosome, or the simpler interpretation of Maynard Smith that both the genetic and the somagenetic anomalies are on the X chromosome and that only one of each is needed. The primary provision of denatured immunoglobulin as a necessary stimulus must have a quantitative and probably a qualitative factor, and the old story of 'septic foci' may have a substratum of truth. Further development of the condition once potentially pathogenic cells have emerged will still be dependent on essentially random factors concerned with sequential mutation of varying degrees of effectiveness plus environmental factors, such as cold and minor trauma, rendering some joints more vulnerable than others. It is highly probable that genetic factors also play a part in determining the vulnerability of joints and the ease with which a vicious circle is initiated. As hinted earlier, the relative balance between titre of circulating antibody and numbers of active immunocytes may be important while, finally, the possibility must not be forgotten that a mutant clone of immunocytes may carry a new antigenic determinant that renders it subject to immune surveillance.

As in every other instance of autoimmune disease we have an immensely complex ecological and micro-evolutionary system at the cellular level.

MYASTHENIA GRAVIS

From the angle of theoretical immunology, autoimmune disease is important only for the light it may throw on the controlling processes which allow the normal functioning of immunity. If the thymus is a key point in immunological homeostasis it is of obvious interest to pay special attention to its involvement in autoimmune disease. Reasons have been given for believing that the thymus might be of importance in the early stages of SLE but more attention has been paid to myasthenia gravis, the only generalized disease in which the thymus is manifestly and regularly involved.

Myasthenia gravis at the symptomatic level is a functional disease of the neuromuscular junction, shown by rapid onset of muscular weakness and fatigue, often limited to some muscle groups, and with drooping of the eyelids the commonest manifestation. The effect is temporarily alleviated by drugs of prostigmine type and at the pharmacological level represents ineffective transfer of acetylcholine across the neuromuscular junction. Biopsy of an affected muscle usually shows very little except for occasional small collections of lymphocytes. Very rarely the lymphocytic infiltration reaches the level of a chronic myositis. In nearly all cases the thymus shows striking changes, either moderate enlargement with conspicuous germinal centres in the medulla, or a low-grade non-malignant lympho-epithelial tumour which may be associated with germinal centres in the uninvolved portions of the thymus. The general consensus of clinical opinion is that thymectomy has a beneficial effect on the disease in the common group of young women with only germinal centre formation in the thymus, while patients with tumour usually show no benefit from removal of tumour and thymus.

No serious attempt to interpret the relationship of the thymic changes to the pathogenesis of myasthenia seems to have been made until we observed the consistent presence of germinal centres in the thymus of the autoimmune strain of mouse NZB. There had, however, already been a recognition that a substantial proportion of myasthenics had circulating antibody reactive with the A band of skeletal muscle and demonstrable by immunofluorescent technique. Later it was shown that, in about half the cases showing muscle reactivity, the same antibody reacted with thymic epithelial or myo-epithelial cells, but other sera reacted only with muscle.

There is no generally accepted interpretation of the pathogenesis of myasthenia gravis but it is not difficult to fit the observations into a pattern similar to that of other autoimmune diseases. The curve of age-incidence and the strong concentration of cases in adolescent and young adult females is in line with a number of other autoimmune conditions. Again, this suggests genetic and somagenetic factors with the initiating event being the emergence of a clone of immunocytes reactive against one or more of a range of antigenic determinants present within a variety of cells. None of these determinants has been chemically defined but they include structures in or functionally related to (a) the neuromuscular apparatus; (b) the A band of skeletal muscle; (c) cardiac muscle and (d) thymic epithelium or myoid cells. There is now a suggestion that the cells involved in the thymus are myoid cells with many of the characteristics of striated muscle cells. Their presence in the thymus remains unexplained. As in every other constellation of autoimmune disease we have again a Darwinian complexity of mutation and opportunity for cellular proliferation, survival and production of antibody. The part played in pathogenesis by antibody on the one hand and by direct cellular action on the other is obscure. In the absence of any record of cellular infiltration or other abnormality at the neuromuscular junction it is possible that the symptoms could be due to antibody becoming specifically attached to an antigenic determinant in neuromuscular junctions, but the possibility that the effect is due to a hormone-like agent rather than an antibody is not excluded.

From our point of view the thymic aspect is of much greater interest. Reverting first to the presence of areas of lymphoid cell proliferation in the thymic medulla, this is best seen in myasthenia gravis but it has also been reported in some of the relatively few biopsies that have been done or cases of other autoimmune diseases. In any extensive series of human thymic biopsies—for example, those obtainable in a variety of surgical procedures in the thorax—an occasional medullary germinal centre will be found. In animals showing autoimmune disease, only the NZB mice and their hybrids have been studied. All show variable but often extensive proliferative medullary lesions.

The least controversial interpretation is that normally the thymus is forbidden ground (because of some peculiarity of the internal environment) for the development of germinal centres or plasma cells and that when these appear they are the progeny of mutant cells resistant to the normal controls. If the antigenic determinant capable of specific stimulation of such cells is present in the thymus this would be an additional reason for the presence of the germinal centres.

Lympho-epithelial tumours of the thymus

Of even more interest than the germinal centres are the lympho-epithelial tumours of the thymus. In general, these are not malignant. A proportion produce or are associated with no general symptoms and are recognized only because of pressure symptoms or from routine X-rays. There are, however, three important conditions associated to a significant degree with such tumours—myasthenia gravis, pancytopenia with aregenerative anaemia and acquired agammaglobulinaemia.

Myasthenia gravis is much the most common. Here several points deserve mention. The cases associated with thymic tumour are, in general, in older patients; are almost invariably associated with demonstrable antibody, and more often show frank myositis. Removal of the tumour has no influence on symptoms and does not change serological reactivity—in both these respects differing from simple myasthenia in young women without tumour. The tumours are always of mixed lymphoid-epithelial type; the two cell types varying in dominance from an almost wholly epithelial and spindled cell tumour to a histological appearance indistinguishable from Hodgkin's disease.

Various interpretations of the relationship of the tumour to the myasthenic syndrome have been suggested. The only one consistent with the approach I have adopted is that in these cases we are concerned with active and widely dispersed clones of reactive immunocytes with capacity to react at a low level with thymic epithelium. The result of that interaction is a chronic proliferative stimulus to the epithelial cells with, as a corollary, a more or less equivalent stimulus to lymphocytic proliferation. There is a real possibility that the type of stimulus is to some extent equivalent to the long-acting thyroid stimulator substance found in thyrotoxicosis.

If this point of view is accepted it is a logical extension to believe that in the target organs or substances previously mentioned are antigenic determinants common to the thymic epithelium. The thymoma would then be a variable concomitant of an autoimmune process, whose significant target was: muscle and neuromuscular junction—myasthenia gravis; haematopoietic stem cell—aplastic anaemia; 'gut-associated' hormone—acquired agammaglobulinaemia. It may be relevant that the branchial cleft epithelium from which the thymus is derived has wide potentialities and gives rise to thyroid, parathyroid and lung. The possibility that among the epithelial cells of the thymus there exists a variety of partially differentiated cells is suggested by the already mentioned myoid cells, and from the well-known fact that when small cysts appear in the mouse thymus the lining cells frequently show typical cilia with the structure of those in the respiratory tract. If this is the case it would have important implications for the censorship function of the thymus.

It would be in accord both with the facts and with this formulation that there should be occasional cases of mixed conditions or of the co-existence with thymoma of types of autoimmune disease outside this group.

ORGAN-SPECIFIC AUTOIMMUNE DISEASES

It has been a curious development in the last decade to find an ever-increasing group of 'diseases of unknown aetiology' being brought into the autoimmune category. One can almost suggest that any disease not of clearly visible genetic, nutritional, infective or traumatic origin which involves a definable function or organ and comes on after a phase of normal health should be regarded as a candidate for interpretation as an autoimmune disease.

Thyroid disease

One of the most interesting aspects of general medicine in the 1960s is the sudden swing of interest toward an autoimmune interpretation of thyrotoxicosis. Frank autoimmune disease of the thyroid, Hashimoto's disease, has been recognized for many years and need only be used here as the classical example of organ-specific autoimmune disease.

Of all the commonly looked-for auto-antibodies, those detected by thyroglobulin-coated tanned cells or complement fixation with thyroid extracts are the most frequently found. In many instances, thyroid auto-antibodies are found with no evidence of thyroid dysfunction but equally, examination of the thyroid *post mortem* in elderly females without history of thyroid disease will show many with significant minor infiltration by lymphoid cells in the thyroid. The serological tests used to measure anti-thyroid antibodies are numerous and several distinct antigenic determinants are probably concerned. The antigens used are thyroglobulin, a second colloid antigen, and a microsomal antigen extractable from thyroids from patients with thyrotoxicosis. Immunofluorescent studies using sections of thyroid tissue differentiate the location of these antigens. Complement fixation and tanned cell methods are also applicable with some, while the thyroid-stimulating antibody (LATS), mentioned below, is detected by *in vivo* tests.

There is quite extensive evidence to indicate a genetic component in thyroid disease. Close relatives of patients with Hashimoto's disease have a higher incidence of positive serological findings, particularly in women, than relatives of matched control individuals. Thyrotoxicosis and Hashimoto's disease are both much more frequent in women than in men but show quite different age incidences. Both patterns of age incidence have, however, analogies with standard autoimmune diseases: thyrotoxicosis with SLE and Hashimoto's disease with rheumatoid arthritis. It is reasonable, therefore, to explore the same general hypothesis of one or more somatic mutations on the background of a genetic deviation from normal. As before, the combination of genetic and somagenetic qualities is responsible for the resistance of the immunocytes involved to the normal homeostatic mechanisms.

What is less clear than in other instances is the distribution of the relevant antigens in the body and their role in controlling the numbers and type of reactive immunocytes. It is relatively easy to produce anti-thyroglobulin antibodies in experimental animals by injection of substantial amounts of thyroid extracts, even without adjuvant. There is therefore no significant tolerance to the specific antigenic determinants. In human adults there are minute amounts of thyroglobulin in the circulating blood and this amount is increased in association with surgical manipulations of the gland. Most individuals do not respond to these concentrations by demonstrable antibody production. It seems the most appropriate initial approach to the human situation to make the following assumptions: (*a*) there is insufficient circulating thyroid antigen of any type in the normal individual to produce tolerance or to induce antibody production, (*b*) small numbers of cells reactive with thyroid antigenic determinants are produced but the position is such that contact with antigen does no more than produce very small amounts of Ig M antibody and no memory cells and (*c*) in persons genetically predisposed, immunocytes of aberrant quality arise by somatic mutation which (i) escape contact with any organ-specific antigen in primary sites of differentiation, (ii) are avid enough to react with thyroglobulin, producing Ig M, Ig G, and memory cells and (iii) have 'invasive' or similar qualities allowing entry into thyroid tissue with production of diffuse lymphocytic infiltration and germinal centres. It is highly probable that such populations of pathogenic immunocytes are heterogeneous and with different functional potentialities.

In earlier discussion the suggestion was raised that an automatic protection of inaccessible antigens from involvement in auto-immune processes could be provided if movement of lymphocytes through the tissues was confined to committed cells, that is, those derived from cells which had already made effective contact with an antigen. Virgin cells would be limited in their movement to entering and leaving peripheral lymphoid tissues. It is difficult to obtain evidence for or against this hypothesis, and it should probably be kept in reserve until a technical approach to testing it is available.

There are considerable numbers of cases on record in which the sequence of thyrotoxicosis, Hashimoto's disease and myxoedema can be recognized. All are strikingly commoner in females. The sequence, however, is by no means invariable and *a priori* it seems unlikely that all cases of thyrotoxicosis have an autoimmune origin. Nevertheless, from our present approach, what is required is simply an interpretation of the part which can be played by autoimmune processes in the sequence.

Interest in thyrotoxicosis as an autoimmune condition arose mainly because of the recognition that LATS present in the blood of some patients with thyrotoxicosis was not, as originally thought, a pituitary hormone of abnormal character but an Ig G. In addition it had long been known that, next to Hashimoto's disease, the highest proportion of sera with antithyroid antibodies came from thyrotoxicoses and, as already mentioned, the age and sex incidence is that to be expected of an autoimmune disease.

Unequivocal demonstration of LATS is possible only in a proportion of cases, but is characteristically present in severe cases with ophthalmic symptoms and pre-tibial oedema. As yet it is not known whether in such cases there is lymphocytic infiltrate in unusual amount in thyroid substance, or whether germinal centres in the thymus are regularly present. Both could be expected and actual demonstration that this was the case would increase our confidence in ascribing thyrotoxicosis to an autoimmune process. An Ig G antibody might well be the primary agent in stimulating excessive activity of the thyroid. The actual antigen or antigenic determinant involved is not yet known and, by implication, it is different in specificity from both thyroglobulin and cytoplasmic antibodies. As in other autoimmune situations the initiation of the process could, by increasing the amount and accessibility of the antigen, generate a vicious circle and also increase the likelihood that other types of immunocyte reactive with thyroid antigenic determinants would be brought into active proliferation.

In all forms of autoimmune disease we find a basically similar situation—the appearance of a wide range of immunocytes reactive against the antigenic determinants involved and a complex and variable ecological situation dependent on the local availability of the antigens concerned and any mutant characters influencing the immunocytes' response. Admittedly this is a very flexible approach which can rather readily be adapted to meet any anomalous circumstance that may arise, but the actual facts of autoimmune disease *are* so individual and only broadly reproducible that any approach must of necessity be a flexible one.

Some special features of the thyroid autoimmune complex call for brief comment. The thymus is regularly enlarged in thyrotoxicosis and when its upper isthmus area is biopsied during surgery of the thymus, about one-third of the specimens show germinal centres. It is unfortunate that there is no safe and convenient way of obtaining biopsy material from the thymus. The sequence of thymic changes associated with a severe case of thyrotoxicosis could be very enlightening and it could well emerge that some of the antigenic determinants were common to thyroid and thymic epithelia.

Other conditions involving specific organs

Another organ of special interest is the adrenal. Non-tuberculous Addison's disease is usually autoimmune in character and organ-specific antibodies are commonly demonstrable. At least half such cases also show thyroid antibodies and there is one reference to the occurrence of germinal centres in the thymus. On the other hand, the great majority of sera positive for thyroid antibodies are negative when tested with adrenal antigens. Of all the organs of the body the thyroid is the most prone to autoimmune disease. In the absence of any reason to the contrary, we can assume that if some human individuals can produce a particular organ-specific antibody others in principle can also give rise to cells with this capacity and, further, that there is no *a priori* reason for believing that any one type of autoimmune pattern will arise with greater frequency than another. It is axiomatic in our approach that any of the mutant forms of resistance to immunological controls arise wholly independently of the immune pattern(s) carried by the cell line. If this is true, then the frequency of different local autoimmune disease types in women must be related to antigen factors, presumably concentration and accessibility. The pre-eminence of thyroid disease would presumably be related to the marked changes in physiological activity associated with emotion, pregnancy, etc., and perhaps an associated leak of antigens into the circulation on a relatively larger scale than other organs.

The next most commonly found antibody is directed toward an antigen present in the gastric parietal cells. This antibody is found in nearly 100 per cent of patients with pernicious anaemia and there is a strong positive correlation with the presence of thyroid antibodies. Using the same type of argument, the accessibility of gastric antigen presumably depends on local trauma and infection, particularly in association with low acid secretion.

The antibodies concerned are each specific so that the positive correlation of antibodies directed against thyroid, gastric cells and adrenal must be more deeply based and at the theoretical level represents the main problem of localized autoimmune disease. Expanding slightly the above interpretation, we assume that in certain individuals, notably females, there is a predisposition for mutant immunocytes to appear in which there is a heightened capacity to induce local autoimmune disease. The exact character of the *cellular* expression of the genotype is unknown, but one or more of the following differences from the normal might be involved: (a) resistance to destruction by antigen in the phase of first differentiation, (b) enhanced capacity to swing from Ig M production to Ig G and (c) capacity to move through tissues in the uncommitted state. Such mutant character will be randomly distributed amongst immunocytes and will be expected to have survival advantage only when the associated immune pattern is reactive with an organ-specific antigenic determinant and when it can meet an adequate concentration of the determinant. With a constant very small influx of mutants of the necessary type, many subjects may escape disease indefinitely unless some initiating trauma or infection allows an abnormally high concentration of accessible antigen. In general the proportion of antibodies for each organ will depend on the various factors relevant to this accessibility of antigen. In fact, the various figures in the literature are not greatly discrepant from what would be expected, on the very simple assumptions that 10 per cent of females in a standard population

Autoimmune disease

will produce significant numbers of mutants and that the chance of these initiating antibody production is 1:3 for both thyroid and gastric parietal cell and 1:200 for adrenal. Then the proportion showing antibody in four different populations would be as in table 6.

TABLE 6. *Occurrence of tissue-specific antibodies in human populations*

Population	Thyroid	Gastric parietal cell	Adrenal
Standard	3·3 (4)	3·3 (7)	0·01 (—)
Hashimoto's disease	100 (97)	33 (27)	0·1 (—)
Pernicious anaemia	33 (33)	100 (83)	0·1 (—)
Adrenal atrophy	33 (52)	33 (—)	100 (60)

Percentages to be expected from the simplified hypothesis given in the text with, in parentheses, approximate percentages observed in series recorded by Mackay and Burnet or Doniach and Roitt.

These fit the published data reasonably well, except for idiopathic adrenal disease, where 60 per cent gave adrenal antibody but 52 per cent gave thyroid antibody. This merely accentuates the point being made by suggesting that a rather higher grade of anomaly is needed to give adrenal damage.

IMMUNOPATHOLOGICAL CONDITIONS ASSOCIATED WITH THE ENTRY OF ENVIRONMENTAL FACTORS

Rheumatic fever

Rheumatic fever has many of the features of an autoimmune disease but it is quite clearly related to streptococcal infection. The connection is currently ascribed to the accidental resemblance or identity of a streptococcal determinant and an inaccessible tissue determinant in cardiac muscle and possibly in synovial tissue. This has been taken by a number of authors as a prototype for all or most autoimmune diseases, so allowing the postulate of an external cause (usually an unidentified virus) instead of the less easily comprehended concept of somatic genetic origin.

The pathogenesis of rheumatic fever is not yet fully understood although Kaplan's demonstration of common antigens in streptococci and cardiac muscle makes it highly probable that the carditis is largely a result of damage by the antibodies and immunocytes that have emerged as a result of the streptococcal infection. The origin of the rheumatic nodule (including the Aschoff body) and of the polyarthritis is controversial, but it seems likely that they represent sites of lodgment of dead or lethally affected streptococci and associated antibodies. The situation is clearly very complex and has a distinct resemblance in some aspects to delayed hypersensitivity. The whole picture suggests that acute or subacute infection of the tonsils provides a situation where antigen, toxic substances and immunocytes are intimately related in a fashion reminiscent of the Freund adjuvant granuloma.

By the time the infection has been present for from 10 to 20 days, a large population of immunocytes, including plasma cells and 'aggressive' lymphocytes, has accumulated and passed to other regions of the body. In one of two possible ways the synovial cells are vulnerable to immunocyte and/or antibody attack. They may have taken up streptococcal antigens circulating in the early stages of the infection or the vicinity of the synovial tissues may be a preferred site for lodgment of antigen–antibody complexes. There is no evidence that an antigenic determinant cross-reacting with a streptococcal product is present in synovia but it cannot be ruled out. Possibly in its favour is the migratory character of rheumatic polyarthritis, indicating that there is some resistance to starting the inflammatory process but that, once started, it involves all the susceptible cells in the joint concerned. If a blood-borne antigen from the streptococcal nidus in the tonsils was concerned it should be readily available to antibody also arriving by the blood. If, however, the antigen is inaccessible until the cell containing it is damaged, the independent build-up of a destructive process in each joint cavity is to be expected.

The process can be pictured as starting with the deposition of antigen–antibody complex in the perivascular region of the joint. This will result in some local damage with leak of antigen from synovial cells and increased local permeability with entry of cells and antibody from the blood. Some of the entering immunocytes will be reactive and the destructive process will continue.

Autoimmune disease

The general problem

This type of action can be considered in a more general form. Inaccessible antigenic determinants as discussed in relation to myasthenia gravis and autoimmune thyroid disease do not provoke tolerance or antibody production in the normal individual. Small numbers of pre-adapted cells are available as for any other random antigen, and when infection by a micro-organism carrying a major antigenic determinant equivalent to one of the inaccessible body antigens occurs, the normal response takes place giving antibody and an increased population of immunocytes. This does not, in itself, give rise to attack on the cells carrying the equivalent body antigen any more than simple immunization of a rabbit with a thyroid extract provokes damage to its thyroid. In both cases some additional 'aggressiveness' of the immunocytes is needed either genetic in origin or invoked by the use of Freund's adjuvant in the experimental situation. It may also be highly relevant how the immune response is distributed among immunoglobulins A, G and M and the various functional forms of immunocyte including those associated with delayed hypersensitivity. A major function of Ig G antibody is to moderate or annul responses in other immunological categories.

It is clear that if a commonly present extrinsic antigen has an accidental cross-over with an inaccessible body antigenic determinant, any tendency of the individual to autoimmune disease will be biased toward the organ in question. Rheumatic fever and glomerulonephritis may well be determined in part by the fact that the region of proliferation of immunologically competent cells is probably at the site of infection where the infected tonsil has many of the qualities of a Freund granuloma. Any anomalous mutants of high survival value and potential pathogenicity will have an abnormally favourable situation to proliferate, a fact that may be responsible for the acute character of rheumatic fever.

In rheumatoid arthritis we have the interesting probability that low-grade streptococcal infection in older people may provide an ever-present opportunity to initiate an immunological process which develops as an autocatalytic one by the appearance of denatured γ-globulin as the bearer of target antigen determinants. This, however, can only happen when the individual has (*a*) the necessary genetic constitution and (b) can allow the appearance by somatic mutation of the abnormal clones which can react pathogenically with denatured γ-globulin.

Non-bacterial antigens, including drugs

The next possibility to be considered is based on the incorporation of a foreign antigen in the cell by a low-grade viral infection. It is essentially immaterial whether the new antigen is a viral protein, or a host protein that has been rendered foreign by the incorporation of a viral episome in the cell genome or some equivalent process. Three experimental examples may be mentioned:

(a) It is generally accepted that polyoma virus fails to produce tumours in animals injected after the neonatal period because antibody or a cellular immune response against a polyoma-induced antigen eliminates neoplastic cells by a process analogous to the homograft reaction (see chapter 13). Here there is nothing equivalent to autoimmune disease since the only cells damaged are neoplastic ones.

(b) Lymphocytic choriomeningitis infection is harmless if there is no immune response normally demonstrable as perivascular cuffing with lymphocytes in the CNS. This can be prevented either by embryonic induction of tolerance by irradiation or by the use of cytotoxic drugs. The actual antigenic determinants concerned are unknown and the effect is rather remote from autoimmune disease, but it is an example of damage by an immune response.

(c) There is available a strain of Rous sarcoma virus which, when injected into neonatal rats, multiplies and gives rise to a curious multicystic disease of the lymphatic system. With complete neonatal thymectomy immediately before inoculation with the virus the rats remain healthy. The lesions affect tissues in which the virus can be shown to multiply and presumably represent a cellular immune response equivalent to delayed hypersensitivity. Here the resemblance to an autoimmune condition is more striking.

There are no established examples of human conditions fitting into any equivalent categories, but there are perhaps hints that hepatitis virus infections may eventually have to be considered as a possible source of something equivalent to group (c). It is known that hepatitis virus infections in man may be long lasting and the range of cells that can suffer non-damaging infection may be more widespread than the liver. Suggestions have been made that lupoid hepatitis and the New Guinean disease kuru (a cerebellar degeneration) may be autoimmune reactions against tissues carrying a new or newly accessible antigen for which hepatitis virus was in some way responsible. Once satisfactory ways of culturing the hepatitis viruses are available, these questions should be readily resolved.

Quite apart from micro-organisms, non-living, potentially noxious material can enter the body and there are two practically important types of immunologically based disease which can result—hay fever and similar allergies and a variety of drug reactions. Like autoimmune disease, these are the reactions of a minority of people though sometimes a large minority. The syndromes cannot be regarded as physiologically normal ones and some intellectual framework, flexible as always, must be found to fit them.

In many ways the best studied and most interesting are the drug reactions which produce haemolytic disease or thrombocytopenic purpura. Here the damage seems to result from the interaction of antigen (hapten) with antibody, producing a complex which attaches to red cells or platelets and with complement leads to their functional destruction. The process can be clearly demonstrated *in vitro*. In a typical case, for example, of stibophen haemolytic reaction, haemolysis of the patient's or anyone else's red cells can be produced in a mixture containing appropriate amounts of drug, patient's antibody, red cells and complement. In addition to the red cells all three components must be present and analysis of the reaction shows that the first effect is the firm union of drug to antibody. This union changes the quality of the immunoglobulin and perhaps after an intermediate stage of aggregation it is 'nonspecifically' attached to red cells if these are present. With complement, haemolysis follows.

In general, if the antibody is principally Ig M, the complexes attach to red cells; if Ig G, to platelets, with production of thrombocytopenic purpura. N. R. Shulman and others have suggested that what are normally regarded as autoimmune haemolytic anaemias or thrombocytopenic purpuras are in fact the response to an undetected virus or other antigen.

Perhaps a more illuminating way to approach the phenomena is to regard them as being based on the same foundation as autoimmune disease in general, the appearance of unusual types of immunocyte. Only a small proportion of persons given the drugs in question develop haemolytic disease or purpura; in some way they differ from the normal. What is probably the simplest answer is that in the susceptible individual there are a few immunocytes with immune receptors of unusual pattern avid enough to bind the hapten directly. Such cells would also produce small amounts of similarly avid antibody. It is possible that the hapten is itself immunogenic in the sense of being able to stimulate such unusual immunocytes directly, but other explanations are possible. In any case, ingestion of the drug in the susceptible individual results in immunological stimulation and significant amounts of the same abnormally reactive antibody are produced and liberated into the bloodstream. The more important factor is the abnormal immunocyte and antibody, not the nature of the drug.

Hay fever and other allergies can be looked at similarly. The main abnormality seems to be in the production of an abnormally high proportion of antibody in the Ig A (Ig E) category. The overwhelming importance of genetic (including somatic genetic) factors is shown by the occurrence of highly allergic subjects who produce almost all their diphtheria antitoxin in the form of Ig A. As yet we seem to have no suggestion as to the nature of any normal homeostatic mechanisms which maintain the ratio of Ig A to Ig G in the plasma, and until this is remedied there is nothing to be said at the theoretical level about the mechanism by which a genetic predisposition to allergic disease is expressed.

13 Immunological serveillance and the evolution of adaptive immunity

In the last decade there has come into being, without either flourish of trumpets or serious controversy, a general current of belief in what I have come to call 'immunological surveillance'. Somatic mutation is constantly occurring in the mammalian body, and on current genetic theory all mutations in structural genes will result, when the gene is activated, in the production of some protein in which the amino acid sequence differs in some respect from the form genetically characteristic of the individual. Theoretically, at least, immune response against the new protein is therefore a possibility. If a sufficient amount of the new antigen is liberated there will appear a clone of immunocytes which could be expected to mount an attack equivalent to a homograft reaction against the mutant cells and eliminate them from the body. One can therefore picture a form of surveillance by which the body is being continually patrolled, as it were, for the appearance of aberrant protein (or perhaps also polysaccharide) patterns.

The idea has arisen from consideration of a variety of immune phenomena associated with clinical or experimental malignant disease. It is in the field of experimental carcinogenesis that we find experimentally verifiable extensions of the idea.

IMMUNOLOGICAL ASPECTS OF NEOPLASTIC DISEASE

Experimental carcinogenesis
When a tumour is provoked by a virus or chemical carcinogen it is reasonable to assume that a process operationally equivalent to a sequence of somatic mutations has occurred, giving rise to at least one protein antigenically distinguishable from any in normal cells. With growth of the tumour, enough of such protein should be produced to allow a demonstrable immune response. This has now been fully established. Tumours produced by injection of polyoma and other 'tumour viruses' in newborn mice or hamsters

contain a new antigen specific for the virus used and currently interpreted as representing the work of a viral episome incorporated into the host cell genome. The immune response to this antigen confers resistance against polyoma tumour cells which are presumably eliminated by the standard method of homograft immunity. Sarcomas produced in mice or rats by intramuscular injection of methylcholanthrene are also antigenic in a similar sense, but here each tumour seems to have a different new antigenic pattern which presumably arises by some form of somatic mutation. It is possible to amputate the leg bearing the primary sarcoma and establish the tumour cells in tissue culture or by passage through syngeneic animals. They can then be used to show that the mouse in which the tumour arose has an active capacity to reject the tumour cells when they are injected, although control mice of the same strain develop tumours.

The most striking characteristic of the tumour viruses is that, except under such special conditions as neonatal thymectomy, tumours are produced only if the virus is administered to newborn mice or hamsters. Injection of virus into older hosts produces antibody to the virus and no tumours. From virus-induced tumours of both polyoma and SV 40 viruses, strains of tumour cells have been obtained that are free of virus and can be transplanted like any other tumour in syngeneic animals. There are two ways by which animals can be rendered resistant to such a tumour. The potential host can be inoculated when more than a week or two old with the cancer virus X or it can be inoculated with a transplant of a tumour induced by virus X in an allogeneic strain of host. In the second case the tumour graft is rejected as a homograft but a few weeks after the immunizing manipulations such mice show a significant resistance to syngeneic tumour which is specific. Tumours produced by polyoma virus have a common antigen which is not demonstrable in the virus but is generally thought to arise by the activity of a viral episome in the malignant cell genome. Similarly, tumours arising after SV 40 virus infection have a common antigen unrelated to that of the polyoma tumours.

The necessity for neonatal infection if tumours are to be produced is currently interpreted as a manifestation of the relative immunological incompetence of very young mammals. Whatever the process of malignant transformation, it takes place rapidly and is associated with a definable antigenic change or addition in the transformed cell and with active proliferative growth. In the neonatal animal the proliferative process is well established before there can be sufficient stimulation by the new transplantation or histocompatibility antigen to produce the immunocytes that could inhibit the growth of the tumours. When virus is given later there is, by hypothesis, transformation and initiation of neoplastic growth but the response is more rapid and enough specifically active immunocytes are mobilized to nip the process in the bud.

The outcome, tumour or no tumour, is dependent on a balance of factors which can be tipped by minor circumstances. An occasional tumour appears when virus is injected into older animals and many more if such animals have been neonatally thymectomized. If, after neonatal injection of virus, a series of further injections is given, either of virus or of irradiated tumour cells, the incidence of tumours can be sharply reduced. Both findings point indubitably to the importance of immunological factors.

In some ways these virus-induced tumours provide an ideal experimental model of the process of immunological surveillance. New tumours with a definable new antigen begin to proliferate. If the immune response is effective they may fail completely to give any symptomatic or pathological manifestation. This is precisely what is assumed to occur in the process of immune surveillance.

Clinical phenomena in man

Malignant disease is proverbially progressive and lethal unless the whole mass of neoplastic cells can be removed by surgery or its equivalent. In fact, however, there are well-known phenomena which point to a significant impact of immunological processes. There are rare but well-documented instances where an established malignancy proven by biopsy and histological examination has retrogressed spontaneously. Most clinicians would agree that unless there was a significant resistance, presumably immunological, against the proliferation of malignant cells and their spread through the body, the results of surgery, radiation and drug therapy of cancer would be much worse than they are.

There are several other aspects of neoplastic disease in man which are or may be relevant. Pathologists concerned with cancer biopsies are aware that there are considerable differences in the extent to which there is a round-celled reaction at the edge of the tumour mass. In some, plasma cells are conspicuous among lymphocytes and histiocytes. Two studies to correlate the intensity of lymphocytic and plasma cellular response with survival showed an inverse correlation. The more extensive the infiltrate the longer the patient was likely to survive. It is a sound rule that where lymphocytes and plasma cells congregate, an immune process of some sort is going on. The correlation with prognosis suggests that the process here is a homograft response against cells which have been recognized as antigenically distinct from normal cells.

It has been of obvious interest to pathologists to seek for early stages in the development of neoplasia by examining tissues that are prone to malignant change but which have been taken from autopsies on persons dying from unrelated conditions. In several such investigations, systematic histological study has shown that areas of apparently malignant change are much more frequent than would be expected from the known age incidence of clinically diagnosable cancer of the organ concerned. There are, of course, uncertainties about the histological diagnosis of cancer, and it may not be wholly legitimate to assume that a nodule with the histological character of a carcinoma would inevitably become clinical cancer if it were not actively inhibited by an immune process. As far as they go, however, results for prostate, thyroid and adrenal point in this direction. Of rather special interest is the quite different shape of the curves of age-specific incidence of histologically diagnosed carcinoma of the prostate and of death from prostatic cancer. The latter rises very sharply with age and only becomes significant 15–20 years after 'malignant' areas begin to appear in the autopsy sections.

Analogous findings are on record in regard to neuroblastomas of the adrenal, which are forty to fifty times more frequent in autopsies on newborn children than would be expected from the later clinical incidence of the tumour. Thyroid nodules classed as malignant on histological criteria are also vastly more common than overt thyroid carcinoma.

One of the recurrent themes of cancer research has been the

search for antigens in human tumours which were specific either for one class of tumours or for malignant cells as against normal cells. In the light of modern work on histocompatibility differences, most such studies were based on naïve ideas and no clear positive conclusions emerged. There are, however, a number of clinical phenomena which, though rare, are directly associated with malignant disease and seem undoubtedly to be mediated by immunological processes. If this is so it is worth while to look at the ways by which abnormal antigens could be produced by malignant cells.

A tumour cell, like any other somatic cell, could in principle produce any antigen to be found in any tissue of the organism in which it developed. It is also in principle susceptible to mutation or its equivalent by which aberrant proteins with new antigenic determinants may be produced. As a tumour develops, 'progression' to greater malignancy with increasing aneuploidy must mean possibilities of gross disturbance of function in the genome. Mutation will be common and, in addition, if de-repression of 'wrong' loci should occur, this could result in the synthesis of proteins normally produced only by specialized cells in particular organs. If a tumour cell developed a metabolic anomaly of this type and concomitantly proliferated freely so as to produce a substantial mass of tumour, abnormal proteins and their characteristic antigenic determinants could be released in significant amounts.

This point of view can be used in an attempt to interpret some of the rarer concomitants of cancer in man.

(a) The abnormal protein may be a potent hormone producing its characteristic effect. The best known example is the occurrence of hypercalcaemia in cancer patients, associated with the presence of parathyroid hormone in the tumour. In a number of cases, removal of the tumour corrected the hypercalcaemia. Other hormonal effects have also been reported. According to Lebovitz these include (in addition to parathyroid hormone) ACTH, antidiuretic hormone and thyroid-stimulating hormone. Tumours of the liver have also been recorded from which excessive symptom-producing amounts of porphyrins were liberated.

(b) The protein may have the antigenic quality of a substance normally present as an 'inaccessible' tissue-specific antigen in some distant tissue. According to the general rule discussed in chapter 12, this antigen can provoke the proliferation of immunocytes and antibody. Under appropriate genetic and perhaps other types of individual circumstances, this could provoke localized autoimmune disease. The standard example which may call for such an interpretation in the carcinomatous neuromyopathy which in one form or another is fairly often associated with oat-celled (anaplastic) bronchial carcinoma. It may be suggested that the symptoms and lesions in the CNS represent an autoimmune attack by immunocytes (and perhaps antibody) directed against antigenic determinants specific for CNS cells and 'inaccessible' in the sense of not being capable of producing normal tolerance. Different antigenic determinants are probably responsible for the anatomical distribution of the lesions. The effect of this fortuitous synthesis and liberation of normally inaccessible antigens will only be visible (i) in individuals capable of giving rise to pathogenic clones of immunocytes, that is, genetically susceptible to autoimmune disease (one component of this susceptibility is female sex), (ii) when the target organ is such that immunological damage produces significant symptoms in a debilitated patient or (iii) when, for one reason or another, antibody is produced which can be detected by available techniques. The hypothesis accounts satisfactorily for (i) the relationship to a specific histological type of tumour, (ii) the limitation to a small proportion of those with the tumour, (iii) a higher incidence in females than males, (iv) a wide variety of localization within the CNS and (v) the presence of tissue-specific antibody in a proportion of cases. Another important condition usually associated with malignant disease, and with all the qualities of an autoimmune process, is dermatomyositis. The same general hypothesis could be applicable here.

(c) The protein is a normal body component and has no detectable effect.

(d) The protein is of aberrant structure and therefore treated as a foreign antigen. In most instances there would be no indication of the existence of either the new antigen or the antibody. It is possible that one particular kind of aberrant protein is produced by a considerable range of malignant tumours. If so, it might be found that a particular tumour extract might react in immunologically

Immunological surveillance and evolution

demonstrable fashion with a proportion of sera from cancer patients but not with normal sera.

Part at least of the characteristic age incidence of cancer probably depends on the progressive weakening of the surveillance function with age. It is well known that elderly patients with cancer will often fail to reject an inoculum of a standard tissue culture line of human carcinoma cells.

There is thus substantial evidence for the contention, first, that new antigens arise in association with the changes which characterize malignant cells and second, that immune reaction to the new antigens occurs under suitable conditions. These are important points when it comes to deciding how the immune mechanism developed in the course of evolution.

MUTATIONAL ORIGIN OF HISTOCOMPATIBILITY ANTIGENS

In this book I have paid much less attention to homograft immunity and organ transplantation than the current volume of work and surgical interest in the field would seem to warrant. This is primarily because its interest for the central theme of the biological significance of immunity is only peripheral. There is no counterpart in nature of blood transfusion or tissue transplantation but it is the object of this chapter to show that two basic mammalian plenomena, placentation of the fertilized ovum and malignant disease, are better understood if the immunological aspect is included in their consideration. In the first instance it is necessary to consider the significance of what might superficially seem to be a surprising finding, namely, that in every type of bird or mammal that has been examined, any two individuals of the same species will reject each other's skin grafts. There are, of course, exceptions, but it must be firmly emphasized that pure line strains of mice or rats are biological monstrosities that could never survive in nature. Nevertheless it has only been by the use of pure line animals that most of our recent understanding of immunity has come, and for the discussion of immunological surveillance and its evolutionary significance the nature of histocompatibility differences is vital.

There are now some hundreds of registered pure line strains of mice, many of which had common ancestors. It is regarded as a reasonable rule that if from a pure homozygous line one develops two parallel lines which are thenceforward kept quite distinct, the two lines will probably begin to show lack of reciprocal acceptance of skin grafts by the time they are separated for ten generations. These histocompatibility changes are genetically based and presumably arise by mutation. Several complex loci are involved and in mice the H2 locus is one responsible for major differences correlated with parallel differences in the agglutinogens of the red blood cells. A number of other loci may also be involved, and there is a particularly interesting set of phenomena based on a histocompatibility gene carried by the small male Y chromosome. In many homozygous strains of mice, male skin grafted to a female will be rejected, since the Y-based antigen is foreign to the XX host. Female skin is, however, accepted by a male host since it contains no antigen foreign to an animal with both X and Y chromosomes.

It seems therefore that the H2 and other histocompatibility loci must be relatively highly mutable and that there is either a premium for survival on diversity or there is no selective advantage of any particular pattern. In discussing the genetic situation one must be careful not to forget that artificial brother–sister mating is specifically designed to avoid conferring any advantage on heterozygosity, so that if a line with histocompatibility genes AA undergoes a mutation by which one allele of A becomes B, then even if AB is more vigorous than AA or BB there will be around a 12 per cent chance that the AA line will, in a few further inbred generations, become BB. However, it is known that wild or pen-bred stocks are highly heterozygous in histocompatibility characteristics and there is at least prima facie evidence of some advantage for survival when the members of a species are heterogeneous in histocompatibility characteristics. The first reason for this that comes to mind is that the absence of such differences would allow the transmission from old to young of malignant disease. If all human beings were antigenically identical, malignant cells, for example, from carcinoma of the skin in an elderly individual, could implant in any abrasion on the skin of an infant. A little thought will show, in fact, that once any sort of malignant tumour developed it would spread probably with steadily increasing invasiveness throughout the community.

To prevent such a calamity we believe that nature, to speak teleologically, invented the mechanism of vertebrate immunity. In some way the body even of the infant must recognize and reject any cell that is not its own. For this there must be differences to recognize and a means of recognizing such differences. It is the central contention of clonal selection theory that the mechanisms of signal and sensor, stimulus and receptor, arose in characteristically biological fashion by making use for a specialized purpose of the already established phenomena of germinal and somatic mutation.

In developing this approach we assume that the regions of the genome coding for histocompatibility antigens are for some reason either more highly mutable than other regions or, perhaps more likely, a much smaller proportion of mutations result in lethal or nonfunctional results. It is logical to assume that this holds for these loci as much in somatic cells as in germinal cells. Since there is evidence that most or all somatic cells produce histocompatibility antigens it follows that the corresponding structural genes must be active in transcription as well as replication with perhaps greater liability to mutation. We can also assume that if historically a certain strain of mouse has given rise to mutant forms carrying histocompatibility antigens A, B, C, D, then it is reasonable that in an A mouse, *somatic* mutation is likely to produce similar results so that occasional cells have antigens B, C or D as well as or in place of A. We should expect, therefore, to find in any homozygous mouse a few cells of alien character, bearing foreign antigens which would in general correspond to the sort that over the history of the species had arisen by germinal cell mutations. In addition, the existence of the foreign antigen would sooner or later allow the proliferation of complementary clones of immunocytes with or without some production of antibody. In this way we should have a highly efficient mechanism to ensure complete protection against the potential calamity of free transmission of cancer cells amongst the population.

There is a good deal of evidence to suggest that this formulation is in fact very near the truth. Simonsen used a fairly elaborate graft-versus-host assay to test the power of strain A to provoke splenic enlargement in F_1 mice in which one parent was A and the other differed in minor or major histocompatibility characters. Where there was only a minor difference it required large numbers of spleen cells from A to produce the standard degree of splenic enlargement in $(A \times A^1)F_1$s, but if A mice were hyperimmunized with A^1 cells and then used as donors, very much smaller numbers were required. When $(A \times B)F_1$s were used in which B differed strongly from A, very few cells from either normal or immunized donors were necessary to produce the standard effect. It was as if in A there were already plenty of immunocytes active against B antigen, while any A^1 antigen which had appeared normally in A was apparently not sufficiently distinctive or in too small amount to provoke a reaction.

Even more impressive results are obtained using the CAM reaction when adult fowl leucocytes are deposited on the chorioallantoic membrane. This is also a graft-versus-host reaction mediated by differences at the B locus. It can be shown that the number of foci produced on the chorioallantois is a measure of the number of cells in the inoculum capable of reacting with the major antigens *not* found in the donor but present in the embryo. Immunization of the donor with antigens of the recipient strain has no significant effect. The number of reactive cells is sometimes quite high (as much as 1 per cent of the large lymphocytes in the inoculum). The most likely interpretation is that this is the result of stimulation by an antigen not present in the genotype of the donor and therefore presumably or necessarily arising by somatic mutation. This, however, has not been properly established and it would be unwise to exclude the alternative possibility that in the region of the genome coding for the combining site there are short stable sequences which ensure that the appearance of a related group of specificities follows change in adjacent labile nucleotides.

A possibility of special interest is that abnormal lymphoid cells (immunocytes) may differ antigenically from normal and therefore be in themselves subject to the surveillance function. This has been suggested on mathematical grounds by Burch and at the clinical level provides a reason, otherwise not easy to find, why autoimmune diseases do not always persist indefinitely. I know of no direct experimental evidence to substantiate the suggestion, but it has been well established that thymic lymphocytes differ antigenically from the majority of circulating lymphocytes.

The picture that emerges then is that in two complementary areas the mammalian organism has made a virtue of mutation as such to evolve, on the one hand, antigenic heterogeneity within the species and, on the other, to create the diversity of immune pattern in the fashions discussed in chapter 6. The existence of antigenic heterogeneity and of a cellular mechanism to recognize and react with it are both necessary to ensure that foreign cells can be recognized and destroyed. This is an adequate answer to the problem of protection against cancer contagion but it has other implications which may be more important.

The whole process of evolution depends on the liability to error of any mechanism for the replication of information and of the indefinite perpetuation of such errors unless they can be corrected. The evolution of genetic systems has given rise to an indescribably elaborate process of chromosomal control to ensure that the organism that arises from the fertilized ovum shall be a fully functional viable being. The processes by which differentiation of, and subsequent maintenance of, bodily function and structure take place make use of the same cellular mechanisms that are concerned with the transmission of inheritable qualities in the germ cells and, in so far as they are exercised in replication and transcription, must be similarly subject to error.

The likelihood of error is usually calculated in terms of the number of replications or generations and the figure of 10^{-8} per nucleotide has been suggested. In the human body there are of the order of 10^{15} cells of which at least 10^{13} are proliferating cells in blood and lymph systems and in expendable epithelial surfaces. Over the whole period of growth and maintenance an average generation time for any cell line of about one day is probably of the right order of magnitude. It must follow, in any large long-lived animal in which maintenance is dependent on a large turnover of cells, that somatic mutation is a highly significant source of potential disaster. For reasons discussed earlier in chapter 6, somatic mutation is only significant when it can be expanded by preferential proliferation of descendant cells and, from the point of view of danger to the individual, the most significant abnormalities are those which initiate or predispose to malignant disease. There are, however, marginal conditions sometimes of great clinical importance which cannot be called malignant but probably depend equally on somatic mutation. From our point of view the most important is autoimmune disease, but there are also Paget's disease of bone, polycythaemia vera, Hodgkin's disease and the various paraproteinaemias.

THE ALLOGENEIC INHIBITION PHENOMENON

It has been recently suggested from the Karolinska Institute that although surveillance of the tissues for 'nonconformist' cells is a reality, the mechanism is not an immunological one.

The primary observation is that a cytotoxic effect on mouse tumour cells can be produced by lymphocytes from a mouse of a different strain which has been immunized either against the tumour or against normal cells of the strain in which the tumour arose. Normal allogeneic lymphocytes have no such effect but if, by the addition of phytohaemagglutinin, aggregation results, cytotoxic action basically similar to that mediated by immune cells is produced. Syngeneic lymphoid cells have no action on the tumour cells under the same conditions. The suggestion is clear that it is the close apposition of two cells differing in histocompatibility antigens which is responsible for the damage. The function of the immune state of the sensitized cell on this view is primarily to ensure intimate contact between the two cells.

The nature of the reactivity of the wandering cells of invertebrates toward foreign structures will be discussed in a later section (p. 302). The existence of such reactivity in the absence of any specific antibody or specifically reactive cells makes it easy to accept Hellström's point of view, but it by no means follows that the immunological component is unnecessary for surveillance. It is a perfectly arguable case that where there is a major histocompatibility difference between a cell in a tissue and all the adjacent cells, allogeneic inhibition could result in the death and removal of the alien cell. With minor antigenic differences such as are present in methylcholanthrene-induced murine sarcomas, however, all the indications are that for these to be differentiated from normal cells an immunological process is essential. Even the immune response may be initially small and require reinforcement to be effective. In general, the mouse or rat in which a tumour arises and is removed is not significantly resistant to the tumour line until it has been immunized with doses of irradiated cells.

Any necessity for serious consideration of the allogeneic inhibition phenomenon seems to have been removed by Mintz's recent description of composite 'allophenic' mice produced by embryological manipulation and fusion of early embryos of two distinct histocompatibility types. These show complete tolerance to and between both types of cell.

SOMATIC CELL HETEROKARYONS AND THEIR SIGNIFICANCE

In connection with this question of the mutual incompatibility of vertebrate cells it is of very great interest that by suitable artifices this incompatibility can be overcome and hybrid cells or, more correctly, heterokaryons produced in which nuclei of quite different origin function normally in a composite cytoplasm. The possibility arose from studies of Japanese workers who found that when Sendai virus, a distant relative of influenza virus, was grown in tissue culture the cells were not obviously damaged but fused into syncytial masses without cell wall demarcation. Subsequently it was found that by inducing infection or even adding heat-killed Sendai virus to a mixed tissue culture of two types of malignant cells, one from a mouse tumour and one of human origin, mixed heterokaryons containing one or more of the two distinctive types of nuclei could be produced. This has been extended in many directions and a number of instances have now been reported where when simultaneous mitosis of two different types of nuclei has occurred the chromosomes have mingled and the two descendant nuclei contained a full complement of chromosomes of each of the two species. Sometimes a viable clone of cells of this double type has developed.

Even allowing for the fact that virus is present in the system this set of phenomena has implications of great importance for many aspects of biology. In a recent review, H. Harris points out that from the immunological angle the important implication is that *there are no intracellular mechanisms for the recognition of incompatibility*. A foreign nucleus appears to be quite at home in the mixed cytoplasm and synthesizes DNA and RNA in normal fashion.

A further observation of great immunological interest is made when human small lymphocytes are added to a culture of HeLa cells. In the absence of PHA or some equivalent agent, small lymphocytes show no DNA synthesis or mitosis in tissue culture. They can, however, produce heterokaryons with HeLa cells and in these the lymphocytic nuclei enlarge, become less heavily stained and actively synthesize DNA. The same enlargement of nucleus and appearance of DNA synthesis is seen even with nucleated erythrocytes from fowl or frog.

Harris, perhaps moving faster than is fully justified, finds that these results suggest that the orthodox view of differentiation as involving a very elaborate process of repression and de-repression in the nucleus is mistaken. In his view the nucleus is subject only to a 'coarse' control of its general synthetic ability, the fine adjustments of protein synthesis and assembly being controlled in the cytoplasm. Should this heterodox approach find experimental support it is going to be of obvious importance to immunological theory. For the present it is the only possible choice to adopt the ruling opinion that vertebrate cells function according to the rules derived from the study of bacteria. This will always be subject to the qualification that conditions are much more complex than in bacteria and that the model we apply may be basically correct yet from its nature divert our interest from other important aspects of the control processes in vertebrate cells.

In the present context of the interaction of body cells with mutant or allogeneic types, it is clear that the process is at a surface level and must involve the generation of signals by the impact of external pattern on surface pattern acting as receptor. This would, of course, be compatible with either of the two alternatives of allogeneic inhibition or immune surveillance.

THE EVOLUTION OF THE IMMUNE PROCESS

Defence processes in invertebrates

Vertebrates evolved from invertebrates, which from the time of the first multicellular organisms must have developed adequate mechanisms to protect them from micro-organismal infection. There are in mammals many signs of defence mechanisms unrelated to recognition of foreignness or antibody production, which represent direct developments from the primitive invertebrate system. It is our contention, however, that as vertebrates evolved, grew larger and more active, the need to counter the internal dangers of somatic mutation provided the frame within which the immune system we know in mammals had to evolve.

There is still much to be done in comparative immunology but it seems possible to make a series of general statements based largely on the writings of Good and his colleagues. The characteristic features of the mammalian immune system are: (*a*) capacity to reject homografts and accept autografts, (*b*) *specific* immune responses either by cellular activity or antibody production, (*c*) the thymus as the initial organ of differentiation, (*d*) lymphocytes and plasma cells as effector cells and (*e*) the immunoglobulins as the vehicle for antibody.

None of these five characteristics is found unequivocally in any invertebrate, though it would be hard to rule out the possibility that a vehicle for antibody, if it existed, could well have very little in common with the mammalian immunoglobulins or that a wandering mononuclear cell might not be equivalent to a lymphocyte. Fairly extensive studies have been made on insects as the most easily handled of the invertebrates. No antibody production has ever been detected and experimental zoologists have no difficulty in transplanting hormone-producing tissues from one individual to another. A striking instance of the absence of immune reaction in invertebrates can be seen in the way certain nudibranch molluscs when feeding on sea anemone tentacles transfer the nematocysts in functional form to their own tissues.

There is of course a fairly elaborate protective response against the entry of foreign organisms or material into invertebrates. After all, it was the classic observation of Metchnikoff on the phagocytic cells of the freshwater crustacean *Daphnia* that initiated the cellular approach in immunology. The evidence appears to be adequate that nothing recognizable as antibody could be detected after the injection of material that would be highly antigenic in mammals into representative insects and marine worms. Nor is there any evidence of homograft rejection although, as would be expected, if one moves too far away there is rejection. A *Cecropia* pupa will accept a tissue from a variety of related species but not from other orders of insects.

There can, however, be no doubt that there is some recognition of foreignness in invertebrates even if it is of a much cruder character than occurs in warm-blooded vertebrates.

In the first place, several authors have found that the body fluids of invertebrates may contain relatively high-titre agglutinins against a range of mammalian red cells and, just as would be the case with 'normal antibodies' of vertebrate origin, appropriate absorption experiments showed that in the coelomic fluid of a Californian lobster a relatively large number of different molecular forms of protein must be present in the fluid. There is no evidence that these 'normal antibodies' are increased by immunization and their existence may mean no more than that any soluble globular protein is likely to carry sequences of amino acids, perhaps in duplex or multiplex form, which have a physical adsorptive action of similar quality to that of an antibody combining site. It is axiomatic that in an organism which has reached a dynamically stable situation, cells must tolerate cells adjacent to them and that mobile cells and proteins must have no harmful effect on cells that are accessible to them. These imperatives would eliminate organisms in which mutation led to a pattern which had a specifically harmful effect but would have no bearing on simple polymorphisms with no significant impact on survival. It means nothing to a lobster whether or not its body fluid will agglutinate rabbit red cells or whether several different (but all harmless) patterns may be present amongst such proteins. But there is material here that could be worked up by mutation and selection till a vertebrate immune system evolved.

At the cellular level the arthropods and most other invertebrates have haemocytes in their body fluids which accumulate around foreign spicules or parasites. At most there is no more than a certain nonspecific increase in the rapidity of such mobilization after 'immunization'. The nature of 'recognition as foreign' still presents a problem. A partial answer may be to adopt the relatively naïve but still legitimate hypothesis that the cell surface has been evolved to be dynamically stable in relation to any other surface or soluble component that it encounters normally. In contact with 'anything else' the consequences have no evolutionary significance. The presence and extent of functional damage to a complex self-renewing surface will depend on straightforward physico-chemical factors impossible to detail but which one can expect to be specially active when the foreign material is remote from normal and especially if it has enzymatically active groupings. Partial denaturation of the surface of contact could well have as a concomitant adhesion to the foreign surface and the development of the typical foreign-body reaction. In the short-term the essential result will be to coat the foreign material, a parasite for example, with a continuous layer of haemocytes which eventually insulates it from providing any further damaging contacts.

The wandering cells of invertebrate body fluids are highly phagocytic and capable of breaking down organic material so that the combination of recognition of grossly foreign character plus phagocytosis and intracellular digestion should be sufficient to provide the basis of an effective protective system against bacterial infection.

Analogies with the invertebrate system in vertebrates

Many of the characteristics of the generalized invertebrate system can be recognized in the mammal and other vertebrates. One of the important *non sequiturs* in much discussion of natural antibodies is to assume that any effect produced by serum in a situation analogous to that used for titrating standard antibody is due to antibody. To be meaningful, that statement requires that the protein responsible should be known to have the standard structure of immunoglobulin M, G or A and that attachment to the substance it reacts with must be by the standard combining site. Many natural antibodies may depend on regular but biologically accidental configurations on a plasma protein that are unrelated to the combining site on immunoglobulins. In reading an excellent recent review on natural antibodies by Boyden, one's chief impression is of the heterogeneity and unrelatedness of the reported facts and the inability to obtain consistent experimental support of any proposed hypothesis relating natural antibodies in a specific fashion to classical immunoglobulin antibodies.

Instead of seeking any unitary explanation of the phenomena I should be content to leave the situation in the plasma of a young normal animal as a basically unanalysable situation. In addition to a vast variety of Ig M molecules with a wide range of specific pattern mostly present in low concentration, Ig G and Ig A antibodies mostly from specifically stimulated clones—there are all the other globulins, haptoglobins, etc., each with their own physiological function. Any of these may show individual reactivity with some arbitrarily chosen reagent, red cell or bacterium, for example, for reasons which will probably never be expressible in more than the general statement that the whole evolutionary function of proteins depends on the capacity of one or other sequence of amino acid residues to combine selectively with almost any conceivable surface configuration. There must be a vast number of biologically meaningless reactions to be detected by any industrious apprentice to immunology which conceivably are related to *any* protein in serum or to other aspects of immunoglobulin than the combining site.

The behaviour of macrophages in mammals has also many resemblances to that of invertebrate cells. Although the results of experiments on the standard source of macrophages, peritoneal exudates in rodents, are often hard to interpret from the presence of large numbers of immunocytes (lymphocytes) as well as of phagocytic cells, the evidence is clear that basically the activity of macrophages is not an immunologically specific one. Macrophages from immune animals are no better at breaking down the substance of the bacteria against which the immunity is directed than those from normal animals. When the macrophages of a mouse develop power to destroy *Listeria* they concomitantly become able to destroy other unrelated organisms such as *Brucella*.

As has been discussed at various places in this book, macrophages of one sort or another are intimately concerned with immune processes in the strict sense, but they are ancillary rather than essential. Opsonization, which may mean the specific or non-specific coating of a particle with partly denatured immunoglobulin often with attached complement components, is a potent and often indispensable adjunct to phagocytosis. Mouse macrophages from peritoneal cavity readily adsorb cytophilic antibody and are so enabled to phagocytose antigenic particles such as red cells. Finally, there is the capacity which may be present in all macrophages but is particularly evident in the dendritic phagocytic cells of the lymph follicles to prepare and retain antigenic determinants in a particularly immunogenic form.

However, there is still evidence that substances such as *damaged* red cells and foreign particles like carbon and starch can be phagocytosed without first being coated with serum protein. Even a pneumococcus can be phagocytosed without opsonization if the macrophage is supported by tissue or some mechanical substitute. There is evidently still present some of the crude ability to recognize foreign material that is essential in the invertebrate.

Immune responses in primitive vertebrates
The most primitive existing vertebrates are the hagfishes and lampreys which appear to be specialized and in part degenerate descendants from the stock that gave rise to the earliest marine vertebrates, the ostracoderms, which appeared in the Upper Silurian. The hagfishes (*Myxinidae*) are parasitic on fish and anatomically appear to be more primitive than the lampreys. Extensive studies made by Good's group in Minneapolis have failed to show any evidence of antibody production or any of the other 'markers' of immune capacity. Lampreys are more advanced anatomically and in their biphasic life history. They have undoubted immune capacity although they produced antibody against only one of the five antigens tested. There are groups of 5–20 cells in the epithelium of the peripharyngeal gutter which could represent a thymus and there was a definite rejection of homografts although autografts were well retained. All the higher fishes show immune responses although elasmobranchs in general give poorer responses than teleosts. Immunoglobulins can be recognized and there are highly specific homograft reactions demon-

strable in scale grafting experiments. In amphibia and reptiles the most interesting feature is the great increase in speed and effectiveness of the immune responses when the temperature is raised.

From the evolutionary point of view then we can probably decide that the evolution of the immune system, essentially in the form known in the higher mammals, took place in the Silurian, perhaps more or less coincidentally with the first development of relatively large ostracoderms or their unarmoured ancestral forms. The application of modern techniques to the structure of the immunoglobulins in the lower vertebrates is just beginning and should eventually provide information of much importance to the understanding of the genetic origins of immune pattern. As yet the most interesting finding is that the immunoglobulin of an elasmobranch, although present in both 7S and 17S form, is antigenically uniform and corresponds almost certainly to Ig M in mammals. In an amphibian, both Ig G and Ig M can be recognized and there is the usual Ig M, Ig G sequence in the standard immune response to an antigen.

Light and heavy chains can be identified in elasmobranchs and all higher vertebrates, so that the need is urgent to look at the fine structure of immunoglobulin in the available cyclostomes if its early evolutionary history is to be unravelled.

A GENERALIZED SKETCH OF THE EVOLUTION OF ADAPTIVE IMMUNITY

In a contribution at present in the press I have tried to draw a self-consistent picture of the evolution of adaptive immune mechanisms, starting with the premise that the process was initially concerned not with defence against infection but with the maintenance of the cellular integrity of the body.

Such an attempt is necessarily more speculative than the generalized approach to the experimental facts with which this book is concerned. I have felt, however, that to present a summary of this picture of how adaptive immunity evolved is the most logical way to round off an exposition of theoretical immunology which claims to have been based throughout on evolutionary principles.

When animals became large enough and lived long enough for somagenetic changes in their cells to become a significant factor in survival, the immune mechanism was initiated as a two-sided exploitation of genetic lability. Histocompatibility antigens became highly modifiable by genetic processes; cell globulins with potential adsorptive power for a variety of organic configurations became increasingly subject to accelerated somatic mutation or some equivalent somagenetic process.

At all stages the immune process is concerned only with the cell surface. As I have already indicated, when cell surface characteristics become inoperative, as when mouse and human cells are grown in mixed tissue culture with Sendai virus, heterokaryons form without any evidence of disability to either nucleus. Histocompatibility differences and the possibility of recognition of foreignness are strictly functions of the cell surface. One can epitomize the immunological situation as a reaction by which one cell, the immunocyte, carries a modified globulin which can 'recognize' an unfamiliar pattern carried on the surface of another cell. That unfamiliar pattern can be a new histocompatibility antigen or a wholly foreign molecule or configuration. Recognition is by reversible union based on steric complementarity of the two patterns.

As has been discussed at some length in chapter 11, delayed hypersensitivity is a relatively primitive reaction in which the antigenic determinant can function as an immunogen only when it is incorporated into the lipoprotein of the surface of one of the mobile cells, lymphocyte or monocyte. Contact of immunocyte and antigen-carrying cell has a stimulatory effect producing as standard response blast transformation of the immunocyte and limited proliferation to a small clone of lymphocytes. Subsequent contact of such sensitized cells by antigen in solution results in more drastic stimulation and the liberation of pharmacologically active substances as described earlier.

Antibody production is a further development on the same essential theme with the casual mobile carrier of antigen replaced by a specialized fixed cell, the dendritic phagocytic cell of the lymph follicles. Recent work suggests also that the differentiation of the stem cells to immunocytes that are potential active producers of antibody is not a function of the thymus but of bursa or bursa-equivalent tissues. The immunocyte, too, has evolved for a more specialized group of functions. There are cell types restricted to the production of one only of the immunoglobulins M, G or A and, for each of these, the corresponding mature plasma cell develops an elaborate lamellate expansion of the endoplasmic reticulum. The standard induction of the immunocyte to antibody production is by contact of its immune receptor with antigenic determinant on the surface of a dendritic phagocytic cell. There are many complexities, diversions and anomalies such as those discussed throughout the body of this book in relation to antibody function and the behaviour of antibody-producing cells. The same central theme of cell surface to cell surface can, however, be discerned almost as clearly as in relation to delayed hypersensitivity.

As we see the picture in mammals, including ourselves, we can summarize immune function against such an evolutionary background as follows.

The primary immune function of surveillance to destroy mutant cells within the body is directly demonstrated in the laboratory models of homograft immunity and graft-versus-host reactions. It provides, too, the master-key to the understanding of delayed hypersensitivity and related phenomena.

Immunoglobulin is synonymous with antibody; this can now be taken as a dogma of the modern approach.

Ig M is the earliest type of antibody produced to any antigenic stimulus and may be the only form which results from nonspecific stimulation of immunocytes. Its main function is as an opsonin to allow phagocytic removal of micro-organisms and to facilitate further antibody production against their antigenic components.

Ig G may have as its main function to damp down the antibody response to a widely present foreign antigen. In mammals with haemochorial placentae it is the main vehicle by which maternal immunity is passively conferred on the newborn.

Ig A is specialized for secretion in glandular products. In ungulates it is concentrated in the colostrum and is the sole vehicle of passive maternal immunity. It appears also to have special qualities in protecting mucous surfaces from infection or in becoming the vehicle of allergic sensitization.

Immunological surveillance and evolution

The evolution of adaptive immunity conforms to the classic pattern. We see a simple theme seized on by the 'master constructors' mutation and selection and progressively moulded and elaborated. From primitive beginnings we reach in the higher mammals a finely tuned process exquisitely adapted to function against what is foreign or abnormal, but equally ringed round with devices to ensure that it will not offend by attacking the normal.

The immune system is a creation of evolution. It has arisen by the exploitation of error in nucleotide replication and it is no more infallible than any other aspect of biological function. It is sound biology to remember that autoimmune disease and myelomatosis are as much part of the universe of immunology as recovery from yellow fever or pneumonia.

Epilogue

A book, even a scientific text, is always liable to develop in a fashion that diverges subtly from what was originally conceived. This one ends without providing that 'definitive' form of clonal selection theory which it was its primary objective to present. Doubts and soft edges continue to abound. I grow more and more doubtful whether we are capable ever of understanding mechanisms that have taken a billion years of evolution to design and prove. Our theories remain crude and naïve.

Any summary can represent only a tentative halt along the road from which we can look forward hopefully or despondently, according to temperament, at the mounting complexities in front of us. Since the days of Ehrlich's side-chain theory there has been a progressive increase in sophistication of the requirements of immunological theory. With each major new development in biology, existent theory necessarily becomes inadequate and with the current applications of molecular biology to the immunoglobulins, the whole theoretical basis of immunology awaits recasting.

The process will go on indefinitely but at every step, as now, it must always be compatible with current understanding of biological processes generally. Now and perhaps permanently there are five levels or categories that have relevance to immunology.

1. The stochastic processes of error in replication which provide the raw material, through mutation and somatic mutation, for all biological change. This applies both to progress or degeneration at the species level and to a significant proportion of physiological and pathological changes in the individual.

2. Stochastic processes by which, from among the many available patterns of biological information, selection is made for some only to reach expression in organism or cell. These include sexual recombination at the level of the organism and phenotypic restriction at the cellular level.

3. The impact of environmental factors in allowing selective

Epilogue

survival and proliferation of certain forms at both the individual and the cellular level.

4. The molecular basis of the storage, replication and expression of biological information as it has been developed from viral and bacterial models, plus what indirect evidence can be gained of its applicability to vertebrate cellular activities.

5. The determinate aspects of biochemical processes as governed by stereochemical patterns in protein structure.

What I have written about the cellular and molecular basis of immune phenomena is a deliberate attempt to keep within those categories to the limit of my knowledge and understanding. Immunology from its very nature, its unique blend of stochastic and determinate processes, is probably better fitted to exemplify the realities of biology than any other major field in vertebrate physiology and biochemistry. Perhaps it is not too immodest to hope, even, that this book, by providing such an example of principles in action, may help toward a broader understanding of biology amongst a group of scientists now over-inclined to limit their interest wholly to the molecular approach.

Bibliography

As a guide to the literature in English bearing on the more academic aspects of immunology, the following notes may be helpful:
Primary publication of new research may be in any one of a hundred journals but a considerable proportion will be found in:
Immunology, Clinical and Experimental Immunology (U.K.), *Journal of Immunology, Transplantation, Immunochemistry, Journal of Experimental Medicine* (U.S.A.), *International Archives of Allergy* (Swiss), *Australian Journal of Experimental Biology and Medical Science.*
Review articles appear in:
Progress in Allergy, Advances in Immunology, Annual Review of Microbiology, Bacteriological Review, Annals of the New York Academy of Sciences.
Recent *textbooks* include:
Humphrey, J. H. and White, R. G. *Immunology for Students of Medicine*, 2nd ed. Oxford: Blackwell Scientific Publications (1964).
Kabat, E. A. *Experimental Immunochemistry*, 2nd ed. Springfield: Thomas (1961).
Raffel, S. *Immunity*, 2nd ed. New York: Appleton-Crofts (1961).
The following are probably the key references for the development of immunological theory:
Metchnikoff, E. *L'Immunité dans les maladies infectieuses.* Paris: Masson (1901).
Ehrlich, P. On immunity with special reference to cell life. *Proc. R. Soc.* **66**, 424 (1900).
Landsteiner, K. *The Specificity of Serological Reactions*, 1st ed. Cambridge, Mass.: Harvard University Press (1936, rev. ed. 1946).
Breinl, F. and Haurowitz, F. Chemische Untersuchung des Präzipitates aus Hämoglobin und Anti-Hämoglobin-Serum und Bemerkungen über die Natur der Antikörper. *Hoppe-Seyler's Z. physiol. Chem.* **192**, 45 (1930).
Pauling, L. Theory of the structure and process of the formation of antibodies. *J. Am. chem. Soc.* **62**, 2643 (1940).
Burnet, F. M. and Fenner, F. *The Production of Antibodies*, 2nd ed. Melbourne: Macmillan (1949).
Jerne, N. K. The natural selection theory of antibody formation. *Proc. natn. Acad. Sci. U.S.A.* **41**, 849 (1955).
Burnet, F. M. *The Clonal Selection Theory of Acquired Immunity.* Cambridge University Press (1959).

INDEX

Adjuvant, Freund's complete (FCA), 182, 203, 209–11, 231
Adrenal, autoimmune disease, 278–80
Agammaglobulinaemia
  congenital, 20, 92
  measles normal in, 28
Allogeneic inhibition, 221, 297–8
Antibody
  bacteriophage, 79
  cytophilic, 251
  definition, 31
  feedback control, 53, 121
  flagellar, 79
  foetal, 196, 222; plasma cells in foetus, 222
  heterogeneity, 7, 35, 36, 102, 126
  immunoglobulin is antibody, 203
  sheep red cell, 165
Antibody plaques (Jerne), 19, 43, 79–80, 165–6
  antigen-coated RBCs, 166
  plaque-forming cells, 166, 215
  in unimmunized animals, 165
Antibody production, 189–212
  to bacterial polysaccharides, 197
  double producers, 199
  foetal production, 196, 222
  genetics of capacity, 143
  Ig M–Ig G change, 196–8, 216
  inhibition by antibody, 120–1, 198, 207, 214
  primary response, 194–9
  secondary response, 191–3
  by single cells, 78–80
Antigen–antibody complex
  adsorption of complement, 161
  immune-adherence, 161
  kidney lesions in SLE, 264
  in rheumatic fever, 281
Antigenic determinant, 117–19
Antigens, 32
  dextran, 34, 118
  'good' antigens, 189, 211
  haptens, 118, 184, 208
  localization *in vivo*, 148
  presentation as stimulus, 205

synthetic polypeptides, 34, 118, 208
Arbovirus infection, 233–6
  neutralizing antibody, 233–4
  pathogenesis, 233
  persistence of antibody, 234
  yellow fever immunity, 28, 235
Aschoff, L., 15, 148
Autoimmune disease, 255–85
  cross-reactive antigens, 256, 282, 283
  dermatomyositis, 291
  experimental allergic encephalomyelitis, 246, 253
  fail-safe system, 255
  forbidden clone concept, 262–3
  heterogeneity, 257
  incomplete antibody and avidity, 262
  organ-specific antibodies, 279–80
  organ-specific types, 257, 274–80
  pernicious anaemia, 279
  somatic mutation, 256
Avidity
  of antibody, 35, 36
  changes during immunization, 184
  and delayed hypersensitivity, 185
  FCA effect, 182
  in immune drug reactions, 285
  of immunocyte receptors, 178–82
  incomplete auto-antibodies, 262

Blood groups, 243–4
Bone-marrow cells
  entry into bursa, 73
  entry into thymus, 65, 66
  origin of macrophages, 153
  stem cells, 37, 60, 69
Bordet, J., 4, 147, 160
Bursa of Fabricius, 71, 204
  bursectomy, 72; effect on immune responses, 72, 92
  entry of stem cells, 73
  hormones, 73

Cancer, 21
  carcinogenic hydrocarbons, 246

Index

Cancer (cont.)
  dermatomyositis, 291
  effect of thymectomy, 287
  neuroblastoma of adrenal, 289
  neuromyopathy, 291
  polyoma virus, 246, 286
  production of abnormal proteins, 290
  spontaneous regression, 246, 288
  SV 40, 287
Clonal selection theory, 11, 12–15, 18, 29
  immune pattern interpretation, 139
Combining site
  affinity labelling, 110
  of antibody or receptor, 31, 105, 108–12
  possible duplex character, 111, 140
  size, 109, 111
  on variable segments, 33, 128, 139
Complement, 147, 160–2
  cf. blood clotting, 160
  components, 161
  in cytotoxic reactions, 177
Coons, A. H., 16, 181
Cyclostomes, 304
  hagfish, 22, 304
  lamprey, 22, 304

Dameshek, W., 74, 163, 218
Darwin, C., 39
Delayed hypersensitivity, 23, 25, 244–54
  cell-surface antigen, 247, 249, 252, 254
  cells concerned, 26, 245, 246, 249
  contact sensitivity, 246
  evolutionary significance, 245
  homograft immunity as, 26, 245
  Lawrence transfer factor, 254
  passive transfer, 26
  relation to infection, 237, 250
  thymus dependence, 253
  tuberculin reactions, 244
Dendritic phagocytic cells (DPC), 86, 155–7
  antibody fixation, 156
  antigen fixation, 89, 149, 156, 207
  in lymph follicles, 155, 192
  in spleen, 155
Differentiation, cellular, of immunocytes, 39, 69
DPC, see Dendritic phagocytic cells

Ehrlich, P., 4, 147, 160
Endoplasmic reticulum, 16, 77, 339
Eosinophils, 147, 157–9
  antigen–antibody, 157–8
  in metazoan infestation, 158–9
Evolution
  cytochrome C, 131
  exploitation of genetic lability, 306
  by gene duplication, 131
  haemoglobin, 131
  histocompatibility antigens, 293
  immunoglobulin, 143, 305
  protein structure, 130–2, 303
  significant immunological needs, 208, 232, 235

Fagraeus, A., 16, 77
Flagellar antigen (flagellin), 79, 211
  distribution in lymph node, 89
  relation to DPC, 156, 211
  response to monomer, 211
Fluorescent antibody, 16, 78
  sandwich technique, 78

GALT, see Gut-associated lymphoid tissue
Gene duplication in immunoglobulin evolution, 39, 114, 141
Genetic factors in immunity, in myxomatosis, 236
Genetic information
  in DNA of genome, 37
  in relation to immune pattern, 13, 68–9
  transfer, 199–202
Germ-free animals, 64
Germinal centres, 15
  antibody in, 17, 148
  lymph nodes, 85
  source of immunocytes, 91, 175
  in thymus, 63
Gm factors
  in human Ig G, 141, 218
  relation to tolerance, 218
Good, R. A., 73, 122, 300, 304
Graft-versus-host reactions, 25
  to assay histocompatibility differences, 295
  on chorioallantois, 19, 295
  in parabiosis, 222
  in rats, 76
  runt disease, 25, 220, 222

Index

Gut-associated lymphoid tissue (GALT)
  appendix, 75
  bursa, 92
  hormone, 92, 204
  plasma cell series, 204

Haemolytic anaemia (autoimmune), 257, 258–63
  Coombs test, 258
  forbidden clone concept, 262
  incomplete antibody, 258, 262
  monoclonal antibody, 258–61
  NZB mice, 259–61
  role of thymus, 261
Haemolytic (Rh) disease of newborn, pathogenesis, 242 [241–3
  prevention by anti-D, 243
Heavy chain, 33, 104
  antigens, 141
  Fc fraction, 112–13
'Heavy chain disease', 101
Histocompatibility antigens, 22, 25
  high level of mutation, 293
  male Y antigen, 293
  relation to immune pattern, 140
  surface function, 299, 306
  tolerance in allophenic mice, 219
Homograft immunity, 23, 25
  absence in invertebrates, 301
  damage to target cells, 252
  as delayed hypersensitivity, 245
  in foetal sheep, 222
  passive transfer, 27
  present in lamprey and fish, 304
  surveillance function, 286
  tolerance, 220–4

Ig A, 98, 115
  carbohydrate, 100
  Ig E subclass, 123, 285
  plasma cells in gut, 123
  in secretions, 100, 122, 154
  summary, 307
  transport piece, 122
Ig G, 32, 98
  genetic markers on, 137
  Gm antigens, 105
  Inv antigens, 105
  LATS in thyrotoxicosis, 277
  placental transfer, 154, 241
  structure, 32, 103–15
  summary, 307

Ig M, 98
  conversion to Ig G, 100, 117, 121–2, 196
  in elasmobranchs, 305
  foetal antibody, 196
  function, 120, 175
  natural antibodies, 119
  in small lymphocytes, 82
  structure, 116, 119
  summary, 307
Immune pattern
  diversity, 30, 31, 39
  origin, 30, 45, 125–46
  polycistronic control, 129
  random character, 39, 45
  somatic mutation, 124, 129
  somatic recombination, 129, 134
  transfer to other cells, 187, 199–201
Immunocyte–antigen interaction, 170–88
  avidity, 171, 178–82
  blast transformation, 84, 174
  cell adhesion, 177, 186, 238
  cell damage and lysosomes, 176–7, 186
  cell death, 212
  commitment, 94
  complement action, 177
  dose relationships, 180, 206
  environmental factors, 182
  influence on adjacent cells, 174, 186, 188
  production of pharmacological agents, 166, 176–7
  range of response, 173, 179, 206, 214
  stimulation to DNA synthesis, 173
Immunocytes, 12, 29, 74–97, 163–88
  aggressiveness, 253
  differentiation from stem cells, 52
  memory cells, 94, 175, 198
  possible somatic hybridization, 200
  progenitor, 181
  receptors, 163–4, 169
  thymus-dependent, 83
  in unimmunized animals, 165
Immunocytes, nonspecific stimulation
  adjacent specific reaction, 166, 193, 204
  in long-lasting immunity, 235
  relation to homeostasis of Ig, 204
Immunoglobulin (Ig), 98–124
  carbohydrate, 114

315

Index

Immunoglobulin (*cont.*)
  electrophoresis, 98, 105
  homeostasis, 204
  nonspecific production, 193, 203, 210
  structure, 40, 99
  synthesis, 13
  types, 8, 190
Immunosuppressive drugs
  azothioprine ('Imuran'), 227
  cyclophosphamide, 230
  Mowbray's factor, α_2-globulin, 217
  6-mercaptopurine, 228
Instructive theories
  experimental refutation, 115
  Haurowitz–Mudd, 5
  Pauling, 6, 115, 127
Invertebrate defence, 300–2
  absence of adaptive immunity, 300
  haemocytes, 302; resemblance to macrophages, 303
  pseudo-antibodies, 301
Isotope labels
  amino acids, 17
  tritiated thymidine, 17, 193

Jenner, E., 3
Jerne, N. K., 9, 43, 73

Koch, R., 25, 244

Landsteiner, K., 4, 5, 31, 118, 128
Light chain, 32
  amino acid sequence, 106–8
  electrophoresis, 105
  Inv antigens, 105, 108
  K and L types, 104
  variable segment, 1, 33, 108, 124, 137–9, 143
Lymph nodes, 49
  embryology, 87
  immune function, 87–92
  movement of cells in, 49, 88, 90
  permeability factor, 89
  structure, 15, 85–7, 88, 97
  thymus-dependent (paracortical) area, 86, 248
Lymphocytes, 46
  action of PHA, 47, 81
  carrier of genetic information, 47, 57, 225
  circulation, 87–8, 90, 93, 152
  immunoglobulins in, 80–2, 167–8

longevity and death, 50, 178
  mobility, 225
  motility, 87, 90
  in non-lymphoid tissues, 95
  origin, 48, 83
  relation to DPC, 156
  source of necleotides, etc., 225
  thoracic duct, 46
  thymus, 46, 49, 83
  vulnerability, 95, 225
Lymphocytes, blast transformation
  by allotypic antiserum, 167–8
  by antigen, 167
  by PHA, 28, 47, 76, 81, 167–9

Macrophages, 18, 148–55
  evolution, 147
  Kupffer's cells, 151, 152
  monocytes, 149
  origin, 152–3
  peritoneal, 150, 152
Mast cells, 147, 159–60
  anaphylaxis, 160
  heteroplastic origin, 159
  histamine liberation, 159, 176
Maternal–foetal relationship, 240–4
  graft-versus-host reaction, 241
  placental passage of Ig G, 241
  Rh disease, 241–3
  selective effect, 244
Metchnikoff, E., 3, 15, 300
Monoclonal immunoglobulins
  haemolytic anaemia, 259
  myeloma proteins, 101–2
  rabbit antibody, 126, 184
  Waldenström's gammopathy, 20, 145
Myasthenia gravis, 271–4
  antibodies, 272
  myo-epithelial cells of thymus, 272
  thymectomy in, 271
  thymic tumours, 273
Myeloma proteins
  of antibody character, 103, 130
  Bence-Jones protein, 101
  in man, 20, 32, 99, 101
  in mice, 45

Nossal, G. J. V., 89

Opsonization, 29, 154
  needed for immunogenicity, 53, 154

Index

Pasteur, L., 3
Pauling, L., 5, 6, 34, 128
Phenotypic restriction, 14, 136
　in immunoglobulins, 114
　Lyon phenomenon, 136
Phytohaemagglutinin (PHA)
　agglutination of red cells, 27
　lymphocyte stimulation, 28, 47, 167
Plasma cells
　as antibody producers, 16, 77-8, 82, 191
　endoplasmic reticulum, 16, 77
　localization, 92
　longevity, 50
　origin, 50, 91, 187, 192
　relation to GALT, 92, 205
Porter, R. R., 33, 103, 104, 119
Porter diagram, 33, 103-4
Postcapillary venules of lymphoid tissue, 49, 87
Protein evolution, 130-2
Protein synthesis, mechanism, 36, 125

Reticulo-endothelial system (*see also* Macrophages), 148
　defined by Aschoff, 15
Rheumatic fever, 257, 280-2
　cardiac muscle antigen, 281
　streptococcal relationship, 280
Rheumatoid arthritis, 257, 266-71
　anti-γ-globulins, 267-9
　Burch's genetic interpretation, 270
　pathogenesis, 268
　rheumatoid factor (RF), 266; in bacterial endocarditis, 267; in macroglobulinaemia, 269
　streptococcal initiation, 282
RNA
　role in antibody production, 202, 207, 209
　transfer of immune pattern, 199, 201-2

Selection theories
　Burnet, clonal selection, 11-12
　Ehrlich, side-chain, 4
　Jerne, 9-10
　Lederberg, subcellular selection, 11, 138
SLE, *see* Systematic lupus erythematosus
Somatic mutation, 40-5
　and ageing, 43

autoimmune disease, 183
fleece mosaicism, 42, 132
frequency of error, 41
magnification of effect, 42, 133
in relation to immune pattern, 124, 135
Spleen
　clonal growth of cells, 19, 146
　plasma cell localization, 92
　thymus-dependent area, 248
Surveillance function, 251, 286-97
　in autoimmune disease, 271, 295
　clinical evidence, 288-90
　cytotoxic actions, 251
　evolution, 293
　new antigens (in malignant cells), 287, 292, (somatic mutational origin), 296
　in polyoma carcinogenesis, 287
　primary immune function, 307
Systemic lupus erythematosus (SLE), 257, 263-6
　antibodies, 264
　model in F_1 mice, 263
　pathogenesis, 265
　thymus as target organ, 265

Thoracic duct
　effects of drainage, 76, 224
　lymphocytes, 46, 75, 187
Thymectomy, neonatal
　change in immune responses after, 60, 65
　in mice, 24, 46, 64
　species and strain differences, 64
　wasting disease after, 64
Thymus, 58-71
　blood-thymus barrier, 223
　cell turnover, 60, 66
　'censorship', 48, 223
　change with age and stress, 62-3
　comparative anatomy, 66, 71
　differentiation of immunocytes in, 52, 59, 68
　enlarged, in thyrotoxicosis, 278
　entry of antigen in neonates, 223
　evolution, 59
　failure to develop, 24, 64
　function, 46, 48, 58-60, 182
　grafts, 60
　hormones, 59, 70, 84
　production of lymphocytes by, 67, 49, 87

317

Index

Thymus (*cont.*)
  structure, 60–73
  target organ in SLE and myasthenia, 265
  thymocytes, 62
  tolerance, chimerism, etc., 48, 69, 71, 221
Thymus-dependent areas in lymphoid tissue, 248
Thymus-dependent immunocytes
  in delayed hypersensitivity, 174, 247–9, 253
  interaction with GALT-dependent immunocytes, 204
  low Ig M production, 190
Thyroid disease
  Hashimoto's disease, 275
  myxoedema, 277
  thyrotoxicosis, 277
Tissue transplantation, 21
  kidney transplants, 227
  requirements for organ transplantation, 227–30
  skin grafts, 23
  use of 6-mercaptopurine and derivatives, 228–30
Tolerance, immunological, 24, 25
  as absence of immunocytes, 30, 54
  acquired, 213, 220–4
  in allophenic mice, 219
  in chickens, 50
  in chimeras, 220, 224
  in congenital infection, 51
  dose relationships, 220
  intrinsic, 219
  as irreversible commitment, 54, 214
  mutual tolerance (parabionts), 223
  neonatal, 213
  to normal body components, 51, 219
  partial, 54
  requiring continued presence of antigen, 55, 218, 220
  role of thymus, 223
  split, 221

  summary, 230–2
  in twins, 51, 217
Trauma and local infection, 236–40
  circulatory reactions, 240
  histamine, 239–40
  inflammation, 239
  relation to delayed hypersensitivity, 237
  staphylococcal infection, 237
  vaccinia lesion, 238
Tuberculin reaction
  cells concerned, 244
  type of delayed hypersensitivity reaction, 244
Twins
  dizygotic, 23; cattle, 51, 217
  identical, 23

Unresponsiveness, immune (*see also* Tolerance, immunological), 213–31
  by depletion of lymphocytes, 224
  immune paralysis, 213
  by immunosuppressive drugs, 226
  by irradiation, 226
  by irreversible commitment, 121
  low-level, 216
  persisting tolerated infection, 217, 219
  physiological, 213, 214–17
  in pyridoxine deficiency, 227

Viruses, immunity to, 233–6
  lymphocytic choriomeningitis, 219, 283
von Behring, E., 4

Wright, Almroth, 4

X-irradiation
  effect on immune responses, 65, 226
  lethal, and rescue by cells, 65, 226
  thymic atrophy, 62